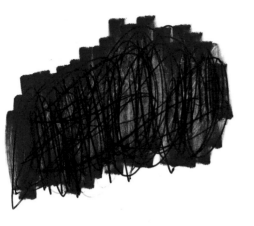

Master Techniques in Facial Rejuvenation

Master Techniques in Facial Rejuvenation

BABAK AZIZZADEH, MD, FACS
Director
The Center for Facial and Nasal Plastic Surgery
David Geffen School of Medicine at UCLA
Audrey Skirball-Kenis Center for Plastic & Reconstructive Surgery
Cedars-Sinai Medical Center
Beverly Hills, California

MARK R. MURPHY, MD
Director
Palm Beach Facial Plastic Surgery
West Palm Beach, Florida

CALVIN M. JOHNSON JR., MD
Clinical Associate Professor
Division of Facial Plastic & Reconstructive Surgery
Tulane University School of Medicine;
Director
Hedgewood Surgical Center
New Orleans, Louisiana

SAUNDERS

ELSEVIER

SAUNDERS
ELSEVIER

1600 John F. Kennedy Boulevard
Suite 1800
Philadelphia, Pennsylvania 19103

ISBN-13: 978-1-4160-0146-1
ISBN-10: 1-4160-0146-8

MASTER TECHNIQUES IN FACIAL REJUVENATION

Copyright © 2007, by Saunders, an imprint of Elsevier Inc.

Library of Congress Control Number: 2006934728

Editor: *Rebecca Schmidt Gaertner*
Editorial Assistant: *Suzanne Flint*
Publishing Services Manager: *Mary Stermel*
Designer: *Louis Forgione*
Marketing Manager: *Kathleen Neely*

Printed in China

Last digit is the print number: 9 8 7 6 5 4 3 2 1

Dedication

Babak Azizzadeh

To Jessica, my beautiful and loving wife. My life would be meaningless without her. To Kylie and Logan for being the most amazing children any father can ask for. To my parents, Yafa and Habib, as well as my loving sister, Katrin, who set the foundation for my personal and professional life.

Mark R. Murphy

This book is dedicated to my wife, Sherry, who has enabled me to fulfill my dreams. To our beautiful children Ned, Nicholas, and Grayson, you are the lights that guide us. To my mother and father, Maureen and Robert, for preparing me for a life of happiness. And to my sister and brother, Diane and David, for sharing in our joy.

Contributors

Editors

Babak Azizzadeh, MD, FACS
Director
The Center for Facial and Nasal Plastic Surgery
Assistant Clinical Professor
David Geffen School of Medicine at UCLA
Audrey Skirball-Kenis Center for Plastic & Reconstructive Surgery
Cedars-Sinai Medical Center
Beverly Hills, California
*The Aging Face Consultation, Short-Flap SMAS Rhytidectomy,
Aesthetic Midface Implants*

Mark R. Murphy, MD
Director
Palm Beach Facial Plastic Surgery
West Palm Beach, Florida
*The Aging Face Consultation, The Open Browlift, The Deep Plane
Facelift*

Calvin M. Johnson Jr., MD
Clinical Associate Professor
Division of Facial Plastic & Reconstructive Surgery
Tulane University School of Medicine;
Director
Hedgewood Surgical Center
New Orleans, Louisiana
*The Aging Face Consultation, The Open Browlift, The Deep Plane
Facelift*

Contributors

Daniel C. Baker, MD
Associate Professor
Department of Plastic Surgery
New York University School of Medicine;
Attending Surgeon
New York University Medical Center;
Attending Surgeon
Department of Plastic Surgery
Manhattan Eye, Ear & Throat Hospital;
Attending Surgeon
Department of Plastic Surgery
Bellevue Hospital
New York, New York
Lateral SMASectomy Facelift

William J. Binder, MD, FACS
Assistant Clinical Professor
Department of Head and Neck Surgery
UCLA School of Medicine

Attending Surgeon
Department of Head and Neck Surgery
Cedars Sinai Medical Center
Los Angeles, California
Aesthetic Midface Implants

Dewayne T. Bradley, MD
Department of Otolaryngology-Facial Plastic Surgery
Virginia Mason Medical Center
Seattle, Washington
Facial Embryology and Anatomy

Andres Bustillo, MD
Facial Plastic & Reconstructive Surgery
Coral Gables, Florida
Blepharoplasty

Mack L. Cheney, MD, FACS
Professor
Department of Otolaryngology-Head and Neck Surgery
Harvard Medical School;
Director of Facial Plastic and Reconstructive Surgery
Department of Otolaryngology-HNS
Massachusetts Eye and Ear Infirmary
Boston, Massachusetts
Short-Flap SMAS Rhytidectomy

Jeannie H. Chung, MD
Associate Staff
Department of Otolaryngology-Head and Neck Surgery
Massachusetts Eye and Ear Infirmary
Boston, Massachusetts;
Active Staff
Department of Otolaryngology-Head and Neck Surgery
North Shore Medical Center
Salem, Massachusetts;
Medical Director
North Shore Dermatology and Cosmetic Surgery Center
Andover, Massachusetts
Facial Suction Lipectomy

Steven C. Dresner, MD
Associate Clinical Professor of Ophthalmology
The University of Southern California Keck School of Medicine
Los Angeles, California;
Director
Fellowship in Ophthalmic Plastic Surgery
Eyesthetica
Santa Monica, California;
Transconjunctival Lower Blepharoplasty

Alvin I. Glasgold, MD
Clinical Professor of Surgery
Department of Surgery
University of Medicine and Dentistry of New Jersey-Robert Wood
Johnson Medical School
New Brunswick, New Jersey
Mentoplasty

Mark J. Glasgold, MD
Clinical Assistant Professor
Department of Surgery
University of Medicine and Dentistry of New Jersey-Robert Wood
Johnson Medical School
New Brunswick, New Jersey
Mentoplasty, Complementary Fat Grafting

Robert A. Glasgold, MD
Assistant Professor
Department of Surgery
University of Medicine and Dentistry of New Jersey-Robert Wood
Johnson Medical School
New Brunswick, New Jersey
Mentoplasty, Complementary Fat Grafting

Ryan M. Greene, MD, PhD
Resident
Department of Otolaryngology-Head and Neck Surgery
The University of Illinois at Chicago
Chicago, Illinois
Rhinoplasty in the Aging Patient

Tessa A. Hadlock, MD
Assistant Professor
Department of Otology and Laryngology
Harvard Medical School;
Division of Facial Plastic and Reconstructive Surgery
Department of Otolaryngology
Massachusetts Eye and Ear Infirmary
Boston, Massachusetts
Short-Flap SMAS Rhytidectomy

Douglas Hamilton, MD
Assistant Clinical Professor
Department of Dermatology
University of California, Los Angeles School of Medicine
Los Angeles, California
Nonsurgical Facial Rejuvenation

Carlo P. Honrado, MD
Assistant Professor
Department of Facial Plastic and Reconstructive Surgery
New York Eye and Ear Infirmary
New York, New York;
Assistant Professor
Department of Facial Plastic and Reconstructive Surgery
New York Medical College
Valhalla, New York
Facial Embryology and Anatomy

Nicanor Isse, MD
Assistant Clinical Professor
Department of Surgery
University of California Los Angeles
Volunteer Faculty

Department of Surgery
University of Southern California
Los Angeles, California;
Professor of Post Graduate Courses and Master Courses
University of Padua
Padua, Italy;
Active Member and Staff
Department of Surgery
Hoag Memorial Hospital Presbyterian
Newport Beach, California;
Provisional Status and Staff
Department of Surgery
Providence Saint Joseph Medical Center
Burbank, California;
Volunteer Faculty Appointment and Staff
Department of Surgery
University of California, Irvine
Irvine, California
Endoscopic Foreheadplasty

Brian P. Kim, MD
Resident Physician
Department of Otolaryngology-Head and Neck Surgery
University of California, Los Angeles School of Medicine
Los Angeles, California;
Fellow
Department of Otolaryngology-Head and Neck Surgery
Stanford University School of Medicine
Stanford, California
Aesthetic Midface Implants

Young Kyoon Kim, MD, PhD
Professor
Department of Dermatology
Cho-Sun University Medical School
Gwangju, South Korea;
Professor
Department of Dermatology
Dong-A University Medical School
Busan, South Korea;
Full Fellowship
Department of Cosmetic Surgery
International Academy of Cosmetic Surgery
Tokyo, Japan;
Director
Department of Cosmetic Surgery
5050 Clinic
Bucheon, South Korea
Asian Blepharoplasty

Samuel M. Lam, MD
Director
Lam Facial Plastic Surgery Center and Hair Restoration Institute
Plano and Dallas, Texas
Asian Blepharoplasty, Complementary Fat Grafting

Wayne F. Larrabee Jr., MD, FACS
Clinical Professor
Department of Otolaryngology-Head and Neck Surgery
University of Washington School of Medicine;
Swedish Hospital;
Director
Larrabee Center for Facial Plastic Surgery
Seattle, Washington
Facial Embryology and Anatomy

Robert E. Levine, MD
Clinical Professor of Ophthalmology
Department of Ophthalmology
University of Southern California Keck School of Medicine;
Co-Founder and Co-Director
Center for Facial Nerve Function
House Ear Clinic
Los Angeles, California
Lateral Canthoplasty

Harry Marshak, MD
Former Clinical Instructor
Ophthalmic Plastic and Reconstructive Surgery
Doheny Eye Institute
Keck School of Medicine of University of Southern California
Los Angeles, California;
Ophthalmic Plastic and Reconstructive Surgery
The Morrow Institute
Rancho Mirage, California
Transconjunctival Lower Blepharoplasty

Norman Pastorek, MD, FACS
Clinical Professor and Director
Facial Plastic Fellowship
Department of Otolaryngology
New York University College of Medicine;
Clinical Professor and Clinical Director of Facial Plastic Surgery
Department of Otolaryngology
New York Presbyterian Hospital-Weill Cornell Medical Center;
Surgeon Director
Department of Otolaryngology
Manhattan Eye, Ear, & Throat Hospital
New York, New York
Blepharoplasty

Oscar M. Ramirez, MD, FACS
Esthétique Internationale
Timonium, Maryland
Tridimensional Endoscopic Facelift

Dean M. Toriumi, MD
Professor
Division of Facial Plastic and Reconstructive Surgery
Department of Otolaryngology-Head and Neck Surgery
University of Illinois at Chicago
Chicago, Illinois
Rhinoplasty in the Aging Patient

Charles R. Volpe, MD
Esthétique International
Timonium, Maryland
Tridimensional Endoscopic Facelift

Edwin F. Williams, III, MD, FACS
Fellowship Director
American College of Surgeons;
Clinical Instructor and Fellow
Department of Otolaryngology-Head and Neck Surgery
University of Illinois
Chicago, Illinois;
Chief
Department of Facial Plastic and Reconstructive Surgery
Clinical Associate Professor of Surgery
Albany Medical Center
Albany, New York;
Medical Director and Founder
New England Laser & Cosmetic Surgery Center;
Medical Director
Williams Center for Excellence
Latham, New York
Facial Suction Lipectomy

Preface

When we decided to embark on this project, there were no books available that presented competing and alternative surgical viewpoints to facial rejuvenation. Most available texts either covered a broad spectrum of plastic and reconstructive surgery methods or presented a single author's surgical technique. This text presents multiple facial rejuvenation procedures from those who do it best. So much of surgery is experience, not just with technique but, more important, with the reasoning and knowledge that have guided surgeons over the years. We have chosen contributing authors from various specialties based on their accomplishments and expertise with facial rejuvenation. Only the most pioneering and time-tested procedures are presented so that both young and experienced surgeons may understand and master the essentials and fine subtleties of facial aesthetic surgery.

With the initial emphasis on anatomy, the pillar of all successful surgery, the text moves forward through the authors' individual preferences and, more important, their rationale for those preferences. Once the reader understands these foundations, the surgical technique is described in detail through text, intraoperative photos, illustrations, and a comprehensive DVD surgical atlas. By providing the reader with these components, we hope to inspire and educate the next generation of masters.

Acknowledgments

There are many people to whom we owe a great deal of gratitude for the completion of the text. First and foremost are our patients, who have entrusted us in the most personal way. We also thank our mentors, Norman Pastorek, Mack Cheney, Keith Blackwell, and Rinaldo Canalis, our family, Ned and Cindy Lautenbach, for their motivation and inspiration, and our current partners, Robert Dattolo, David Lehman, Carolyn Agresti, Carlos Heaton, John Murray, David Alessi, Babak Larian, Lance Wyatt, and Kami Parsa, whose unflinching support has aided us in the pursuit of our passion. Finally, we must acknowledge the unbelievable amount of work that Rebecca Gaertner, Suzanne Flint, Krystyna Srodulski, and Stasia Droze put forth in making this book a reality.

Contents

CHAPTER ONE

The Aging Face Consultation

Mark R. Murphy, MD • *Calvin M. Johnson Jr., MD* • *Babak Azizzadeh, MD, FACS*

HISTORY

The elusive features of beauty have been studied for millennia. The facets of beauty change with time, and with every era new components take on a greater or lesser importance. Alhough this quest leads to many definitions, it has also identified certain specific features that define beauty. We must search through the art or writing of an era to understand what constituted beauty at that time. From ancient Egyptian depictions of Queen Nefertiti to the paintings of Leonardo da Vinci, the pursuit of facial beauty has been attempted by history's greatest artists (Fig. 1-1). Through their work, we can glean the details that, when brought together, create beauty. In ancient times, combinations of facial features, body proportions, hair color, and skin tone could remain popular for centuries. As time progressed, however, these preferences began to change more quickly, first by decades, later by seasons, and now by weeks.

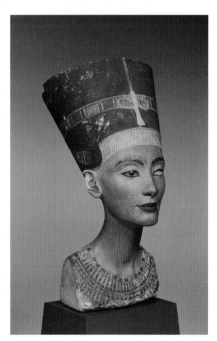

Figure 1-1 The classical beauty of the Egyptian Nefertiti continues to be seen as an ideal image of beauty and elegance. Copyright © Bildarchiv Preussischer Kulturbesitz/Art Resource, NY.

The ideal of universal beauty is just that, an ideal. Differences in epochs, cultures, and ethnicity dictate that a unanimous definition of beauty will be ever elusive. However, there are common threads in the proportions and harmony of the face that throughout time and civilizations confer an overall sense of attractiveness.[1] Beauty can be defined and measured.[2] It has also been shown that attractiveness plays a covert but significant role in the way people behave and how they react to another.[3] Through the centuries we can see the ever-changing definition of beauty, and recognizing its perception is an innate human trait.[4] Indeed, infants have been shown to prefer faces that have been deemed more attractive.[5] This tendency continues through adulthood. Faces that deviate the least amount from standard averages have been found to be more attractive among older study participants.[6] The traits that subjects have found to be consistently more attractive in females are high cheekbones, large eyes, a smaller vertical third of the face, and a narrow jaw.[7]

ANCIENT GREECE

The ancient Greek civilization is considered by many to be the progenitor of modern facial analysis. The Greek artist Praxiteles (370–330 BC) provided a model of beauty with his sculpture of Aphrodite. His work, and that of others influenced by him, displays the evolution of beauty by incorporating human expression into the classic context of a goddess (Fig. 1-2). With her triangular forehead and eyes that express warmth, innocence, and sadness, she conveyed components of reality that had been overlooked by Praxiteles's predecessors. Her features were regular and depicted imperfections that added to her beauty by making her more human. In creating the sculpture of Aphrodite, Praxiteles emphasized subtlety versus the more rigid, precise expressions popular at that time. Her facial features emanated beauty without overwhelming the observer. Aphrodite became a standard of beauty passed on to subsequent generations.[3,8,9]

The origin of the pursuit of beauty is often associated with the ancient Greeks, and their effect still permeates our modern conceptions of desirability. It was the Greek civilization, Plato specifically, that defined beauty as an

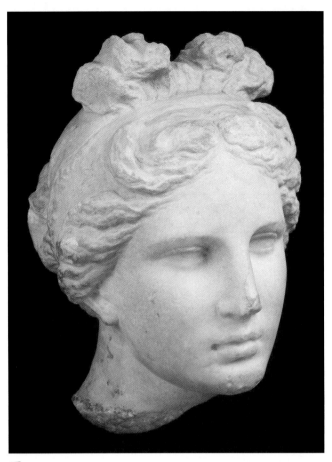

Figure 1-2 The face of Aphrodite serves as a model of facial proportion and beauty. Copyright © 2004 Museum of Fine Arts, Boston, MA.

RENAISSANCE

The Greek influence reemerged in the late 14th century at the birth of the Renaissance. The Renaissance covered many aspects of human endeavor and included the search, definition, and expression of beauty. The goal of the artists of the time was not merely the depiction of objects, but the creation of them from various forms to attain an ideal. The positive tone of this time is echoed in its artistic impressions. No longer were women depicted in the harsh terms of earlier times. They emerged as independent and intelligent.[3] Peter Paul Rubens (1577–1640) depicted vigorous female forms that were once seen as the ideal portrayal of female beauty, perhaps due to the spirit they emanated as opposed to the forms themselves. The women Rubens created were intelligent and alert, with dark eyes, long necks, and round heads (Fig. 1-3). This ideal evolved as Rubens aged and the vigor of his early paintings was slowly displaced by softness in form in his later works.[3,13]

Although the Renaissance is noted for its humanistic approach to art, it valued the mathematical method that dated back to the Greeks. The artists of the era desired to discover scientific explanations of beauty. The science of beauty intrigued the artists of this age as never before. The theories of Vitruvius Pollios (first century BC), a Roman architect, on using the human form to derive

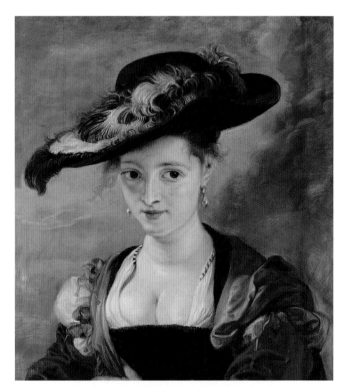

Figure 1-3 The societal evolution of the perception of beauty is evidenced in Rubens' portrait of the young women whose dark eyes and manner belie an advanced intelligence. Copyright © Erich Lessing/Art Resource, NY.

appropriate balance. We see this concept mirrored today as we analyze the face into fifths, vertically, and thirds, horizontally. To the Greeks the concept of balance went beyond physical characteristics and included wealth, health, and beauty.[3] Indeed, the Greeks considered physical beauty to be worthy of fame. They delved into the meaning of these factors in the context of an orderly universe. In this vein, they attempted to understand the concept of beauty as they sought to define it through mathematical terms.[10] The Greeks, and others throughout history, also realized beauty is attained when good taste, balance, and proportion are in harmony.

This sentiment was echoed by Polyclitus (fifth century BC). He defined a series of proportions that he believed would produce an image of faultless beauty. For his doubters, he would create two sculptures, one naturalistic and one according to his proportioned principles. Viewers of the works agreed the statue following strict proportions was more beautiful by far.[3,11] This balance, known as the elusive "golden mean," has been the topic of debate for centuries as artists, architects, and philosophers have sought to define beauty through mathematical terms.[12]

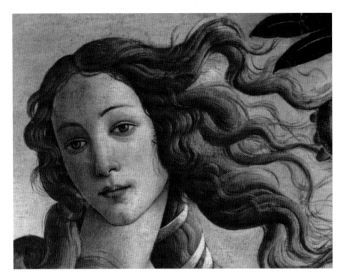

Figure 1-4 The flowing, obvious beauty of Venus epitomizes the Renaissance ideal of beauty. Copyright © Erich Lessing/Art Resource, NY.

perfect proportions in building sacred edifices were not merely taken as reference but as foundation.

Perhaps no other artist is more closely defined by this period than Leonardo da Vinci (1452–1519). Da Vinci's passionate pursuit of proportion is seen throughout his copious works. Da Vinci was relentless in his pursuit of the balance between science and beauty. His numerous studies of the face and head stand as masterpieces of the human form. Da Vinci first broke the face into thirds to assess their individual contributions to the whole.

The Renaissance artist Sandro Botticelli (1444–1510) again illustrated the desire to place classic concepts in a modern format.[3] By combining the traditional features of beauty with the partialities of his time, Botticelli epitomized the Renaissance ideal. In *The Birth of Venus*, Botticelli depicted a traditional subject with current features. Her long, angular face had previously been depicted as a standard oval. Her emotions emanate from her geometrically regular and perfectly calm facial expression (Fig. 1-4).[3] The two common threads in the pursuit of beauty are adherence to classic forms and a modern manipulation of those forms to meet the taste of the times.

The Romantic period was heralded by Prud'hon's interpretation of female beauty. In his images of his mistress this ideal woman merges dream and sensuality. The woman in the painting titled *The Happy Mother* gazes adoringly at her nursing infant (Fig. 1-5). Prud'hon stressed the natural beauty of maternity—and with this physical and emotional bond, the beauty of feminine tenderness is skillfully portrayed.

HISTORY OF FACIAL REJUVENATION

Aesthetic surgery is the pursuit of what is described by the Greek word *aisthetikos*, meaning a passion for that which

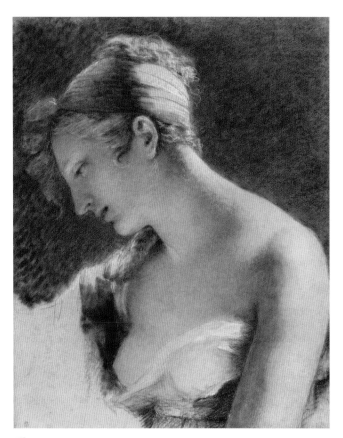

Figure 1-5 The soft, feminine portrait of this mother gazing at her child depicted the Romantic sense of beauty. Copyright © The J. Paul Getty Museum.

is beautiful. The surgical enhancement of appearance was roundly dismissed until the late 1800s. Before this time, such perceived vanity was socially unacceptable and the procedures themselves were considerably dangerous. As the constraints of the Victorian era receded, women became empowered to alter their appearance as they chose. Makeup and hair styling became commonplace and the shroud surrounding the world of cosmetic surgery began to slowly unravel. Surgery, however, was a perilous endeavor at the beginning of the 20th century. Anesthesia methods were crude at best and antibiotics were not in existence yet. It would not be until the middle of the century that these two vital components to surgical management of complex problems came into common use.[3]

The surgeons during this time had little to no appreciation of the challenges they faced. The knowledge of facial anatomy and function was marginal. Little was known about the complex interplay of skin, muscle, fat, cartilage, and bone. Manipulation of these components could not be confidently addressed until the physiology of blood supply, lymphatic drainage, and flap dynamics was more completely understood.

This field has rapidly evolved over the past 20 years as aesthetic surgery has blossomed to the forefront of

American culture. The final barriers to cosmetic alterations have been removed with the advent of less invasive methods and glamorization of plastic surgery in the media. Cosmetic surgery has indeed become commonplace with magazines and television shows promoting it on a daily basis.

CONSULTATION

HISTORY

A complete history and physical examination must be performed prior to the analysis of the patient's cosmetic desires and possibilities. This is especially true in cosmetic surgery. There can be no excuse for an overlooked medical issue that can compromise the health of a patient undergoing an elective procedure. General issues that should be investigated include previous surgeries, medications, alcohol use, allergies, and any coexisting medical conditions. Specific issues to facial rejuvenation such as the use of aspirin and other nonsteroidal anti-inflammatory medications, hypertension, and smoking history should be thoroughly explored.

If the patient plans to undergo eyelid rejuvenation, a complete ophthalmologic history should be obtained with emphasis on dry eye symptoms. There is significant controversy for the role of a formal ophthalmologic consultation.[14-16] Each patient should be individually evaluated in order to determine the need for an ophthalmology evaluation. A history of dry eyes usually requires formal testing of tear production using the Schirmer test. Thyroid-related diseases, facial palsy, and prior blepharoplasty are also important conditions that increase the risks of eyelid malposition in the postoperative period.

PHYSICAL EXAMINATION AND FACIAL ANALYSIS

The physical examination is specific to each surgeon and there is no right or wrong way to examine the patient. However, certain components of the physical examination should always be included. We prefer to analyze the overall appearance of the face. The ethnicity, body habitus, and general proportions of the face should be considered. A three-dimensional approach must be considered to account for the patient's facial volume, skin texture, muscular activity, and bony skeletal support. Several landmarks and known relationships should be appreciated by all surgeons performing aesthetic surgery (Table 1-1; Fig. 1-6). The face is generally broken down into fifths vertically, based on the width of an eye, and thirds horizontally, as measured from the hairline to the glabella, glabella to the subnasale, and subnasale to menton (Fig. 1-7). Any facial asymmetry should be noted at this time. All normal faces have some level of asymmetry, which should be conveyed to the patient.

Table 1-1   Standard Facial Angles

Angle	Description
Nasofrontal angle	Angle between the nasion, glabella, and the dorsal line of the nose (~115 to 135 degrees)
Nasofacial angle	Angle between the dorsum of the nose and the facial plane (~30 to 40 degrees)
Nasomental angle	Angle between the dorsal line of the nose and a line from the pogonion to the nasal tip (~120 to 132 degrees)
Mentocervical angle	Angle between a line from the menton to the cervical point and the facial plane (~80 to 95 degrees)
Nasolabial angle	Angle between the line of the nasal columella and tangent of the upper lip (~90 to 105 degrees)

Facial rejuvenation procedures must create an overall harmony to the face without any major discrepancies. All facial regions must therefore be assessed during the consultation. The upper third of the face encompassing the forehead, brow, and eyes is generally evaluated jointly. The middle third of the face is composed of the midface, malar eminence, submalar soft tissue, nasolabial fold, and nose. The lower third of the face is assessed by evaluating the perioral, jowl, and neck regions. Specific aspects of the evaluation will be discussed in the following sections.

Skin

Our preference is to first examine the condition of the patient's skin. Whether for facial rejuvenation or rhinoplasty, the status of the skin will have profound ramifications on the result of the planned procedure. The texture, thickness, pigmentation, degree of sun exposure, and smoking-related skin changes should be completely evaluated. The youthful face has smooth elastic skin with ample subcutaneous tissue. Subcutaneous fat and muscle begin to atrophy with time and the skin becomes less elastic. For facial rejuvenation, the skin should be manipulated in vectors similar to those of the proposed procedure to assess its mobility. Dynamic and gravitational rhytids must be evaluated and the surgeon should note any previous procedures, scars, or skin lesions. Fitzpatrick scale can be utilized to evaluate appropriate candidates for skin resurfacing (Table 1-2).[17,18]

The surgeon should at this time educate the patient as to the consequences of certain skin types and conditions. Thick, oily, porous skin tends to mask fine irregularities

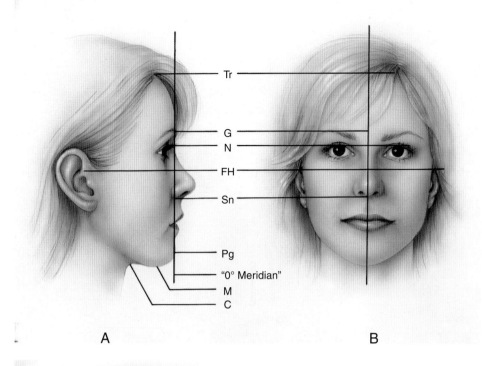

A   B

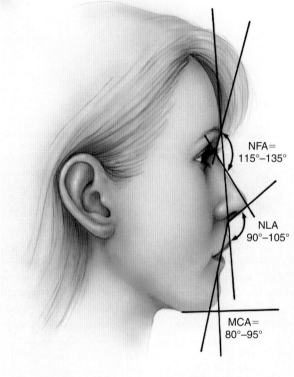

NFA=
115°–135°

NLA
90°–105°

MCA=
80°–95°

C

Figure 1-6 Facial landmarks (**A** and **B**). The *Frankfort horizontal plane (FH)* is determined by drawing a straight line from the supratragal notch to the infraorbital rim. The *cervical point (C)* is the junction of the submental area and neck. The *glabella (G)* is the prominence of the forehead at the level of the supraorbital rim in the lateral view. The *menton (M)* is the lowest point of the chin. The *nasion (N)* is the deepest depression at the superior aspect of the nose. The *pogonion (Pg)* is the anteriormost projection of the chin. The *subnasale (Sn)* is the junction of the nasal columella and upper lip. The *trichion (Tr)* is the anterior border of the hairline in the midline. The *0° meridian* determines chin and facial projection; a line is drawn at the level of the nasion and perpendicular to the Frankfort horizontal plane. The *nasofrontal angle (NFA)* is the angle between the nasion, glabella, and the dorsal line of the nose (**C**). The *mentocervical angle (MCA)* is the angle in between the facial plane and a line drawn from the menton to the cervical point. The *nasolabial angle (NLA)* is the angle between the nasal columella and the tangent line of the upper lip.

but at the cost of increased scarring. Thin skin generally heals better than thick skin at the expense of the patient's perceiving slight irregularities that might otherwise go unnoticed. This is especially true when the surgeon performs rhinoplasty, a procedure increasingly popular with the aging population. The ideal skin type lies between these two extremes.

The patient's facial volume also needs to be thoroughly assessed. This is an area which has been historically undervalued in facial rejuvenation. During the

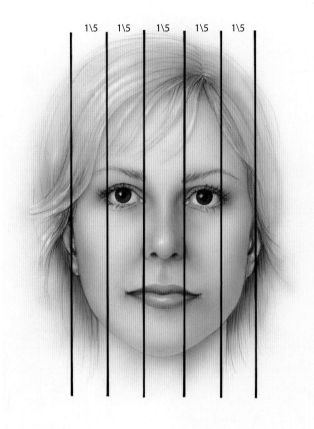

A

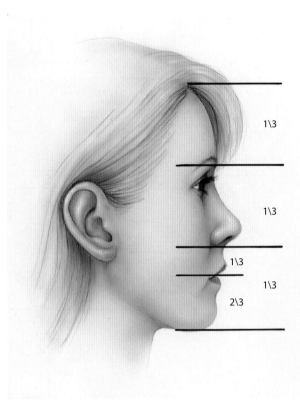

B

Figure 1-7 *Facial* proportions. The vertical facial proportions are generally broken down into fifths based on the width of an eye (**A**). The horizontal facial proportions are divided into thirds as measured from the hairline to the glabella, from the glabella to the subnasale, and from the subnasale the menton (**B**). The lower third can be further broken down to the upper one third, from the subnasale to the junction of the lips, and the lower two thirds, from the junction of the lips to the menton.

Table 1-2   Fitzpatrick Skin Evaluation

Skin Type	Skin Color	Reaction to Sun
Type I	Very white or freckled	Always burns
Type II	White	Usually burns
Type III	White to olive	Sometimes burns
Type IV	Brown	Rarely burns
Type V	Dark brown	Very rarely burns
Type VI	Black	Never burns

aging process, the subcutaneous fat and muscles not only shift secondary to gravitational forces, but also deflate and atrophy. Furthermore, the skeletal framework may also recede in the edentulous patient.

Forehead and Brow Complex

The upper third of the face is initially evaluated by looking at the relationship of the forehead, brow, and eyes. This region of the face is often overlooked by patients. Outside observers, however, tend to focus on the forehead and eyes to a greater degree than the lower face. We feel it imperative to highlight this region and educate the patient on its importance. The exact configuration of the brow is a topic of debate, though the general shape is agreed upon.[19,20] Ellenbogen used the following criteria for the ideal brow position: the brow usually begins medially through a vertical line drawn perpendicularly from the alar base; the lateral aspect of the brow should terminate laterally at a line drawn obliquely through the lateral canthus of the eye and the alar base; the medial and lateral portions of the brow should lie at the same horizontal level; the brow should be fuller medially and gently taper as it progresses laterally; and the apex of the brow should lie on a vertical line drawn from the lateral limbus (Fig. 1-8).[19] Others argue that the apex should lie farther laterally at a similar line drawn through the lateral canthus.[20] In females, the brow should lie just above the orbital rim, especially laterally. The ideal position of the brow for men is along the superior orbital rim itself.[21]

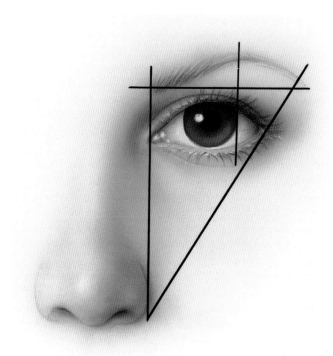

Figure 1-8 The ideal eyebrow position. The brow begins medially through a vertical line drawn perpendicularly from the alar base. The lateral aspect of the brow should terminate laterally at a line drawn obliquely through the lateral canthus of the eye and the alar base. The brow should lie at the same horizontal level and be fuller medially, gently tapering while progressing laterally. The apex of the brow should lie on a vertical line drawn from the lateral limbus.

The aging forehead is highlighted by dynamic rhytids and ptotic tissue. The soft tissues of the brow complex are continuously drawn inferiorly by gravity and depressor muscle activity. These forces are exacerbated in the aging population owing to the loss of soft tissue volume and skin elasticity. Young patients can also present with brow ptosis secondary to overactive depressor muscle activity. Brow ptosis can have a significant impact on accentuating upper eyelid dermatochalazia. A manual lifting of the brow and upper lid complex with a gentle upward sweep makes this point evident to the patient. Asymmetries are common and should be conveyed to the patient after the evaluation of the brow complex. Patients are usually not aware of these irregularities at the time of the consultation. It is very common, however, for the patient to notice them postoperatively.

In addition to the static examination of the patient, the dynamic movements of the upper third must be fully understood. There are four key muscles to consider: frontalis, procerus, corrugator supercilii, and the orbital portion of the orbicularis oculi. The frontalis muscle is the primary elevator of the brow complex contributing to the horizontal forehead rhytids. The contraction of the corrugators serves to bring the brow inferior and medial. This movement causes the patient to have a rather menacing appearance that, when coupled with the ptosis

of the aging brow, gives the look of a tired, unpleasant individual. These muscles also contribute to the formation of vertical rhytids in the glabella. The procerus, like the corrugators, also causes the medial aspects of the brows to move inferiorly. However, the procerus's slightly different vector of action causes horizontal glabellar rhytids. The orbital portion of the orbicularis oculi muscle also significantly impacts the appearance of the brow by causing an inferomedial movement of the brow.

Alopecia should be discussed with all men considering brow rejuvenation. Personal and family history of hair loss should be obtained in all cases. Women also have unique concerns that arise when considering brow manipulations. The hairline, style, and volume of the hair are but a few of these topics that dictate the approach to the brow.

Treatment Considerations: Forehead and Brow Complex

The aging process of the forehead and brow complex has been historically undertreated. In the treatment protocol, rhytids and ptotic tissue should be seen as two independent processes that each require specific management. Neuromuscular paralytic agents such as botulinum toxin type A (Botox) should be utilized to treat the dynamic forehead and glabellar rhytids. Fillers can augment the results of botulinum toxin type A in cases of deep glabellar and forehead rhytids. Free fat transfer and injectables such as stabilized hyaluronic acid can also improve the volume deflation of the brow region. Brow ptosis is almost always treated surgically. The coronal and endoscopic browlifts are the most commonly used techniques. The pretrichial foreheadlift should be considered in patients who present with high hairline.

Eyelids and Periorbital Region

Dermatochalazia and pseudoherniation of the orbital fat are the most common reasons patients present for eyelid rejuvenation. Other conditions seen in the periorbital area include festooning secondary to excess skin, soft tissue, and orbicularis muscle; malar bags due to edematous sagging soft tissue containing fluid or fat; and orbicularis hypertrophy.

The physical examination of the periorbital region is vital. Basic ophthalmologic examination must be performed. This includes the evaluation of the extraocular muscles, visual acuity, and Bell's phenomenon (upward rotation of eye with attempted eyelid closure). Other key components of the assessment include the outline and size of the palpebral fissure, the relative positions of the medial and lateral canthi, the intercanthal distance, skin lesions, asymmetry, exophthalmos, enophthalmos, crow's-feet, and signs of previous surgery. In the Caucasian patient the intercanthal distance should be equal to the interalar width. The lateral canthus should be about 2 mm superior to the medial canthal angle. The periorbital area should be assessed individually and as a component of the midface and forehead.

The upper eyelid examination usually focuses on the level of brow ptosis, dermatochalazia, and extent of lateral hooding. The brow should be elevated manually so that the patient may fully understand its contribution to upper lid dermatochalasis. A gentle sweep of the upper lid excess skin, if present, will also provide the patient with a firm grasp of the potential postblepharoplasty outcome. If patients are complaining of peripheral visual loss secondary to excess dermatochalazia, they should have a formal ophthalmologic evaluation and testing. Other conditions such as lagophthalmos and eyelid ptosis (blepharoptosis) should also be ruled out at this time. The superior eyelid margin should lie about 1.5 mm below the superior corneal limbus in a neutral gaze. Blepharoptosis (Fig. 1-9) can be quantitatively determined by measuring the margin reflex distance-1 (MRD_1), which is the distance between the corneal reflex and the upper eyelid lash line (normal range 4–4.5 mm).

In the lower eyelid, careful attention is needed to evaluate eyelid laxity, pseudoherniation of orbital fat, and double convexity deformity as well as conditions that may lead to postblepharoplasty complications. The degree of lower lid fat pseudoherniation can be assessed by gently pressing on the globe while the patient is looking up. Lower eyelid skin excess should also be determined by having the patient look up, thereby stretching the skin and revealing the exact amount of redundancy. Double convexity deformity occurs when the malar fat pads and suborbital orbicularis oculi fat (SOOF) descend inferiorly while the orbital fat pads herniate through a weakened septum (Fig. 1-10).[22] Retaining ligaments in the lower eyelid also cause characteristic creases and hollows in patients with ptotic soft tissue, decreased skin elasticity, and volume atrophy.[23]

Postoperative blepharoplasty complications such as ectropion and lower lid retraction can be avoided if the surgeon properly evaluates the resting position and strength of the lower lid. The margin of the lower eyelid should lie just above the inferior limbus (see Fig. 1-9). The margin reflex distance-2 (MRD_2) can be used to objectively determine the extent of lid retraction. Excess scleral show in this area is a sign of eyelid malposition, which needs be addressed at the time of blepharoplasty. The lid distraction and snap tests are performed to evaluate the integrity of the lower lid (Fig. 1-11). During the snap test, gentle inferior traction of the lower lid from the globe is performed to assess how quickly it returns to its normal position. The eyelid should normally "snap"

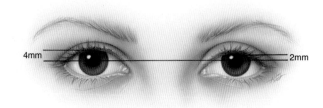

A

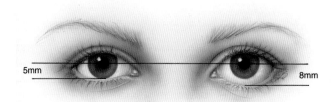

B

Figure 1-9 Margin reflex distance (MRD) –is used in the evaluation of upper eyelid ptosis and lower lid retraction. Eyelid ptosis can be quantitatively determined by measuring the margin reflex distance-1 (MRD_1) (**A**). The MRD_1 is determined by measuring the distance between the corneal reflex and the upper eyelid lash line and has a normal range of 4.0 to 4.5 mm. The margin reflex distance-2 (MRD_2) is utilized to determine the amount of lid retraction (scleral show) by measuring the distance between the corneal light reflex and the lower eyelid lash line during a neutral gaze (**B**). The lash line should normally be adjacent to the lower limbus with an MRD_2 of 5 mm. In patients with lower lid retraction with scleral show, this distance is usually greater than 7 mm.

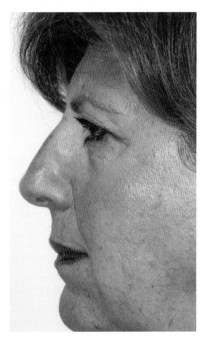

Figure 1-10 Double convexity deformity. Double convexity deformity results from the descent of the malar fat pad and suborbicularis oculi fat pad (SOOF) coupled with herniation of lower eyelid orbital fat through a weakened septum.

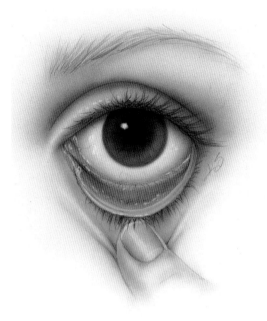

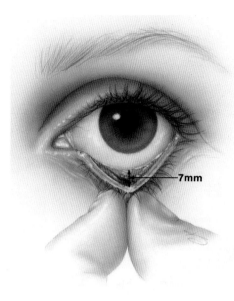

7mm

Figure 1-11 Lower lid laxity evaluation. In the snap test, the lower lid is pulled downward and away from the globe and the patient is asked not to blink (**A**). Lid laxity is present if the puncta is displaced by more than 3 mm from the medial canthal tendon. The lid should return to its normal position in less than 1 second. The lid distraction test is performed by grasping the lid and pulling it away from the globe (**B**). Distraction of more the 7 to 10 mm indicates a lax lid.

A

B

back to its normal position in less than 1 second. Excess lid laxity is noted if the puncta is displaced by more than 3 mm from the medial canthal tendon, if the lid is slow to return to its normal position, or if blinking reflex is needed to bring it back to its resting location.[24] In the lid distraction test, the lower lid is grasped and pulled away from the globe. Distraction of more than 7 to 10 mm indicates a lax lid.[25] Patients with a negative orbital vector are also at an increased risk for untoward surgical complications such as lower eyelid malposition and hollowed appearance. The orbital vector is determined by drawing a straight vertical line between the cornea and the inferior orbital rim from the lateral view; if the orbital rim falls behind this line, then the patient is diagnosed with a negative vector. Proptosis secondary to thyroid-related ophthalmic disorders are a leading cause of a negative orbital vector. A hypoplastic malar eminence may also contribute to, or magnify, a proptotic eye.

If the patient has signs and symptoms of dry eye syndrome, a formal ophthalmologic evaluation should be considered. The Schirmer test is the preferred method for evaluating patients who are at risk of developing postoperative dry eye syndrome. After the placement of topical anesthetic, a Schirmer strip (Cooper Laboratories, Puerto Rico) is positioned in the lateral fornix. Normal individuals will have more than 10 mm of moisture after a 5-minute placement.

The Midface

The midface is the region medial to the preauricular crease and lateral to the nasolabial fold. This area has gained increasing attention over the last two decades. Multiple approaches to mid-face rejuvenation are now available. The main components of the aging process in

Treatment Considerations: Eyelid and Periorbital Region

Eyelid rejuvenation can yield dramatic results. Dynamic rhytids in the crow's-feet can be successfully treated with botulinum toxin type A. Upper blepharoplasty has become standardized, although recently there has been a movement toward orbicularis- and fat-sparing procedures. Lower blepharoplasty can be performed using the skin-muscle flap or transconjunctival techniques. Patients with tear-trough deformity may need to undergo fat transposition and limited resection of orbital fat. Significant double convexity deformity should be treated with midface lifts and volume restoration utilizing soft tissue fillers. Canthoplasty procedure should be considered in patients with lower lid laxity. The treatment considerations in eyelid rejuvenation should always include addressing the aging changes affecting the eyebrows and midface.

this region include the descent and atrophy of the cheek soft tissue. This ptotic and atrophic midface tissue not only accentuates the nasolabial fold and other retaining ligaments but also creates depressions and hollowness in the submalar and lower eyelid region. One of the most important aspects of the midface examination is the relationship of the malar skeletal framework to the submalar soft tissue (see Chapter 12). Prominent malar eminence is of great assistance to the surgeon in providing the patient with excellent surgical results. The layman's "high cheekbones" are classically associated with youth and beauty. They serve as the scaffolding that enables the surgeon to suspend the ptotic tissues of the aging face. However, high cheekbone with significant submalar

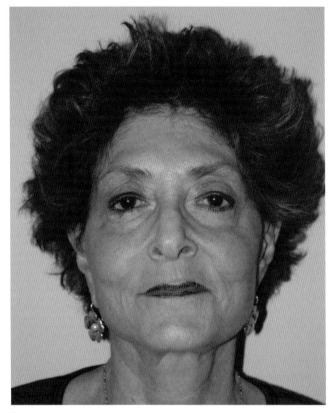

A

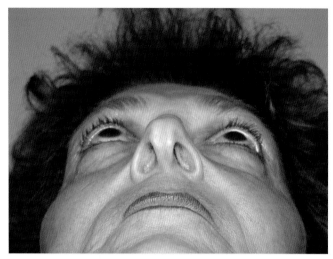

B

Figure 1-12 Frontal (**A**) and base (**B**) views of a patient with an aging nose.

volume loss may increase the "skeletonization" of the face, which is associated with an aged appearance.

The contribution of the nose to the aging face has also gained increased attention. The importance of the nose to the overall facial appearance is evident by its central location and often overwhelming effect on the patient's sense of facial beauty. The skin, cartilage, and soft tissue of the mid and lower thirds of the nose are malleable unlike the nasal bone. Just like the rest of the midfacial region, the nose is significantly affected by decades of shearing forces and decreasing skin elasticity. Patients are often under the impression that noses "get bigger" or "continue to grow." This is not completely incorrect. Aging forces do cause the nasal tip to droop with time, giving the impression that the lower third is indeed "getting larger." The nasal support structures also lose strength over time. As such, the nasal base may widen and buckling may become evident in noses that have not had preceding trauma or surgery (Fig. 1-12). Rhinoplasty in this patient population requires unique techniques to address the complex anatomical changes of the nose.

Lower Face and Neck

The key elements of the lower third of the face are the perioral region, jowls, chin projection, and neck. The perioral region encompasses the lips, chin, and soft tissue from the menton to the nasal base bordered by the nasolabial folds. Several aging changes are noted here. First, there is a loss of volume in the lips as they become thinner over time, usually with the upper lip being more affected. Vertical perioral rhytids form in a radial pattern around the oral orifice secondary to the orbicularis oris hypertrophy and decreased skin elasticity. These rhytids are more common and difficult to treat in smokers. Marionette furrows also emerge during this time as the inferior extensions of the oral commissure and the nasolabial lines. These furrows result from the descent of the lower and midfacial tissue as they abut the rather static soft tissue of the perioral area.

Treatment Considerations: The Midface

As a result of the complex three-dimensional anatomy, facial analysis plays a vital role in the protocol for midface rejuvenation. Aesthetic surgeons must utilize multiple techniques to achieve satisfactory results in this difficult region. Patients with early signs of aging can be treated with soft tissue fillers to restore facial volume, efface the nasobalial fold, and improve depressions near the lower eyelid. Individuals with moderate midface ptosis without significant volume loss can be surgically treated with deep plane rhytidectomy or endoscopic midface lift. Patients with advanced volume loss will additionally require volume enhancements via fat grafting, submalar implants, or volumizing fillers such as injectable poly-L-lactic acid. Individuals with double convexity deformity may require endoscopic midface lift, lower blepharoplasty, or soft tissue fillers in order to efface the infraorbital rim and improve the cavitary depression in the region.

Table 1-3   Edward Angle Dental Occlusion Classification

Angle Class	Description
Angle class I (normal)	The mesiobuccal cusp of the maxillary first molar articulates within the mesiobuccal groove of the mandibular first molar
Angle class II (overbite)	The mandibular first molar articulates distal to the mesiobuccal cusp of the maxillary first molar
Angle class III (underbite)	The mesiobuccal groove of the mandibular first molar is mesial to the mesiobucccal cusp of the maxillary first molar

Table 1-4   Dedo Classification of Cervical Abnormalities

Class	Description
Class I	Minimal deformity Well-defined cervicomental angle Normal platysmal tone Minimal fat accumulation
Class II	Cutaneous laxity Normal platysmal tone
Class III	Accumulation of fat
Class IV	Platysmal banding
Class V	Retrognathia
Class VI	Low positioned hyoid

Chin projection is another key component of the lower third of the face. Similar to the malar eminence in the midface, a strong mandible provides an advantageous anatomic feature for facial rejuvenation. In addition to congenital microgenia and orthognathic malocclusion, the aging population can also develop soft tissue atrophy and bony erosion of the symphyseal region leading to a decreased chin projection. During the assessment, the patient's occlusion must be first evaluated (Table 1-3). The chin position is then assessed from the lateral view. Gonzalez-Ulloa developed a simple method based on the Frankfort line to analyze facial and chin projection.[26] The Frankfort plane is a straight horizontal line drawn from the supratragal notch to the infraorbital rim (see Fig. 1-6). A perpendicular line, designated as the 0° meridian, is then drawn from the Frankfort plane at the level of the nasion to determine the amount of chin projection. If the pogonion is posterior to this line, the patient has microgenia. In women, the 0° meridian is generally 1 to 2 mm anterior to the pogonion.

The jowls are perhaps the most prominent feature of the aging face. The prejowl sulcus specifically results from soft tissue and bony atrophy of the anterior mandibular groove inferior to the mental foramen. Mandibular erosion in edentulous patients can lead to an exaggeration of the jowls and prejowl sulcus.

The last area of the lower face examined during the consultation is the neck. In the appropriate candidate, tremendous gains can be attained in the neck, ensuring a satisfied patient. The young, attractive neck is one with scant soft tissue in the submental area and a defined, strong mandibular line. Several components of the aging neck should be evaluated. The amount of submental fat (superficial and deep to the platysma), platysmal banding, hyoid position, skin redundancy and ptotic submandibular glands should all be taken into account. The Dedo cervical classification is a useful tool for neck analysis (Table 1-4; Fig. 1-13).[27] The hyoid should

Treatment Considerations: Lower Face

The lower face and neck require a combination of surgical and nonsurgical methods to achieve the best possible aesthetic outcome. The perioral region, for example, is a very difficult area to treat surgically. Soft tissue fillers as well as skin resurfacing are indispensable tools in the management of this area. The marionette furrows are also not significantly improved with facelift techniques and almost always require fat grafting or injectable fillers.

Patients with microgenia and class I occlusion are candidates for chin augmentation. Alloplastic chin implants are straightforward procedures and represent an excellent technique for chin augmentation in patients with mild to moderate microgenia and shallow labiomental sulcus. Sliding genioplasty is a technically more demanding operation that should be reserved for patients with vertical microgenia or deep labiomental sulcus. Individuals with class II or III occlusion should be referred for orthognathic surgical evaluation. If patients with severe malocclusion do not desire orthognathic surgery, they should be educated as to the limitations of facial rejuvenation.

The jowls are very well treated with most types of facelifts including the deep plane rhytidectomy, lateral SMASectomy, and short-flap SMAS (superficial musculoaponeurotic system) rhytidectomy. The prejowl sulcus is difficult to address even with aggressive facelifting techniques. Extended chin implants can successfully address this region and should be considered if this is an aesthetic complaint the patient wants remedied.

Suction-assisted lipectomy, corset platysmaplasty, chin augmentation, and cervicofacial rhytidectomy are indispensable techniques for neck rejuvenation. Isolated platysmal banding can be successfully treated with high doses of botulinum toxin type A in patients who do not desire surgical intervention.

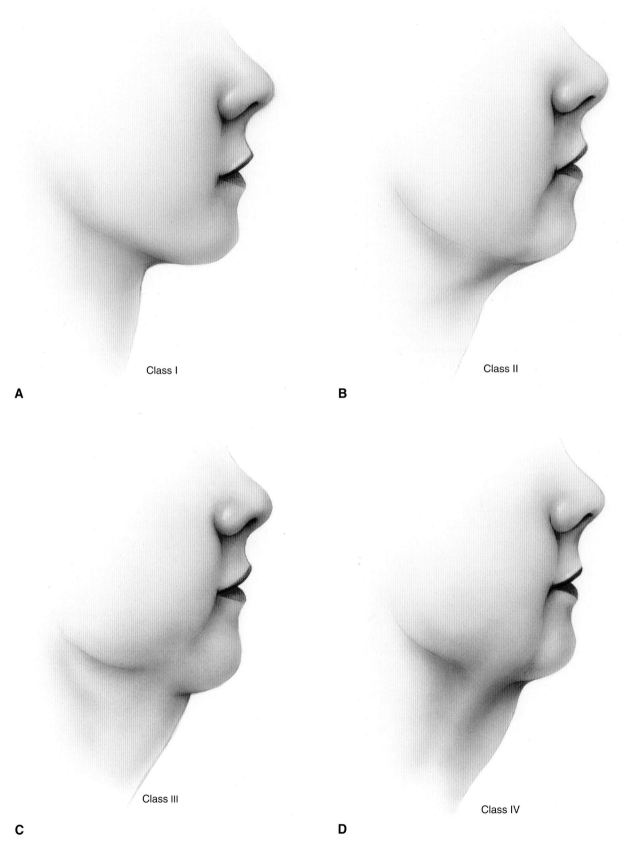

A   Class I

B   Class II

C   Class III

D   Class IV

Figure 1-13 Dedo neck classification system. Class I patients have minimal deformity with well defined cervicomental angle, normal platysmal tone, and minimal fat accumulation. Class II patients have cervical skin laxity with normal platysmal tone. Class III patients show signs of fat accumulation. Class IV patients have platysmal banding.

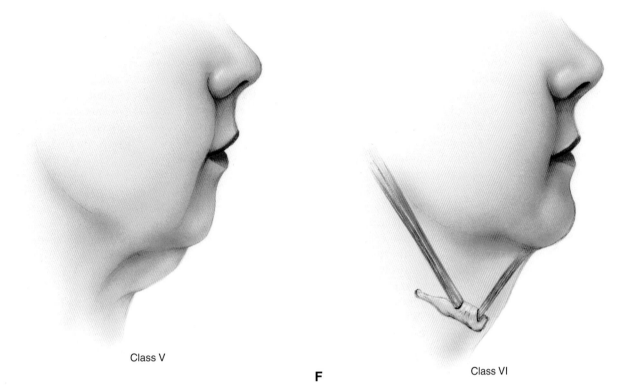

E   **F**

Class V   Class VI

Figure 1-13 *Continued.* Class V individuals have retrognathia. Class VI patients have an anterior and low positioned hyoid bone.

ideally be situated at the level of the fourth cervical vertebra. The hyoid at this position serves to create a sharp demarcation of the cervicomental angle providing the patient with an attractive angular appearance. Individuals with anteriorly positioned hyoids do not obtain satisfactory cervicofacial rhytidectomy results and therefore should be appropriately consulted. The appearance of the neck is also greatly affected by the surrounding anatomy such as microgenia and excessive jowling.

IMAGING

PHOTOGRAPHY

Photography is an essential component of the consultation process. Excellent standardized photographs allow better communication between the surgeon and patient. Patient photographs assist the surgeon in several different ways. In the planning stages, photographs can display facial features not readily obvious on the initial physical examination. In the operating room, they act as a guide when the patient is in the recumbent position and local anesthesia has distorted the anatomy. Postoperatively, the images serve as a reminder of the improvements gained for both the patient and the surgeon. They enhance communication between colleagues and are required for medicolegal documentation.

In the last decade digital photography has overtaken standard 35-mm film photography in many practices. The images with digital photography are arguably not as precise as those of film; however, the ease and economy of this method have allowed it to become the preferred medium for patient documentation. One of the key advantages of digital imaging is the potential for savings. There are three main costs involved with digital photography: initial set-up, photograph development, and storage. Although the initial set-up is more expensive than standard photography, the processing, printing, and storage of digital photographs can save a practice thousands of dollars over the long term. Digital photographs can be printed in the office, stored on a hard drive, and backed up on a server for a nominal cost, whereas standard photographs must be developed at an outside facility and then stored, incurring additional physical space and labor overhead. The printing of quality digital photographs is relatively expensive at this point. But, in a similar pattern to the costs of digital cameras, we expect this cost to decrease over time. In addition, retrieval of digital images for medicolegal, research or other reasons is far simpler than for standard photographs, which are often stored in cumbersome file cabinets. The accelerated evolution of single lens reflex (SLR) digital photography will continue to improve the quality of digital photographs.

There are several other advantages to choosing digital over 35-mm film format. Standard 35-mm photographs age poorly compared to the electronic format. There is also the increased security of this medium, which allows for remote storage to avoid loss from fire or other disaster. Digital medium allows the surgeon to better present his or her work during Power Point presentations. Last, the digital medium allows the visualization of the images in real time and permits instant communication with other physicians when one is faced with complicated cases.

Two predominant factors determine the quality of digital images: resolution and dynamic range. Resolution is determined by the size and number of the individual pixels. Dynamic range refers to the extent of the range of color choices that exist for each pixel. When a camera creates a digital image it converts the captured image into numbers. This process divides the subject into distinct numeric units. In digital photography, these units are named pixels. The precision of replicating the captured image relies on the number of pixels. Within each pixel the camera assigns a particular value to represent the color of the image. This function is dictated by the hardware employed to take the photograph. Increasing the color depth, referred to as the bit depth, increases the dynamic range of the camera. Storage of full-color images requires 24 bits of information per pixel. At this range, the photographer can represent nearly 16 million colors, allowing for film quality images.[28]

When the digital camera obtains an image, it focuses light onto a specialized device called a charge-coupled device (CCD) versus the film of standard photography. The CCD then takes the light and converts it into electrical signals. These signals are then processed by an amplifier and sent to an analog-to-digital converter that digitizes these signals. These digits are then processed by a computer within the camera. The processed image is then stored on a memory card.[28] Two primary file formats are employed by digital photographers for storage: TIFF and JPEG. JPEG compresses images whereas TIFF does not. Compression can save a significant amount of space, at the cost of image quality. High-quality compression ratios are generally in the 3:1 to 4:1 range. We prefer the JPEG format for its ease of use in retrieving files and minimized storage space. TIFF formats are uncompressed and thus consume a significant amount of storage space. Their advantage is superior preservation of data and lack of compression artifacts seen with JPEG formats.

Currently, there is no general consensus on the number of pixels required for digital cameras to match the resolution of a 35-mm film. For most surgeons, resolutions between 1.5 and 2.7 million pixels are more than adequate. We prefer digital SLR systems for the flexibility and greater image quality. In brief, the SLR system is actually defined by its viewing system. Light enters the SLR camera via the lens and strikes a mirror. This mirror then directs the light to a focusing screen where the image is resolved. A prism then inverts the image to the viewfinder so that the photographer can view the image properly. Owing to the dynamics of this system, any slight change in focus, essential for excellent photographs, can be viewed directly through the viewfinder as opposed to an image on an LCD screen in non-SLR digital cameras. In addition, parallax errors, seen in cameras that use a viewfinder that does not look through the lens, are alleviated in SLR systems. SLR cameras also provide superior depth-of-field perception.

A 1:1 aspect ratio, the ratio of an image's length to its width, is ideal. Most digital cameras use a 4:3 aspect ratio, while some higher end cameras employ a 3:2 ratio.[28] To ensure a 1:1 image the size of the CCD must be known. Consultation with the manufacturer should be undertaken prior to purchasing a lens, a vital component of all SLR systems.

Before purchasing digital equipment, the reader is advised to consult with a local professional and the latest publications because this technology is rapidly progressing. The key to excellent, dependable digital photography is the continual use of the same camera in an identical fashion. Digital cameras are individually unique in the way they capture images and thus it is recommended to use the same camera in a dedicated photography room for consistency. The photography room should be isolated from daily light fluctuations and other variables that can alter the image. The lighting methods, flash or lamps, is an individual decision. This is true for either digital or 35-mm film. We prefer a tripod-mounted camera to minimize shake and the slight movements that invariably arise with handheld photographs. A fixed tripod also minimizes the variable distance between the photographer and subject. Markings should be placed in the room to ensure consistency. The patient should sit on a rotating stool that allows for the recommended positions without excessive manipulations. A light blue background provides for a greater depth of field and thus a more three-dimensional appearance than darker colors. The background should be a solid color with a nonreflective surface. All forms of glasses should be removed. In addition, hair should withdrawn from the field either via ties or headbands to ensure adequate evaluation of the brow and upper lid complex. Standard reference points should be created to further ensure consistent photographs.[29] Several standard views are required for patient evaluation: frontal, left and right lateral, left and right oblique, and close-up views of certain areas of concern, predominantly the eyes (Fig. 1-14). The Frankfort line should be parallel to the floor and is utilized to obtain

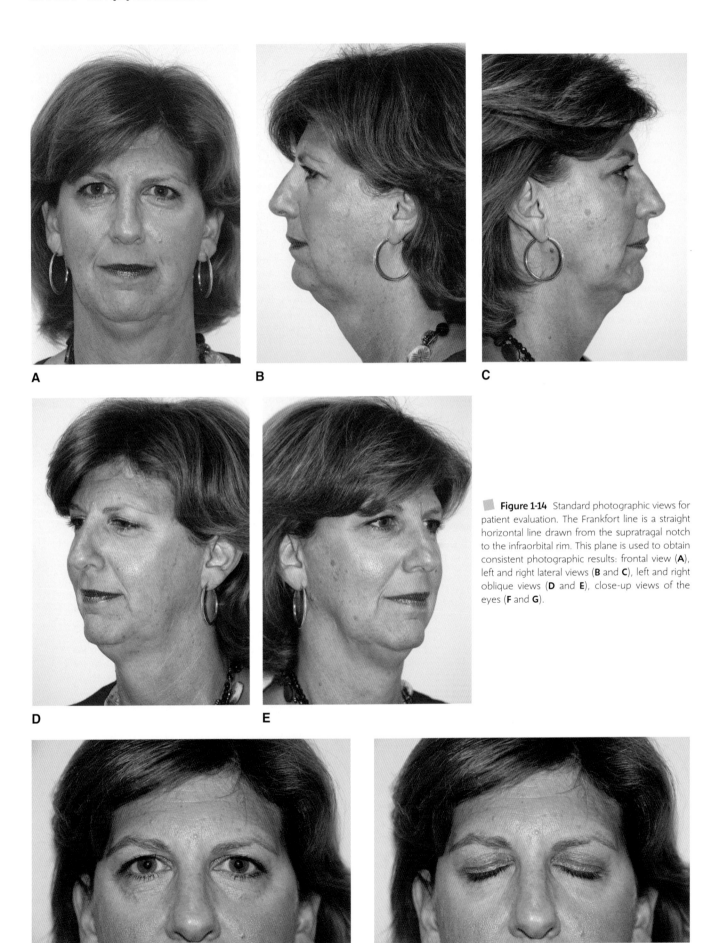

Figure 1-14 Standard photographic views for patient evaluation. The Frankfort line is a straight horizontal line drawn from the supratragal notch to the infraorbital rim. This plane is used to obtain consistent photographic results: frontal view (**A**), left and right lateral views (**B** and **C**), left and right oblique views (**D** and **E**), close-up views of the eyes (**F** and **G**).

constant photographs. The Frankfort line is a straight horizontal line drawn from the supratragal notch to the infraorbital rim. The surgeon should be sure to obtain the oblique view in a consistent manner as it can be acquired from a variety of angles. Some have argued that the tip of the nose should be in line with the opposite cheek.[30] Others recommend less rotation, aligning the medial canthus with the oral commissure.[31]

MORPHING SOFTWARE

Another component of digital photography that merits discussion is that of morphing software programs. With the use of these complex tools, patients can actually view the proposed changes that are being discussed. These programs assist in planning the procedure and guide patients in exactly what they desire and the limitations of what can be achieved. By employing these devices the patient and surgeon can clearly articulate to one another their respective goals. It also allows the surgeon to reveal certain aspects of facial appearance that the patient may not have fully appreciated. For example, patients are often uninformed of the effect of chin projection on the appearance of the nose. Obviously, such a powerful tool must be used with caution. The patient must be consistently reminded that these are computer images and should not be taken as a guarantee of results. This technology also has its shortcomings. It excels at two-dimensional manipulations such as dorsal hump reduction but does not perform as well with three-dimensional changes. Other components of the program, such as facial resurfacing, are also not optimal. In summary, this tool has several unique advantages that must be employed wisely by the facial cosmetic surgeon.

REFERENCES

1. Gonzales-Ulloa M: A quantum method for the appreciation of the morphology of the face. Plast Reconstr Surg 1964;36:241.
2. Patzer GL: The Physical Attractiveness Phenomena. New York: Plenum Press, 1985, p 16.
3. Romm S: The Changing Face of Beauty. Baltimore: Mosby Year Book, 1992.
4. Ricketts RM: Divine proportion in facial esthetics. Clin Plast Surg 1982;9:401.
5. Langlois JH, Roggman LA, Casey RJ, et al: Infant preferences for attractive faces. Dev Psychol 1987;23:363.
6. Langlois JH, Roggman LA: Attractive faces are only average. Psychol Sci 1990;1:115.
7. Perrett DI, May KA, Yoshikawa S: Facial shapes and judgment of female attractiveness. Nature 1994;368:239.
8. Richter GMA: The Sculpture and Sculptors of the Greeks. New Haven: Yale University Press, 1970, p 200.
9. Gardner EA: Six Greek Sculptors. London, Duckworth, 1910.
10. Tolleth H: Concepts for the plastic surgeon from art and sculpture. Clin Plast Surg 1987;14:585.
11. Richter GMA: The Sculpture and Sculptors of the Greeks. New Haven: Yale University Press, 1970, p 212.
12. Seghers MJ, Longacre JJ, de Stefano GA: The golden proportion and beauty. Plast Reconstr Surg 1964;34:382.
13. Brophy J: The Face in Western Art. London: Harrup, 1963.
14. Pastorek N: Preoperative ophthalmic evaluation is a personal choice. Arch Otolaryngol Head Neck Surg 2001;127(6):724.
15. Tarbet KJ: Ophthalmic evaluation should be a preoperative requirement prior to blepharoplasty. Arch Otolaryngol Head Neck Surg 2001;127(6):723.
16. Burke AJ, Wang T: Should formal ophthalmologic evaluation be a preoperative requirement prior to blepharoplasty? Arch Otolaryngol Head Neck Surg 2001;127(6):719.
17. Fitzpatrick RA: Facial resurfacing with the pulsed carbon dioxide laser. A review. Facial Plast Surg Clin North Am 1996;4(2):236.
18. Fitzpatrick TB: The validity and practicality of sun-reactive skin types I through VI. Arch Dermatol 1988;124(6):869.
19. Ellenbogen R: Transcoronal eyebrow lift with concomitant upper blepharoplasty. Plast Reconstr Surg 1983;71:490.
20. Cook TA, Brownrigg PJ, Wang TD, et al: The versatile midforehead browlift. Arch Otolaryngol Head Neck Surg 1989;115:163.
21. Rafaty FM, Brennan G: Current concepts of browpexy. Arch Otolaryngol 1983;109:152.
22. Goldberg RA, Edelstein C, Balch K, et al: Fat repositioning in lower eyelid blepharoplasty. Semin Ophthalmol 1998;13(3):103.
23. Muzaffar AR, Mendelson BC, Adams WP Jr: Surgical anatomy of the ligamentous attachments of the lower lid and lateral canthus. Plast Reconstr Surg 2002;110(3):873, discussion 897.
24. Beehuis GJ: Blepharoplasty. Otolaryngol Clin North Am 1982;15:1979.
25. Holt JE, Holt GR: Blepharoplasty: Indications and pre-operative assessment. Arch Otolaryngol 1985;111:394.
26. Gonzalez-Ulloa M, Stevens E: The role of chin correction in profileplasty. Plast Reconstr Surg 1968;41(5):477.
27. Dedo DD: A preoperative classification of the neck for cervicofacial rhytidectomy. Laryngoscope 1980;90:1894.
28. Long B: Complete Digital Photography, 2nd ed. Hingham, Mass: Charles River Media, 2003, p 485.
29. Powell N, Humphrey B: Proportions of the Aesthetic Face. New York: Thieme-Stratton, 1984.
30. Zarem HA: Standards of photography. Plast Reconstr Surg 1984;74:137.
31. Ellenbogen R, Jankauskas S, Collini FJ: Achieving standardized photographs in aesthetic surgery. Plast Reconstr Surg 1990;86(5):955.

CHAPTER TWO

Facial Embryology and Anatomy

Carlo P. Honrado, MD • Dewayne T. Bradley, MD • Wayne F. Larrabee Jr., MD, FACS

EMBRYOGENESIS

Embryogenesis is a dynamic multiple-step process that begins when an oocyte from a female is fertilized by the sperm from a male (the *pre-embryonic* period). The first 2 weeks after fertilization focuses on rapid proliferation and differentiation of the embryo with subsequent implantation of the egg into the wall of the uterus. Also, the development of the amniotic cavity and the embryonic disc gives rise to the three germ layers of the embryo during this period.

The start of the third week marks the beginning of the embryonic period (weeks 3 through 8) and is characterized by the formation of the primitive streak, notochord, and the three germ layers (ectoderm, endoderm, and mesoderm) from which all embryonic tissues and organs develop.[1] The *ectoderm* gives rise to structures such as the epidermis and nervous system. The linings of the respiratory system and gastrointestinal tracts as well as certain glandular organs arise from the *endoderm* layer. The *mesoderm* is the source of muscle, bone, connective tissue, and blood vessels. The embryonic period is of particular importance because most organ systems develop during this time, and by the end of the eighth week the embryo has a distinctly human appearance. However, because the origins of major structures are established during this critical phase, congenital abnormalities may first appear at this time if there is any teratogenic exposure to the embryo.

The fetal period spans from the ninth week after fertilization to the birth of the fetus. This period is characterized by rapid growth and maturation of the developing organ systems. Head growth slows significantly in comparison to growth of the fetal body.

This chapter focuses on aspects of embryogenesis that pertain to facial plastic and reconstructive surgery. Embryology of the branchial/pharyngeal arches and their derivatives, orbit/eyelid complex, auricle, face, nose, and palate will be discussed in detail. A description of facial anatomy will follow.

EMBRYOLOGY

THE BRANCHIAL/PHARYNGEAL APPARATUS

The branchial, or pharyngeal, apparatus greatly contributes to the formation of the head and neck and begins to form during the fourth week of gestation.[2] This apparatus consists of branchial arches, pharyngeal pouches, branchial grooves, and branchial membranes. By the end of the fourth week of gestation, four well-defined arches are visible on the external surface of the embryo. The fifth arch (also referred to as the sixth arch, depending on the theory one follows) is also present but is not visible externally (Fig. 2-1A). Each arch is composed of mesoderm-derived mesenchymal tissue and contains an aortic arch artery, a branchiometric nerve, a cartilaginous bar, and a muscle component.[3] These arches are separated by prominent grooves, or clefts, which are derived from ectoderm, and pharyngeal pouches that are lined by endoderm. As the grooves develop, they push medially through the surrounding mesenchyme and approach the medially positioned pharyngeal pouches.

The first branchial arch is often referred to as the mandibular arch and plays a significant role in the development of the face. This arch develops one small prominence, which forms the maxilla, zygoma, and squamous portion of the temporal bone, and one large prominence, which forms the mandible. Important structures that arise from this arch are the muscles of mastication, the maxillary artery, and cranial nerve V3 (CN V3). Other derivatives from the first arch are listed in Table 2-1.

The second branchial arch is also known as the hyoid arch. Around the fifth week of development, this arch will overgrow the third and fourth arches, resulting in the formation of the cervical sinus of His (Fig. 2-1B). This sinus and the second, third, and fourth branchial grooves subsequently obliterate, resulting in the smooth contour of the neck. Failure of this area to fully obliterate may possibly lead to the formation of a branchial sinus.[4] Table 2-1 lists the second through fifth arch derivatives.

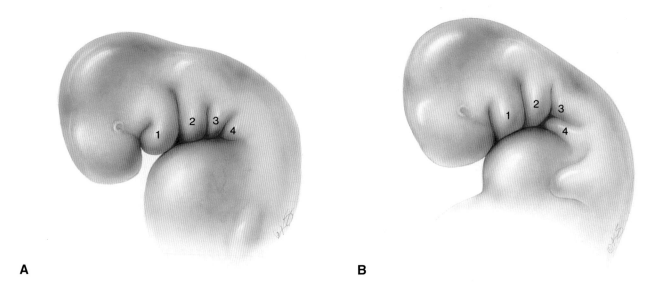

Figure 2-1 Lateral view of a human embryo at approximately 4 weeks (**A**). During the fifth week of development, the second arch overgrows the third and fourth arches, forming the cervical sinus of His (**B**).

Table 2-1　Structures Derived from the Branchial (Pharyngeal) Arches

Arch	Cranial Nerve	Skeletal Structure	Muscles	Ligaments
I (mandibular)	Trigeminal (V3)	Meckel's cartilage: malleus head and neck, incus short process and body, mandible	Muscles of mastication, tensor tympani, tensor veli palatini, stylohyoid, anterior belly of digastric	Anterior ligament of malleus, sphenomandibular ligament
II (hyoid)	Facial (VII)	Reichart's cartilage: malleus manubrium, incus long process and lenticular process, stapes, styloid process, lesser cornu of hyoid, upper part of hyoid body	Muscles of facial expression, stapedius, stylohyoid, posterior belly of digastric, buccinator	Stylohyoid ligament
III	Glossopharyngeal (IX)	Greater cornu of hyoid, lower part of hyoid body	Stylopharyngeus, superior and middle constrictors	
IV	Superior laryngeal (X)	Thyroid cartilage, cuneiform cartilage	Inferior constrictor, cricopharyngeus, cricothyroid	
V/VI	Recurrent laryngeal (X)	Cricoid, arytenoid, and corniculate cartilages, trachea	Intrinsic laryngeal muscles (except cricothyroid)	

Corresponding to each branchial groove are pharyngeal pouches, which represent outpouchings of the primitive pharynx. These pouchings are lined by endoderm and also push through the surrounding mesenchyme during the fourth and fifth weeks of the embryonic period. Each pouch contains a ventral and dorsal wing and gives rise to several important organs such as the parathyroid glands and thymus.[5]

EMBRYOLOGY OF THE EXTERNAL EAR

The first sign of the developing ear is seen by the presence of the otic disc, which appears as a thickening on the surface of the ectoderm at the end of the third week of gestation.[6] The disc soon invaginates and is called the otic pit.

Six small elevations known as hillocks develop at the dorsal ends of the first and second arches (Fig. 2-2). The

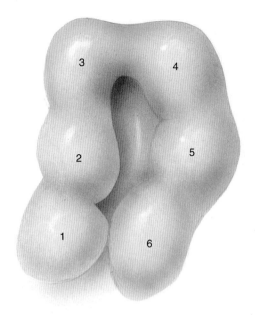

A

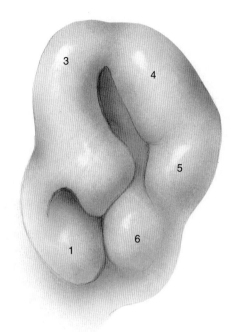

B

Figure 2-2 Formation of the external ear during the sixth week of development (**A–C**). Shown are the six hillocks.

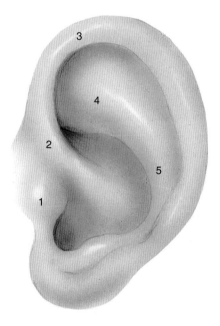

C

first branchial groove, which is located between the first and second arches, deepens and canalizes to form the external auditory canal. The first three hillocks arise anteriorly from the mandibular arch, and the other three hillocks develop from the hyoid arch.[7] These hillocks will gradually fuse to form the auricle of the external ear. Although there is much controversy, it is generally accepted that the tragus, helical crus, and helix are formed from the mesodermal components of the first arch, corresponding to the first, second, and third hillocks, and that the fourth through sixth hillocks from the second arch give shape to the antihelix, antitragus, and lobule, respectively. By the 20th week of development, an anatomically complete ear can be seen. The final shape of the auricle is determined by the intrinsic and extrinsic muscles of the ear that cause plical folding of the cartilage.[8]

Initial positioning of the auricle lies in the ventro-caudal part of the neck region.[1] But as the mandible develops, the developing ear is pushed in a dorsocranial direction and subsequently lies on the side of the head at the level of the eyes by approximately the 32nd week of gestation.

Most abnormalities of the ear, such as anotia or microtia, arise from insults that occur during the first 7 weeks of gestation.

EMBRYOLOGY OF THE EYE

Eye formation is evident by the beginning of the fourth week and has its origins from neuroectoderm, ectoderm, and mesoderm. Thickening of the surface ectoderm in the area of the future eye occurs in response to signals produced by the optic vesicles, which are evaginations from the brain. This thickening results in the formation of the lens placodes. The central portion of the placode invaginates to form the lens pit, which subsequently separates from the surface epithelium to form a spherical lens vesicle, the precursor of the lens of the eye.

During the fifth week of embryogenesis, small depressions develop above and below the eye, forming the primitive upper and lower eyelids.[9] As they become more distinct during the embryonic period, the lids approach each other and subsequently fuse by the ninth week. Prior to fusion, the lacrimal gland and its ducts also develop. Mesodermal components are responsible for the formation of the ocular muscles, orbicularis oculi muscle, and tarsus, which develop while the eyelids are fused. Separation of the eyelid complex begins during the 20th week in an anterior to posterior fashion and takes approximately 3 weeks.[3]

EMBRYOLOGY OF THE FACE AND NOSE

The embryology of the face begins early in the fourth week around a large stomodeum, which becomes the future mouth. Proliferation of neural crest cells occurs in the developing brain and migrate to form, together with mesodermal cells, the facial primordia. These neural crest cells play a major role in forming the bone, cartilage, and ligaments of the facial region. Five facial primordia appear as prominences around the stomodeum: the single median frontonasal prominence and the paired maxillary and mandibular prominences (Fig. 2-3).

Facial development continues until around the eighth week of gestation. The frontonasal prominence is primarily responsible for forming the forehead and the nose. However, the first part of the face to form is the mandible and lower lip. This occurs from the medial migration and fusion along the median plane of the two mandibular prominences. Toward the end of the fourth week, bilateral thickenings, called nasal (olfactory) placodes, occur on the surface of the ectoderm on the ventrolateral part of the frontonasal prominence. The nasal placodes initially are convex but subsequently invaginate during the sixth week. Mesenchymal proliferation also occurs around the rim of the placodes, creating elevations known as the medial and lateral nasal prominences. The depressed nasal placodes are now referred to as nasal pits, which are the primordia of the nostrils and nasal cavities (Fig. 2-4). Owing to the continuing proliferation of the nasal prominences, the nasal pits deepen and are called nasal sacs.

Proliferation of the paired maxillary prominences also occurs during this period. They migrate medially and contact the medial and lateral nasal processes. Lying between the maxillary prominence and the lateral nasal process is the nasal groove, which marks the future site of the nasolacrimal duct. Merging of the medial nasal process and maxillary prominences results in continuity of the lip and upper jaw with formation of the philtrum, premaxilla, and primary palate (Fig. 2-5). Separation of the nasal pits from the stomodeum also occurs. Failure of

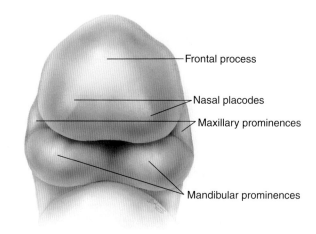

Frontal process

Nasal placodes

Maxillary prominences

Mandibular prominences

Figure 2-3 The five facial primordia comprise the frontal prominence, the paired maxillary prominences, and the paired mandibular prominences. The nasal placodes are also shown.

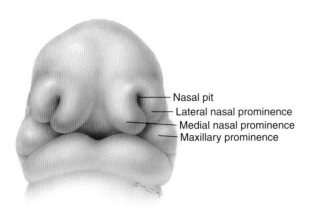

- Nasal pit
- Lateral nasal prominence
- Medial nasal prominence
- Maxillary prominence

Figure 2-4 Appearance of the nasal pits from growth of the medial and lateral nasal processes.

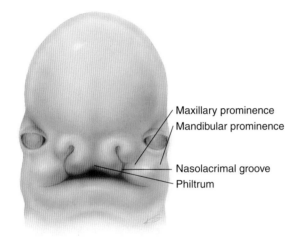

- Maxillary prominence
- Mandibular prominence
- Nasolacrimal groove
- Philtrum

Figure 2-5 The nasolacrimal groove forms between the lateral nasal process and maxillary prominence.

the maxillary prominences to fuse results in cleft lip and palate deformities.

Proliferation of mesenchyme from the first and second branchial arches results in formation of the muscles in the face. Mesenchyme from the first arch differentiates into the muscles of mastication, which are innervated by the fifth cranial (trigeminal) nerve. The muscles of facial expression arise from mesenchyme from the second branchial arch with their nerve supply coming from the seventh cranial (facial) nerve.

EMBRYOLOGY OF THE NASAL CAVITY AND PARANASAL SINUSES

As mentioned in the earlier section, the nasal placodes become depressions called nasal pits. Proliferation of the mesenchyme around the pits results in formation of the medial and lateral nasal prominences and deepening of the pits to form nasal sacs. The nasal sacs lie ventral to the developing forebrain and they migrate in a dorsal-caudal direction. An oronasal membrane separates the sacs from the oral cavity. This membrane subsequently ruptures, allowing the oral cavity to communicate with the nasal cavity in the area of the nasopharynx.

The inferior, middle, and superior turbinates arise from elevations on the lateral nasal wall. Diverticuli also occur along the lateral nasal walls, which will give rise to the future sinuses, which are pneumatic extensions of the nasal cavities. Only the maxillary and ethmoid sinuses are present at birth. The frontal sinus develops from an anterior ethmoid air cell at about 2 years of age. The sphenoid sinus also develops around age 2 and arises from a posterior ethmoid air cell.

The nasal septum arises from portions of the merged medial nasal prominences. In addition, ectoderm along the roof of the nasal cavities differentiates to form the olfactory epithelium. Some of these cells become receptor cells and form the olfactory bulb of the brain.

EMBRYOLOGY OF THE PALATE

The formation of the palate occurs between the 6th and 12th weeks of gestation. The primary palate, also known as the median palatine process, begins to form from the innermost portion of the intermaxillary segment of the maxilla. This segment is formed by the fusion of paired median nasal processes and maxillary prominences. The primary palate ultimately forms the premaxilla and represents only a portion of the hard palate that lies anterior to the incisive foramen.

The secondary palate is embryologically distinct from the primary palate and begins to develop during the eighth week. Formation of the secondary palate results from inferior and medial growth and migration of the mesenchymal projections called the lateral palatine processes of the maxilla, also known as the palatal shelves. The palatal shelves are initially separated by the tongue. With growth of the mandible, the tongue moves anteriorly, allowing the shelves to assume a more horizontal orientation.[10]

The sequence of normal palatal formation begins when the nasal septum and the palatal shelves come into contact. Closure occurs in an anterior to posterior direction starting at the incisive foramen. Bone formation also occurs during this period, completing the rest of the hard palate. Posteriorly, this area does not become ossified, resulting in the soft palate.

The degree of clefting that can occur from failure of proper fusion can range from a bifid uvula to a complete cleft of the secondary palate.

FACIAL ANATOMY

Considerable effort has been made over recent years to understand facial anatomy. Anatomy traditionally taught in medical school has failed to describe the complex relationships that are of interest to surgeons and does not highlight aspects relevant to surgical approaches. Several texts have approached the topic of surgical facial anatomy, as it forms the foundation of all facial plastic surgical procedures. Nowhere in the body is the anatomy as complex as in the head and neck region. In this section of the chapter we have summarized the relevant anatomic relationships for facial rejuvenation, highlighting critical features for each of the anatomic regions. The areas critical to the aging face are presented as the following regions: eyelid/orbit, forehead/brow, hair/scalp, cheek/midface, lip/chin, and neck. Each region is reviewed based on its underlying skeletal framework, skin and soft tissue covering, motor innervation, sensory innervation, and lymphovascular supply to facilitate understanding of complex anatomic relationships. Areas such as the nose and ears have not been covered to allow a more complete review of areas most relevant to the aging face.

EYELID AND ORBIT

Skeletal Framework

The orbit forms a roughly conical structure with the base surrounded by the orbital rim. The orbital rim is primarily composed of the frontal, zygomatic, and maxillary bones (Fig. 2-6). The remainder of the orbit has contributions from the maxilla, sphenoid, frontal, ethmoid, zygomatic, and lacrimal bones. The orbital rim is relatively thick bone and is the site of circumferential periosteal attachment called the arcus marginalis and is clinically relevant as encountered during endoscopic forehead lifts with release being essential for mobilization. Additionally, the orbital rim is the site of orbital septal attachment. The floor and medial walls, in contrast to the rims, are thin and easily fractured. Whitnall's tubercle is

an anatomically important area as it is the site of lateral canthal tendon attachment. This area is not easily identified intraoperatively, and its position must be estimated clinically. Anatomically, it forms a prominence approximately 5 mm posterior to the lateral orbital rim and is important when reconstructing the lateral canthal tendon, as when performing a canthopexy or tarsal strip procedure. The lateral orbital rim is also a useful landmark during numerous surgical procedures and in assessing eye position. For example, the eye is described as exophthalmic or enophthalmic, based on the distance from the lateral orbital rim to the apex of the cornea. Normally, the apex of the cornea is 12 to 16 mm from the rim. The bony foramina for the ethmoid arteries are present on the medial orbital wall. The anterior ethmoid is approximately 24 mm from the anterior lacrimal crest. The posterior ethmoid is 12 mm from the anterior ethmoid. The orbital apex is found 6 mm from the posterior ethmoid.[2]

Myocutaneous and Soft Tissue Covering

The skin of the eyelid is very thin and elastic, covering the orbicularis oculi muscle with little intervening subcutaneous fat (Fig. 2-7). The underlying orbicularis muscle is divided into the palpebral and orbital portions. The palpebral portion is further subdivided into the pretarsal and preseptal portions (Fig. 2-8). The orbital septum is encountered deep to the orbicularis and extends from the orbital rim down to where it fuses with the levator

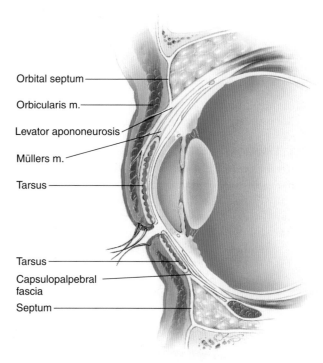

Orbital septum
Orbicularis m.
Levator apononeurosis
Müllers m.
Tarsus

Tarsus
Capsulopalpebral fascia
Septum

Figure 2-7 The skin of the eyelid and its relationship to the orbicularis oculi muscle.

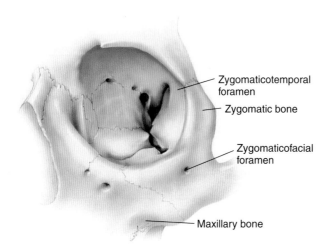

Zygomaticotemporal foramen
Zygomatic bone
Zygomaticofacial foramen
Maxillary bone

Figure 2-6 The orbit is composed of several facial bones.

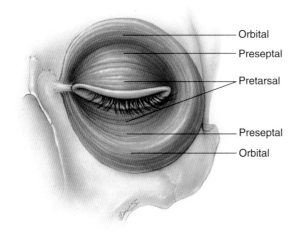

Orbital
Preseptal
Pretarsal
Preseptal
Orbital

Figure 2-8 The orbicularis oculi has several constituent components.

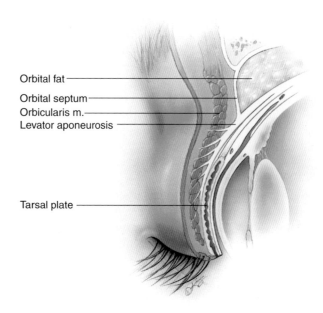

Orbital fat
Orbital septum
Orbicularis m.
Levator aponeurosis

Tarsal plate

Figure 2-9 The upper eyelid and the relationship of the orbital septum, orbicularis oculi, and orbital fat are illustrated. Note the tarsal plate and levator aponeurosis relationship with the levator attaching to the anterior surface of the tarsus and interdigitating with the skin at the lid crease.

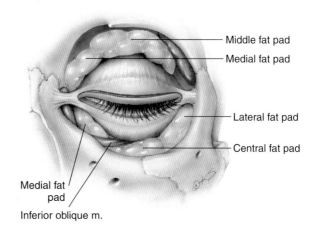

Middle fat pad
Medial fat pad

Lateral fat pad

Central fat pad

Medial fat pad

Inferior oblique m.

Figure 2-10 The fat components of the upper and lower lids. Please note the upper lid contains only two pockets, whereas the lower contains three.

palpebrae aponeurosis (see Fig. 2-7). The levator attaches near the orbital apex and extends to insert on the front face of the tarsal plate. The levator does not insert on the superior edge of the tarsus, and thus exposure of the tarsus, as in a gold weight procedure, requires reconstruction of this layer to prevent ptosis. Deep to the levator is Müller's muscle, which assists in upper lid elevation (see Fig. 2-7). As mentioned previously, the fusion of the levator muscle and orbital septum along with levator fibers interdigitate with the dermis of the eyelid skin, forming the lid crease (Fig. 2-9). The configuration of the levator insertion into the overlying skin and muscle shows racial variability.[11] The absence of dermal attachments of the levator contributes to the absence of a supratarsal crease seen in Asian eyelids. Deep to the orbital septum are the orbital fat compartments. The upper lid has a medial and central compartment with the lacrimal gland occupying the lateral compartment. The superior oblique muscle divides the medial and central compartments (Fig. 2-10).

The lower eyelid has a similar structure with a few notable differences. The lower lid retractors comprise the inferior tarsal muscle and capsulopalpebral fascia (see Fig. 2-7). The lower lid retractors fuse with the orbital septum 2 to 3 mm below the edge of the tarsus, which is crucial when approaching the orbital fat via a transconjunctival approach or the orbital rim in a preseptal approach. The orbital fat in the lower eyelid is separated into lateral, medial, and central compartments with the inferior oblique separating the latter two (see Fig. 2-10).

The canthal tendons are fascial condensations that extend medially and laterally. Laterally the canthal tendon attaches to a bony region called Whitnall's tubercle, which has been reviewed. Medially the canthal tendon has an anterior and a posterior leaf that insert anteriorly and posteriorly on the lacrimal fossae, respectively. This arrangement is thought to create a pumping action and facilitate tear drainage.

Several anatomic areas of the periorbital region are relevant to the management of the aging face and worthy of specific mention. First, is the SOOF (suborbicularis oculi fat), which is a fat pad that lies beneath the orbicularis oculi; its descent leads to skeletonization of the rim. ROOF (retro-orbicularis oculi fat) lies deep to the superior orbicularis oculi; in this supraorbital position it is encountered when the surgeon is performing the inferior dissection during a brow lift and releasing the arcus marginalis. The superior portion of the malar fat pad can also contribute to aging as additional hollowing of the orbital rim is noticed with its descent. Normally its superior portion lies over the malar eminence and smooths the contour with the SOOF of the orbital rim. The nasojugal fold region corresponds to the fold formed by the eyelid, cheek, and nose in the medial orbit. When this area is deep it is referred to as a tear trough deformity. Last, festoons represent hypertrophied orbicularis oculi muscle that manifests as folds seen over the lower eyelid into the malar region.[2]

Innervation

Motor innervation of the orbicularis oculi is supplied by branches of the facial nerve. Müller's muscle is controlled by sympathetic fibers, and interruption of these fibers causes ptosis, as in Horner's syndrome. The levator palpebrae is innervated by the oculomotor nerve. Sensory supply consists of branches from V1 and V2, including the supraorbital, infraorbital, and supratrochlear nerves.[12]

Lymphovascular Supply

The eyelid has extensive blood supply with contributions from multiple sources. The tributaries include the angular, transverse facial, ophthalmic primarily through the supraorbital, supratrochlear and dorsal nasal extensions, infraorbital, zygomaticofacial, and lacrimal arteries. The main result of these numerous blood supply sources is the formation of a superior and inferior marginal arcade. The marginal arcade parallels the lid margin and is supplied by the medial and lateral palpebral arteries, which receive blood from many sources as just named. The venous drainage parallels the named arterial supply. Particularly notable is that the venous drainage occurs via both a superficial and a deep route. The deep route occurs via the orbit and ends in the cavernous sinus. This valveless system is a possible route of infectious spread. As a result, infections in this region are taken very seriously to avoid the dreaded complication of cavernous sinus thrombosis. Lymphatic drainage occurs primarily to the parotid area and it is not unusual to see preauricular lymphadenopathy with severe conjunctivitis. A small portion of lymphatic drainage from the medial portion of the lower lid and medial canthal region occurs to the submandibular region.[12]

FOREHEAD AND BROW

Skeletal Framework

The underlying calvarium is composed of the thick frontal bone centrally and the thinner temporal fossae. The temporal region has contributions from the frontal, greater wing of the sphenoid, parietal, and temporal bones. The supraorbital rim varies in prominence and thickness and contributes to the overall contour of the brow. The frontal bone is very strong and has a thick outer table, intervening frontal sinus, and thin inner table.[12]

Myocutaneous and Soft Tissue Covering

The frontal bone is covered centrally by periosteum that is adherent at the superior temporal line and at the supraorbital rim in an area referred to as the arcus marginalis. The surgeon must release the arcus marginalis when performing a subperiosteal browlift in order to adequately mobilize the brow. The galea is a facial sheet that splits and envelops the frontalis muscle, which is the primary elevator of the brow. The galea sends dermal attachments just above the brow, which forms its origin. Laterally, the galea attaches to the superior temporal line forming an area of confluence with periosteal attachments and temporalis muscle fascial attachments referred to as the conjoint tendon or fascia. The frontalis muscular action is to elevate the brows and can contribute to transverse forehead rhytids. Laterally, multiple layers contribute to the temporal fossae and are of critical importance when both open and endoscopic browlift procedures are performed. This area can be confusing partially because of inconsistencies and variability in nomenclature. Starting superficially the skin is encountered, followed by the temporoparietal fascia (TPF) with superficial temporal arterial branches running within it. Just deep to the TPF is a thin layer of fat sometimes referred to as the *superficial temporal fat pad*. The frontal branch of the facial nerve runs in the superficial temporal fat pad and clinically is found on the undersurface of the TPF in this thin layer of fat. The temporalis fascia proper or deep temporal fascia attaches to the superior temporal line anchoring the temporalis muscle to the skull. The temporalis muscle extends inferiorly from its superior fan shape to insert on the coronoid process. The deep temporal fascia lies on the surface of the temporalis muscle and extends inferiorly, splitting into two leaves, the superficial layer and the deep layer of the deep temporal fascia. Between the two layers is the intermediate temporal fat pad (Fig. 2-11). The temporal fat pad sits on top of the zygomatic arch and is enveloped by the superficial and deep layer of the temporalis fascia as it attaches to the anterior and posterior edge of the arch, respectively. This relationship is important to appreciate because the frontal branch of the facial nerve lies just superficial to the superficial layer of the deep temporal fascia at the level of the zygomatic arch. Therefore, it is important to stay in the immediate subcutaneous plane or deep to superficial layer of the deep temporal fasciae when dissecting in the area of the arch.[2]

Please note that the TPF is sometimes referred to as the *superficial temporal fascia* and the deep temporal fascia as the *temporalis fascia proper*. In addition, the fat pad between the layers of temporalis fascia as it envelops the arch is also referred to as the temporal fat pad, as the thin layer of adipose tissue just deep to the TPF is not very distinct, and many authors do not refer to it as a separate structure.

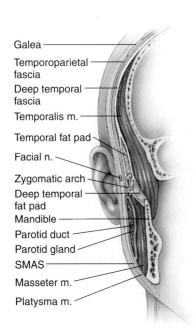

Galea
Temporoparietal fascia
Deep temporal fascia
Temporalis m.
Temporal fat pad
Facial n.
Zygomatic arch
Deep temporal fat pad
Mandible
Parotid duct
Parotid gland
SMAS
Masseter m.
Platysma m.

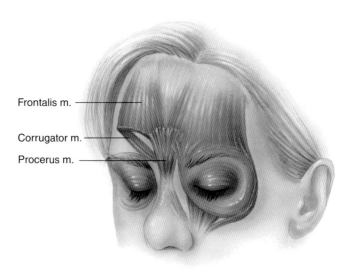

Frontalis m.
Corrugator m.
Procerus m.

Figure 2-12 The musculature of the brow is responsible for creation of rhytids in this area, depending on the vector of muscle contraction.

Figure 2-11 The SMAS (superficial musculoaponeurotic system) is a fibrofatty layer that transmits the actions of the muscles of facial expression to the overlying skin. This coronal section illustrates the relationship of the SMAS with the parotid gland, zygomatic arch, temporalis fascia, and temporoparietal fascia (TPF). Note that the frontal branch of the facial nerve is intimately associated with the TPF.

Several muscles play important roles in the aging forehead and include the procerus and the corrugator supercilii muscle. The procerus extends in an upside-down pyramidal shape from the nasal bones up to where it inserts into the overlying subcutaneous tissue. The corrugator begins at the superior medial orbital rim and travels in an oblique direction to its dermal attachments. During the corrugator's course it pierces the orbicularis oculi and frontalis muscle. The corrugator runs through a small fat pad just on the undersurface of the galea enveloped frontalis muscle, the retro-orbicularis oculi fat pad. Both the procerus and the corrugator function as brow depressors. The corrugator action leads to vertical rhytids in the glabellar region and horizontal rhytids are created by the procerus (Fig. 2-12). The corrugator has an intimate relationship with the neurovascular supply of the forehead as well. The supratrochlear and supraorbital neurovascular bundles exit the orbit and travel superficial to the corrugator before piercing the frontalis muscle approximately 1.5 cm above the rim.

Innervation

Multiple nerves serve both sensory and motor functions that come into play in the forehead and temporal regions. The frontal branch of the facial nerve proceeds obliquely over the arch to provide motor supply to the frontalis muscle. Because the frontal division is a terminal branch

with little cross innervation, as seen in the buccal region, injury can lead to significant loss of function. The pattern of facial nerve branching is quite variable; however, several landmarks can be used to guide the surgeon as to the location of this branch. One method described by Correia and Zani is that the temporal division lies in the triangular region marked by the inferior attachment of the ear lobe, brow, and superior forehead crease (Fig. 2-13).[13] Additional landmarks use the halfway point between the lateral edge of the lateral orbital rim and the root of the helix. Three to five branches generally traverse the arch in this region. Last, all the branches run anterior to the superficial temporal vessels and approximately 2 cm posterior to the anterior end of the zygomatic arch (Fig. 2-14).[14]

The sensory supply to the forehead region is primarily from the ophthalmic division of the trigeminal nerve via the supraorbital and supratrochlear nerves. Laterally, the auriculotemporal and zygomaticotemporal nerves make smaller contributions. The relationship of the supraorbital and supratrochlear nerves to the corrugator has already been described as they run with the arteries of the same name and has clinical relevance when sectioning the corrugator muscle during a brow lift. The supraorbital nerve emerges either from a notch or foramen that lies roughly in the midpupillary line. The supraorbital nerve divides into a superficial and deep branch, supplying the medial and lateral forehead, respectively. The supratrochlear nerve runs vertically approximately 2 cm lateral to the midline, which corresponds closely to the medial brow. The supratrochlear nerve then pierces the

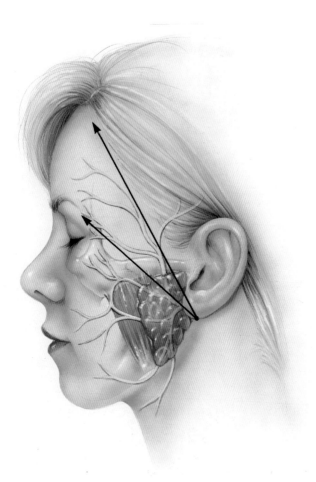

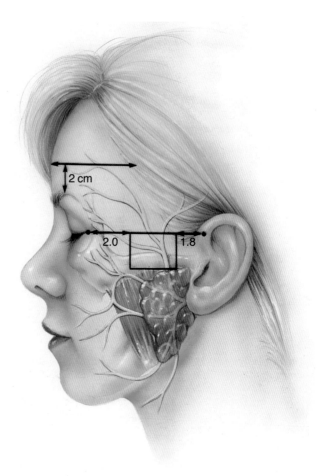

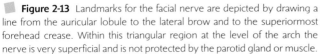

Figure 2-13 Landmarks for the facial nerve are depicted by drawing a line from the auricular lobule to the lateral brow and to the superiormost forehead crease. Within this triangular region at the level of the arch the nerve is very superficial and is not protected by the parotid gland or muscle.

Figure 2-14 Landmarks for the frontal branch of the facial nerve. Note that the anterior rami runs approximately 2 cm posterior to the anterior end of the zygomatic arch.

orbicularis oculi and frontalis obliquely starting at the superior brow and then running just superficial to the frontalis.[2]

Lymphovascular Supply

The blood supply to the forehead and brow comes from multiple sources including the supraorbital, supratrochlear, dorsal nasal, infratrochlear, and superficial temporal arteries. The vascular pattern of the supraorbital and supratrochlear arteries parallel the pattern just described for the corresponding nerves. The venous drainage is by named veins that correspond to the arterial supply. The so-called sentinel vein is a prominent venous tributary found in the region of the zygomaticofrontal suture and is a branch of the zygomaticotemporal vein. Other branches can often be appreciated as the dissection is carried inferiorly past the zygomaticofrontal suture. Lymphatic drainage occurs primarily to the parotid region, postauricular nodes, and occipital and submandibular nodes.

SCALP AND HAIR

Skeletal Framework

The skeletal framework is described by overlapping terms that include the calvarium, cranium, and skull. The skull includes the bones of the head, face, and mandible. In contrast, the cranium includes the skull without the mandible and the calvarium includes the cranium without the skull base and generally is considered to be the region above the supraorbital rim. The underlying calvarial bone is membranous bone with a thicker outer table of cortical bone and a thinner inner table of cortical bone sandwiching an intervening layer of cancellous bone. The frontal bone, occipital bone, and paired parietal bones make up the calvarium.[12]

Myocutaneous and Soft Tissue Covering

The scalp consists of layers that start with the skin superficially and overlie subcutaneous tissue. The galea is the next layer encountered and is a thin, fibrous aponeurosis that surrounds the frontalis and occipitalis anteriorly and posteriorly, respectively. The galea is separated from the adherent periosteum by loose areolar tissue, providing a convenient and easily dissected plane. The temporalis and frontalis muscles have already been discussed and the occipitalis does not play an important role in facial rejuvenation. The skin is rather thick with a firm, dense subcutaneous layer that is highly vascular and can bleed profusely, as it is inelastic, preventing vessel contraction. Hair follicles in the scalp do not emerge at right angles to the scalp but emerge at angles that vary with the region of the scalp. The pattern of hair follicle angulation progresses inferiorly at the vertex and follows a centripetal pattern. The anterior scalp hair is oriented in a more linear pattern and is angled anteriorly and inferiorly.[15]

Innervation

The neural supply to the anterior scalp has been covered in the previous section. In addition to the supraorbital and supratrochlear nerves, the auriculotemporal, great auricular (C2 and C3), and lesser occipital (C2) nerves provide sensation laterally. Posteriorly, sensation is supplied by the greater occipital nerve with C2 and C3 contributions. The greater occipital nerves supply the scalp to the interauricular line and thus transverse incisions posterior to this can denervate the scalp. Similarly, transverse incisions anteriorly can disrupt the supraorbital

and supratrochlear nerves. Vertical incisions along the superior temporal line lie roughly between the greater and lesser occipital nerves.[12]

Lymphovascular Supply

The scalp has an extensive blood supply with contribution coming from the external carotid artery and includes the occipital, superficial temporal, and postauricular arteries. The arterial supply to the temporal region has previously been partially reviewed in discussion of the forehead. However, the vascular supply in the scalp is important for various flap reconstructions in the treatment of alopecia. The superficial temporal artery originates from the external carotid artery and continues superiorly to give off the transverse facial artery that runs along the zygomatic arch. Shortly thereafter, a middle temporal branch is given off and supplies the temporalis muscle. The superficial temporal artery continues superiorly, running in the TPF and branching into an anterior and posterior branch. The posterior branch supplies a wide area over the parietal region with the anterior branch forming collateral connections with the supraorbital and supratrochlear arteries.[16] This configuration allows for the creation of two separate flaps: the temporalis muscle flap based on the middle temporal artery and the TPF flap drawing from the superficial temporal artery (Fig. 2-15). Further, the posterior branch is the supply for the Juri and related flaps in hair restoration. The venous drainage generally follows the named arterial supply. Of clinical

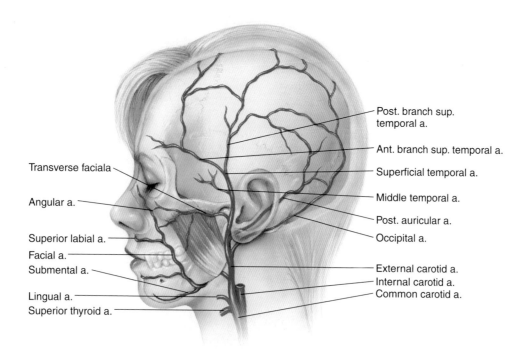

Transverse faciala

Angular a.

Superior labial a.

Facial a.

Submental a.

Lingual a.

Superior thyroid a.

Post. branch sup. temporal a.

Ant. branch sup. temporal a.

Superficial temporal a.

Middle temporal a.

Post. auricular a.

Occipital a.

External carotid a.

Internal carotid a.

Common carotid a.

Figure 2-15 The primary blood supply to the face is from the external carotid artery and its branches.

importance are the intracranial venous connections, which provide potential routes for spread of infection. The first has already been described in the forehead anatomy section and involves drainage of the ophthalmic tributaries to the cavernous sinus. Second are the emissary veins, including the parietal vein with connections to the superior sagittal sinus and mastoid vein with connection to the sigmoid sinus. The scalp lymphatics drain to the parotid, postauricular, and occipital nodes.[12] Additional drainage to the posterior triangle and jugulodigastric region occurs. Adenopathy in these regions during infection is not uncommon.

MIDFACE AND CHEEK

Skeletal Framework

The zygoma, maxillae, and zygomatic arch with its temporal bone contribution largely make up the contour of the midface. This area is important in terms of facial support and is described as a series of vertical and horizontal buttresses. The lateral buttress is the zygomaticomaxillary buttress and the medial buttress is referred to as the nasomaxillary buttress, based on the bones that contribute to them. The horizontal buttresses include the maxillary alveolus, zygomatic arch, and the infraorbital rim. The buttress system represents an area of thicker and stronger bone that supports the facial skeleton. The arch is important in helping to determine the anterior posterior dimension of the midface.

Myocutaneous and Soft Tissue Covering

The layers of the face are deceptively complex and have particular relevance to facial rejuvenation and facelift surgery in particular. The overlying skin is supported by the underlying fat and SMAS (superficial musculoaponeurotic system). The importance of facial fat is seen in patients with atrophy leading to a hollow appearance. One striking example of this is in patients treated with highly active protease inhibitors for human immunodeficiency virus (HIV). The importance of facial fat is also seen as patients age, with the formation of jowls. Several fat pads are particularly important and include the malar, nasolabial, and pre- and subplastysmal fat pads. Soft tissue fillers to augment these areas are becoming increasingly popular in the management of the aging face. Two areas of particular interest are the melolabial crease and the oromandibular fold, representing the junction between the cheek and perioral aesthetic units.

An understanding of the SMAS is essential for rejuvenation of the lower two thirds of the face. SMAS represents a fibromuscular layer that is continuous with the platysma inferiorly and the galea and TPF superiorly (Fig. 2-16). The SMAS is less distinct over the zygoma and in the perioral regions. The SMAS, as it proceeds toward the melolabial fold and oromandibular crease,

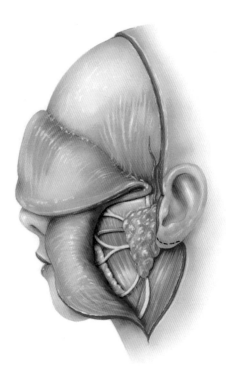

Figure 2-16 The SMAS (superficial musculoaponeurotic system) has been reflected in this drawing, highlighting its continuous nature with the galea, temporoparietal fascia, and platysma. The SMAS is relatively discontinuous at the zygoma. The facial nerve can be seen in relation to the masseter, Stensen's duct, and buccal fat.

forms an area of relatively dense attachment to overlying skin. These two areas represent regions of confluence with cutaneous attachments contributed by the perioral musculature and SMAS, which tether these areas. These relatively fixed points deepen and become conspicuous as the malar fat pad and nasolabial fat pad descend. This process leads to a deep melolabial crease and marionette lines inferiorly. Related to this process is the formation of jowls, which result largely from the descent of the malar fat pad over the edge of the mandible and dense attachments in the region of the oromandibular fold. The SMAS is distinct from and superficial to the parotideomasseteric fascia underlying the midface. The SMAS invests the zygomaticus major and is superficial to the buccal fat that is found anterior to the parotid (Fig. 2-17). The facial nerve branches lie deep to the SMAS and will be discussed shortly.[17]

The soft tissue of the midface is further anchored by various osseocutaneous retaining ligaments. In these areas dissection during facelift surgery is more difficult because the skin is anchored to the underlying periosteum. The so-called McGregor's patch or zygomatic retaining ligament is encountered at the junction of the zygoma and zygomatic arch (Fig. 2-18). The buccomaxillary ligament is found in the region of the zygoma and infraorbital rim near the attachment of the zygomaticus major muscle. The orbital ligaments suspend the forehead and eyebrow and are found at the zygomaticofrontal suture. The dense

The facial muscles comprise the muscles of facial expression, including the buccinator, which arises at the ptyergomandibular raphe and attaches to the orbicularis oris. The zygomaticus minor, levator labii superioris, levator labii superioris alaeque nasi, risorius, and zygomaticus major are elevators of the lip (Fig. 2-19).[18,19] The masseter provides bulk and fullness to the angle of the mandible region, functioning as a muscle of mastication.

Innervation

The facial nerve constitutes the main motor supply to the face. It supplies the muscles of facial expression, and the anatomic considerations are paramount during procedures to rejuvenate the aging face. The facial nerve exits the stylomastoid foramen and the main trunk can be found just deep to the tympanomastoid suture.[20] It enters the parotid gland and travels through the substance of the gland, separating it into anatomically arbitrary superficial and deep lobes. There is no distinct plane of separation in the parotid. The main trunk splits at the pes anserinus into a superior and inferior division. The branching pattern is complex and variable from patient to patient with the general pattern consisting of temporal/frontal, zygomatic, buccal, marginal mandibular, and cervical divisions. The branches of the nerve exit the parotid gland running on top of the masseter muscle and associated parotideomasseteric fascia. The zygomatic branch roughly parallels Stensen's duct. As the nerve travels anteriorly it supplies the facial musculature from the undersurface. This point is essential when performing deep plane facelifting techniques to ensure that the surgeon stays superficial to the zygomaticus major to avoid nerve transection. The natural tendency when dissecting in the region of the zygomaticus major is to follow the plane deep to the muscle as the SMAS invests the muscle. However, staying on top of the facial musculature protects the facial nerve. The marginal mandibular nerve has a variable course and can lie as inferior in the neck as the submandibular gland, usually 1 to 2 cm but up to 3 or 4 cm below the edge of the mandible. After looping below the body of the mandible it proceeds superiorly, anterior to the facial vessels. The marginal branch is deep to the platysma. The posterior facial vein is a useful landmark and the nerve is superficial to it.[14,21,22]

The infraorbital nerve supplies the sensory innervation to the central face from the orbital rim to the commissure. From the commissure to the mandible buccal branches of cranial nerve V3 provide sensation. The auricular temporal nerve innervates the preauricular area.

Lymphovascular Supply

The external carotid artery and its branches are the major blood supply to the superficial layers of the face. The contribution by the superficial temporal system has been covered in the forehead and periorbital sections. The facial artery travels over the mandible at the anterior

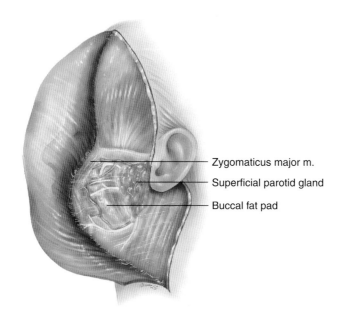

Figure 2-17 The vital structures on the face are depicted in this illustration with attention paid to the relationship of the buccal fat pad.

Zygomaticus major m.

Superficial parotid gland

Buccal fat pad

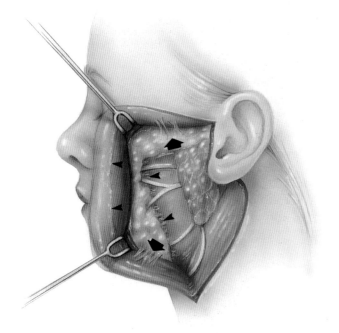

Figure 2-18 The major retaining ligaments of the face are depicted. These osseocutaneous ligaments are rather strong in the area of the zygoma, McGregor's patch, and mandible. Weaker attachments are seen at the anterior edge of the masseter.

attachments at the zygomaticofrontal suture are particularly important, as they must be released to adequately mobilize the brow during a forehead lift. Last, the mandibular ligaments are found at the junction of the anterior and middle thirds of the mandibular body.

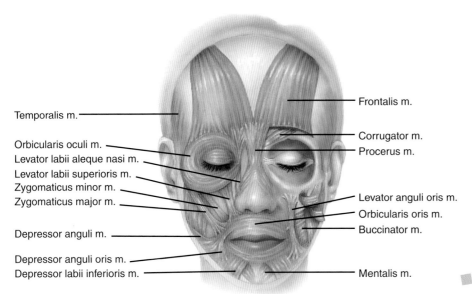

Temporalis m.

Orbicularis oculi m.
Levator labii aleque nasi m.
Levator labii superioris m.
Zygomaticus minor m.
Zygomaticus major m.

Depressor anguli m.

Depressor anguli oris m.
Depressor labii inferioris m.

Frontalis m.

Corrugator m.
Procerus m.

Levator anguli oris m.
Orbicularis oris m.
Buccinator m.

Mentalis m.

Figure 2-19 The muscles of facial expression.

border of the masseter muscle, continuing an oblique course and becoming the angular artery along the side of the nose as it continues until the medial canthal region. The first branches of the facial artery are the inferior and superior labial arteries. As the facial artery becomes the angular artery, there is significant anastomosis with branches of the infraorbital artery. These branches form a transverse nasal artery that supplies the nasal sidewall. The majority of the blood supply to the midfacial skin is via the facial and the infraorbital arteries. They supply the subdermal plexus, which provides a rich supply and is the basis for facial flaps. Therefore, protection of the subdermal plexus is important for flap viability. The venous drainage is extensive and parallels the named arterial supply. The facial vein parallels the facial artery and empties into the internal jugular vein. The retromandibular or posterior facial vein drains the region of the parotid and empties either directly into the internal jugular vein or forms a confluence with the anterior facial before emptying into the internal jugular vein. The infraorbital vein drains into the pterygoid plexus, which is responsible for draining the deeper layers of the face.

The lymphatic drainage from the central face has its first echelon in the parotid and periparotid nodes. The lower face and second echelon of the central face drain to submental and submandibular regions (level I). Drainage from the temporal and infratemporal fossae is to the upper cervical nodes (level II).

LIP AND CHIN

Skeletal Framework

The perioral region is supported by the teeth, respective maxillary and mandibular alveolar ridges, and the mentum, which corresponds to the symphysis of the

mandible. The position of the chin must be determined in relation to the occlusion to accurately describe deficiencies in chin projection. If the chin is small but the occlusion is normal (class I occlusion), then the patient has microgenia. If the size of the mandible is normal, as is the chin, but the chin is retruded due to occlusal problems (class II occlusion), then the patient is retrognathic. If various parts of the mandible are small and the patient has class II occlusion, then the patient has micrognathia.

Myocutaneous and Soft Tissue Covering

The skin and subcutaneous tissue, unlike the cheek, are closely adherent to the underlying orbicularis oris muscle. This attachment along with the attachment of the SMAS in the region of the melolabial fold contribute to the aged appearance as the more mobile and abundant cheek fat falls over this relatively fixed area.[23] The perioral region is divided into the chin and lips. The lips have a white and a red portion. The white portion extends from the melolabial crease to the vermilion and the labiomental crease inferiorly to the vermilion. The red portion has wet and dry components. The junction is where the two meet, and the appearance is based on the dry portion having a keratinizing epithelium. The shape is described as a cupid bow with a central philtral segment. The lips are surrounded by a white roll at the junction of the white and red portions of the lip just outside the vermilion border. The underlying muscular support is by the orbicularis oris with insertions into the modiolus at each commissure. The mentalis supports the chin portion of the perioral region. The lip elevators have been mentioned in the cheek portion as they originate in the midface and insert into the orbicularis sphincter. These muscle elevators of the lower third of the face are counterbalanced by the depressor muscles: platysma, depressor anguli oris, and depressor labii inferioris.

Innervation

The motor supply is via the facial nerve. Sensation superiorly is via the infraorbital branches and inferiorly by the mental nerves. The supraorbital, infraorbital, and mental nerves all exit via foramina roughly in the same sagittal plane at the midpupillary line. The mental nerve can be found between the first and second bicuspids.

Lymphovascular Supply

The main blood supply is via the inferior and superior labial arteries, which are supplied by the facial artery. The labial arteries run on the intraoral surface of the orbicularis muscle. Lymphatic spread is bilateral in the central portion of the lip to the submandibular region and mental areas. The lateral aspects of the lip drain into the ipsilateral level I nodes.[12]

NECK

Skeletal Framework

The soft tissues of the neck are supported by the mandible superiorly and clavicle inferiorly, along with the cartilaginous structures of the larynx and trachea.

Myocutaneous and Soft Tissue Covering

The platysma is continuous with the SMAS and has two flat bellies with a raphe centrally forming an inverted V shape. Laxity in the central region with the associated raphe forms platysmal bands. Two fat pads are of note in rejuvenation. The preplatysmal fat pad generally plays a lesser role, as it tends to atrophy with age. However, fat deposition into the subplatysmal fat pad with dehiscence of the platysmal and resultant pseudoherniation leads to this fat being superficial and resulting in the submental waddle.

Innervation

The platysma is innervated by the cervical branch of the facial nerve. Multiple cervical plexus branches provide sensation. The great auricular nerve provides sensation to the ear and superolateral aspect of the neck and is the most frequently injured nerve during facelift surgery. It emerges at the lateral border of the sternocleidomastoid in a region referred to as Erb's point and runs on top of the sternocleidomastoid.[12]

Lymphovascular Supply

The blood supply to the platysma includes the submental branch of the facial artery as the dominant supply with minor contributions from the transverse cervical artery. The relevant vessels include the external jugular found on the surface of the sternocleidomastoid. The facial vessels are seen anteriorly and cross the mandible obliquely into the cheek.[12]

CONCLUSION

The anatomy of the face is the foundation upon which procedures for rejuvenation of the face are laid. Detailed knowledge of the facial embryology has led to a better understanding of the layered anatomy of the face. This knowledge is most clearly of value in facelift surgery and has enabled the increased success of the deep plane technique. The SMAS and its relationship to the facial nerve and facial musculature illustrate the central role anatomy plays in surgical procedures. Although not exhaustive by any means, this review is intended to provide a platform on which the remainder of the text can rest.

REFERENCES

1. Moore KL, Persaud TVN: The Developing Human: Clinically Oriented Embryology, 5th ed. Philadelphia: WB Saunders, 1993.
2. Larrabee WF, Makielski KH, Henderson JL: Surgical Anatomy of the Face, 2nd ed. Philadelphia: Lippincott Williams & Wilkins, 2004.
3. Goding GS, Eisele DW: Embryology of the Face, Head and Neck. In Papel ID (ed): Facial Plastic and Reconstructive Surgery, 2nd ed. New York: Thieme, 2002.
4. Davies J: Embryology of the Head and Neck in Relation to the Practice of Otolaryngology. Rochester, Minn: American Academy of Ophthalmology and Otolaryngology, 1965.
5. Lee KJ: Essential Otolaryngology: Head and Neck Surgery, 7th ed. Norwalk, Conn.: Appleton & Lange, 1999.
6. O'Rahilly R: The timing and sequence of events in the development of the human eye and ear during the embryonic period proper. Anat Embryol (Berl) 1983;168:87-99.
7. Siegert R, Weerda H, Remmert S: Embryology and surgical anatomy of the ear. Facial Plast Surg 1994;10(3):232-243.
8. Zerin M, van Allen MI, Smith DW: Intrinsic auricular muscles and auricular form. Pediatrics 1982;69:91-93.
9. Pearson AA: The development of the eyelids. I: External features. J Anat 1980;130(1):33-42.
10. Sykes J: Diagnosis and treatment of cleft lip and palate deformities. In Papel ID: Facial Plastic and Reconstructive Surgery, 2nd ed. New York: Thieme, 2002.
11. Liu D, Hsu WM: Oriental eyelids. Anatomic difference and surgical consideration. Ophthal Plast Reconstr Surg 1986;2:59-64.
12. Janfaza P, Nadol JB, Galla R, et al: Surgical Anatomy of the Head and Neck. Philadelphia: Lippincott Williams & Wilkins, 2001, pp 1-150.
13. Correia P de C, Zani R: Surgical anatomy of the facial nerve, as related to ancillary operations in rhytidoplasty. Plast Reconstr Surg 1973;52:549-552.
14. Bernstein L, Nelson RH: Surgical anatomy of the extraparotid distribution of the facial nerve. Arch Otolaryngol 1984;110:177-183.
15. Tolhurst DE, Carstens MH, Greco RJ, Hurwitz DJ: The surgical anatomy of the scalp. Plast Reconstr Surg 1991;87:603-612; discussion 613-614.
16. Abul-Hassan HS, von Drasek Ascher G, Acland RD: Surgical anatomy and blood supply of the fascial layers of the temporal region. Plast Reconstr Surg 1986;77:17-28.

17. Jost G, Levet Y: Parotid fascia and face lifting: A critical evaluation of the SMAS concept. Plast Reconstr Surg 1984;74:42-51.

18. Matthews TG: The anatomy of a smile. J Prosthet Dent 1978;39:128-134.

19. Philips E: The anatomy of a smile. Oral Health 1996;86:7-9, 11-13.

20. Tabb HG, Tannehill JF: The tympanomastoid fissure: A reliable approach to the facial nerve in parotid surgery. South Med J 1973;66:1273-1276.

21. Anson BJ, Donaldson JA, Warpeha RL, et al: Surgical anatomy of the facial nerve. Arch Otolaryngol 1973;97:201-213.

22. Celesnik F: Surgical anatomy of the intraglandular portion of the facial nerve. J Maxillofac Surg 1973;1:65-73.

23. Jost G, Levet Y, Wassef M: Superficial musculoaponeurotic system in the upper lip. Plast Reconstr Surg 1986;77:161, 160.

CHAPTER THREE

The Open Browlift

Mark R. Murphy, MD • Calvin M. Johnson Jr., MD

HISTORY

The brow has historically been overlooked in the rejuvenation of the aging face. The focal procedure of facial rejuvenation has always been the rhytidectomy. Surgical forehead rejuvenation began at the turn of the 20th century.[1] Passot has been generally recognized as a pioneer in the field.[2] Several other surgeons described their work over the subsequent years.[3-6] The interest in these procedures waned, as the effects were often found to be transitory. However, as with most plastic surgery procedures, interest in brow rejuvenation was renewed in the latter half of the 20th century, when new techniques evolved and results improved.[7-9]

There has been, and continues to be, significant controversy as to the "correct" technique to rejuvenate the brow, for example, whether to use an open versus an endoscopic approach. Although this controversy is now spilling over to rhytidectomy, the contention that one operation is superior to the other has left many surgeons unsure of the appropriate approach. This confusion has contributed to the subjugation of the browlift to the less controversial rhytidectomy and blepharoplasty procedures, and thus choosing to avoid addressing the aging brow in lieu of correcting the aging face and periorbital regions.

Historically all brow rejuvenation procedures were performed via the open technique. And although this procedure has excellent long-term results, patients and surgeons were often hesitant to undergo such an involved procedure with extensive incisions and recovery time. With the advent of the endoscopic techniques in the early 1990s, surgical rejuvenation of the upper third of the face became increasingly popular.[10-14] This trend, coupled with the advent of noninvasive paralytic agents, brought brow rejuvenation to the forefront of facial rejuvenation.

PERSONAL PHILOSOPHY

Comprehensive facial rejuvenation merits an appraisal of all components of the face. This is especially pertinent for the upper third of the face. This is the focal region of the face during communication with others. The importance of the periorbital area is seen in everyday life. Indeed, it is so common in our observations of others that it is often overlooked. When speaking to or meeting someone for the first time, attention is immediately brought to the periorbital area, much more so than the jowls or the neck that so bothers the aging patient. Patients with brow ptosis subconsciously raise their brows when viewing themselves in the mirror. This cannot be done on the ptotic, sagging tissue of the middle and lower thirds of the face. Thus, the patient masks an issue that others see at all times. Though simple, this is an often-overlooked point that must be discussed with the patient.

The importance of brow rejuvenation is vital to facial rejuvenation. In our practice, this procedure is often seen as *the* primary operation to rejuvenate the face. In addition, if the middle- and lower-third rejuvenation is performed without addressing the brow, the patient may be left with an overall disharmonious appearance.[15]

The primary reason for brow rejuvenation in our practice is to address the patient's concern about looking heavy, tired, or angry, especially in the glabellar area. The goals of any browlifting procedure are to eradicate the depressing effect of the musculature of the glabellar region and to raise the lateral aspects of the brow. A key benefit of the open approach is the excellent exposure, which allows for precise handling of these problems. There is no need for overcorrection with the open approach because the surgeon can be confident that the results will be long-lasting. This is due to excision, rather than suspension, of the ptotic tissues.

There have been concerns over the side effect profile of the open browlift techniques. Likewise, the endoscopic techniques are being questioned as to the quality and longevity of the results. Despite the variety of methods to surgically, or nonsurgically, address this area, it often remains neglected.

The endoscopic techniques have done a tremendous amount to reinvigorate interest in the aging upper third of the face. Surgeons have noted the advantages of smaller incisions; less downtime; reduced scarring, numbness, and alopecia; and minimizing the loss of blood.[12,16] However, the endoscopic techniques do have selected disadvantages. For example, there is still no method of fixation that is clearly superior to others.[17-24] The technique has a limited ability to correct severe eyebrow ptosis and must be utilized only in certain patients.[24,25] In addition, the endoscopic record is not yet defined.[26] A recent report in the literature has confirmed many surgeons' trepidations about this technique. Only 50% of plastic surgeons surveyed felt that their results were satisfactory more than 2 years after the operation.[27]

In addition to the longevity concerns regarding endoscopic browlifts, there have also been questions regarding its impact on the contour of the brow. It has been found that the greatest impact of the endoscopic browlift is medially not laterally, thus contributing to the dreaded "surprised look" and not affecting the lateral brow where the lift is generally desired.[28,29] This highlights another advantage of the open browlift technique. The coronal approach allows for more control of the brow contour by way of its differential scalp incision.[30]

Although the emphasis in the last decade has been on endoscopic and less invasive methods such as the use of botulinum toxin-A, the open browlift has a proven record of providing excellent, lasting results with minimal side effects. The open browlift maximizes the optimal removal of the corrugators and excess skin that accumulates with time.[31] In our opinion, the main role for the endoscopic approach is in young patients with a minimal amount of ptosis. In our practice, however, we often suggest deferring the procedure in younger patients until the concerns have truly manifested themselves, at which point we perform what we believe to be the procedure of choice, the open browlift. We feel the open browlift is the optimal operation in patients with severe ptosis of the brows, deep glabellar or midforehead wrinkles, or a preexisting high forehead, when a trichophytic lift is selected. The results achieved with this forehead lift are predictable, natural appearing, long lasting, and aesthetically pleasing with minimal morbidity.[15]

Other surgeons have also reported that the open technique is more effective in achieving the three main goals of brow surgery: brow elevation, reduction of transverse lines, and reduction of glabellar lines.[32] In addition, even those who favor the endoscopic technique state that some patients will benefit from the open approach.[33]

The negative side effects of the open browlift techniques seem to have been unduly emphasized in the literature. In a recent, unpublished report on the significance of the side effects of the open browlift techniques, the authors found an overwhelming percentage of patients would recommend the procedure to a friend or relative.[34] Recent reports have also thrown light on various vague detractions of the open technique. The difference in the rate of alopecia between the two techniques is small, and sensory loss has been noted to be higher with the endoscopic techniques.[32,35] In summary, the open browlift technique has a similar complication rate, a comparable rate of sensory loss, and a higher patient satisfaction rate.[32] The other issue commonly mentioned when discussing the open approach to forehead rejuvenation is the extent of the incision. We feel that this is predominantly a matter of proper patient education. Certainly, if patients feel that they are going to be "scalped," they will not consent to the procedure.[14,33]

The coronal incision can be completely camouflaged with the patient's hair. In the case of the trichophytic incision, only the anterior aspect is exposed, and this component of the incision can also be masked with hair when the patient wears her bangs combed forward. In both instances the incision generally heals imperceptibly when proper beveling is employed during the incision and meticulous technique is applied during the closure. The patient must be counseled as to the amount of time it requires for the wound to heal completely. If the patient does not wish to have an open procedure because of the incision, the endoscopic approach should be explored with the patient.

The open technique via the pretrichial route enables the surgeon to manipulate certain situations in unique ways. For example, the pretrichial lift allows for shortening of an elongated forehead. A long forehead disrupts the harmony of the face and adds to the patient's age.[36] The forehead shortening capabilities of the trichophytic browlift are unobtainable with the endoscopic technique.[37,38] Detractors argue that the incision placement prohibits the use of this technique, but many feel that with proper planning, technique, and execution this approach yields an excellent aesthetic result.[39] This is not to say that this procedure may be used in all patients with an elongated forehead. If the patient is overly self-conscious of scarring or has a hairstyle that positions the hair posteriorly the surgeon would be wise to avoid this technique.

The decision-making process for the coronal vesus the pretrichial approach has been reported on in the literature.[15,40] We generally agree with these parameters but do make exceptions in certain cases to the 5 cm rule.

The purpose of this chapter is not to determine which technique is superior. That is a decision to be made during the consultation. The open browlift technique should be familiar to all plastic surgeons rejuvenating the upper third of the face. Endoscopic and open techniques should be discussed with all patients. As with any procedure, the risks and benefits should be fully explained to the patient.

ANATOMY

To appropriately rejuvenate the brow, the surgeon must be knowledgeable of its anatomy. The position and movement of the brow are determined by several factors. First among these are the paired frontalis muscles. The frontalis is the sole elevator of the brow. These paired muscles have a definitive midline separation[41] (Fig. 3-1). Each of these muscles originates from the galea aponeurotica. This fascia also encases the muscles, and inserts into the

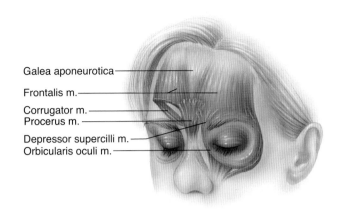

Galea aponeurotica —
Frontalis m. —
Corrugator m. —
Procerus m. —
Depressor supercilli m. —
Orbicularis oculi m. —

Figure 3-1 The musculature of the brow.

orbicularis oculi muscles, which then insert into the eyebrow dermis. Only the lower 20% of the frontalis muscle is mobile.[42]

The brow has four depressor muscles: the procerus, corrugator, depressor supercilii, and the orbital portion of the orbicularis oculi[14] (see Fig. 3-1). The depressor supercilii is located on the medial arc of the orbicularis and is considered by some to be part of the orbicularis.[43] This muscle aids the corrugator in depressing the medial head of the brow. The corrugator musculature originates from the frontal bone near the superomedial orbital rim and inserts into the dermis of the forehead skin behind and immediately superior to the middle third of the brow.[41] Contraction of the corrugator complex results in depression of the brow and deep vertical glabellar rhytids. The procerus originates from the nasal bone and inserts into the lower medial skin of the forehead. Its contraction leads to the most inferior horizontal rhytid over the radix of the nose.[43]

The galea is contiguous with the superficial temporalis fascia laterally. The periosteum of the frontal bone is contiguous with the temporalis fascia. These respective fascia layers converge just medial to the temporal fusion line of the skull.

The sensory innervation to the scalp is relatively straightforward. The two major nerves are the supraorbital and supratrochlear, with the supraorbital nerve supplying the majority of the scalp. The supraorbital nerve has two main divisions, superficial (medial) and deep (lateral).[44] The deep division of the supraorbital nerve runs under the deep galeal plane and over the periosteum toward the superior temporal line before taking a turn superficially through the galeal fat pad on its way to the skin of the frontoparietal scalp.[14] The superficial division courses from the orbital rim and over the frontalis muscle and terminates in the anterior scalp.[42] The superficial branch supplies the sensation to the forehead skin and anterior scalp. The superficial branches of the supraorbital nerve and the supratrochlear nerve

both travel over the superficial surface of the frontalis muscle. The frontal branch of the facial nerve runs within the superficial temporalis fascia on its way to innervate the frontalis muscle.

PREOPERATIVE ASSESSMENT

Numerous studies have considered the ideal appearance of the female eyebrow.[45-51] A variety of factors determine the aesthetically pleasing brow. An individual's ethnicity, age, sex, culture, and adjacent structures all influence the perceived beauty of the brow. Though opinions differ on certain facets of the brow, certain desirable traits commonly recur: (1) the medial brow should lie at, or below, the level of the supraorbital rim, (2) the brow should have an apex lateral slant, (3) the medial brow should begin in the vertical plane of the inner canthus and lateral extent of the ala, (4) the brow ends laterally in line with a tangent drawn from the lateral ala through the lateral canthus, and (5) the apex of the brow should lie above either the lateral limbus or lateral canthus.[45,46,47-49,52] Another key feature of brow beauty is the relationship to the dorsal line of the nose (Fig. 3-2). When the brow continues this gentle slope (brow-tip aesthetic line) it adds to the inherent attractiveness of the face.[7,45,53]

The decision of trichophytic versus coronal incision will be discussed with the patient during the preoperative

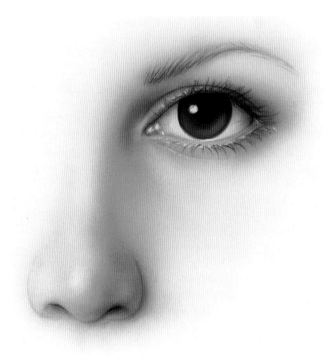

Figure 3-2 The ideal aesthetic of the brow depends on individual preferences. The goal is to provide the patient with an elegant slope of the brow as it evolves into the contour of the nose.

assessment. This judgment is based on the position of the hairline, low versus high, and the manner in which the patient wears his or her hair.[54] Of course, the personal preferences of the patient must also be taken into account.

The key to an accurate preoperative assessment is the relaxation, manual if necessary, of the brow. It is in repose that the patient must objectively view the resting position of the brow. As mentioned earlier, the patient reflexively raises his or her brow when placed in front of a mirror or when a photo is taken. The surgeon can manually position the brow as it appears at rest with the patient's eyes closed and then instruct her to open her eyes slowly. This maneuver enlightens the patient as to the issues at hand and furthers confidence in the surgeon as an expert who truly sees the face in a different manner from the layman.

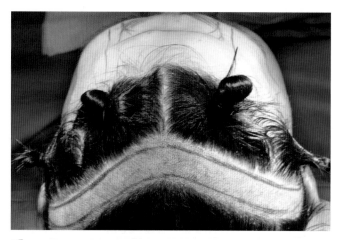

Figure 3-3 The standard coronal markings.

TECHNIQUE

The sequence of procedures for facial rejuvenation usually begins with the forehead lift. We rarely perform a solitary procedure on the brow. Most often it is in conjunction with an upper and lower lid blepharoplasty and deep plane facelift. We choose to do the brow first because it allows for a more conservative, and accurate, upper lid blepharoplasty. In select cases, such as patients with deep-set eyes, previous blepharoplasty, or limited redundancy of upper lid skin, the browlift is all that is needed for upper third facial rejuvenation.

Marking and shaving of hair can be performed prior to or after the administration of the anesthetic. Patients are often very anxious during this time, and the marking and shaving of hair amplifies these feelings. We prefer to do these tasks after the administration of general anesthesia. In an arena in which cost management is a priority this can be done prior to administering the anesthetic.

When a coronal approach has been chosen, a fusiform segment of tissue is shaved and marked for excision (Fig. 3-3). The markings for the excision should lie 5 to 6 cm posterior to the anterior hairline. The lateral extent of the incision should terminate approximately 1 to 2 cm above the superior insertion of the auricle to the skull in an attempt to incorporate the superficial temporal vessel within the flap (Fig. 3-4). If this vessel is compromised, however, the blood supply to this flap is substantial. The surgeon should ensure that an adequate amount of temporal hair is left behind. This is particularly important when this procedure is being performed in conjunction with a facelift in which a portion of the sideburn is shaved as well. The incision should parallel the anterior hairline tapering at the lateral aspects to a point. We prefer to mark and excise the amount of tissue to be removed at the beginning of the case rather than making one incision, anterior or posterior, mobilizing the scalp, and then deciding on the appropriate amount to excise. We have

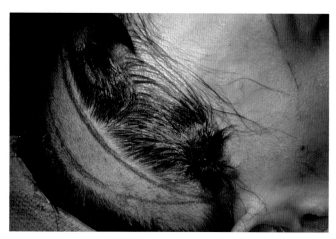

Figure 3-4 The coronal markings mimic the anterior hairline and taper laterally.

found we can reliably gauge the amount to be resected by assessing the mobility of the scalp and its associated effect on brow position prior to incision. It is acceptable to decide on the exact amount of skin to be excised after raising the flap. However, we have found that precise incising of this thick tissue, as is mandated when trying to preserve as many hair follicles as possible, is very challenging after it has been mobilized. With adequate experience the surgeon is highly successful in anticipating the total skin excision prior to the initial incision. Generally speaking, the amount of skin lies between 1 and 2 cm. If the surgeon discovers that he or she has miscalculated and resected too much tissue, the posterior scalp elevation can be performed to aid in the closure. Obviously, it is better to err on the side of caution and remove less excess skin if the surgeon is uncertain as to the exact amount to be removed.

The trichophytic incision is more difficult to plan and perform but yields a tremendous result when attention is paid to the details. The marking begins with a trimming,

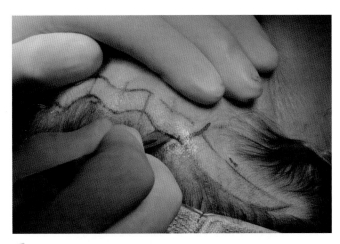

Figure 3-5 The markings for the trichophytic lift are similar to those for the coronal lift but have undulations in the center and the angles are slightly different; note the beveling of the incision.

with scissors, of the first two to three rows of hair in the anterior aspect of the hairline. Laterally the hair is shaved as an elongated, curved triangle with its apex above the superior insertion of the auricle to the scalp (Fig. 3-5). This area is generally 4 to 5 cm in length and should not be placed too inferiorly to avoid encroaching on the temporal hairline. This termination point varies from patient to patient depending on the position of the hairline and the contour of the patient's skull. Once the incision is created a flap must be mobilized to allow access to the glabellar musculature. This procedure often requires folding the flap upon itself, and thus, an adequate rotation point must be chosen laterally. In the midline, the incision has gentle undulations closely following the hairline. This undulation allows improved camouflage of the incision over a simple straight line. The posterior aspect of the incision should be placed in the transition zone between the thick posterior hair of the scalp and the fine hairs that constitute the anterior hairline (see Fig. 3-5).

The hair is secured with rubber bands anteriorly and with a circumferential band of tape posteriorly. In the trichophytic browlift the only hair that is secured with rubber bands is the lateral temporal hair. The hair is shaved in the fusiform ellipse in the coronal approach and as described in the previous paragraph for the tricophytic approach. The surgeon should be mindful not to place the posterior tape too tightly around the circumference of the head, thus creating a "false" lift that results in under-resection.

The incisions are re-marked and injected with local anesthetic. We prefer a mixture of equal parts of 0.5% lidocaine with 1:200,000 epinephrine and 0.5% bupivacaine with 1:200,000 epinephrine. The injection should be in the galeal plane where most of the vessels run their course. Local anesthetic should also be injected into the subgaleal plane as well. Bilateral supraorbital and supratrochlear blocks are administered. And last, the corrugator and procerus muscles are directly injected to aid in pain management as well as for vasoconstrictive purposes. The patient is then prepped and draped in the standard fashion. We prefer to staple a sterile towel around the head in a parallel course to the taping, being mindful not to place the towel too tightly.

The incisions are then performed with a No. 10 blade. We prefer this blade for its increased surface area, which reduces the need to change blades frequently. Excessive use of smaller blades leads to increased cost and operating time. The forehead skin is thick and will quickly dull smaller blades. The blade must be sharp and the surgeon should not hesitate to use several blades in making these incisions. A dull blade will cut imprecisely, which should never occur in cosmetic surgery. Proper beveling of both the pretrichial and coronal incisions is vital to attaining maximal hair regrowth and scar camouflage. In the coronal incision the bevel parallels the follicles throughout the length of the incision (Fig. 3-6). The entire amount of shaved hair is removed, leaving a hair to hair closure. Thus, the patient may be reassured preoperatively that he or she will not have a noticeable region of alopecia postoperatively. The coronal incision traces further laterally than the pretrichial incision and the orientation of hair at the end point of the incision is almost perpendicular to the skin; the blade must mimic this orientation.

The pretrichial incision requires alternating beveling techniques. In this technique, the surgeon must be cognizant of three separate areas of the planned incision (Fig. 3-7 to 3-10). The first is the anterior, visible, aspect of the incision. In this area the beveling transects the follicles to allow them to grow through the incision as it heals over time. The hair in this area generally grows in an anterior direction, and the incision is almost perpendicular to the follicles. The bevel must be at an angle that transects the shaft of the follicle while maintaining the base of the follicular unit, which has

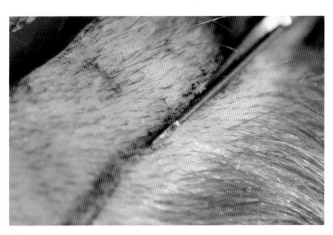

Figure 3-6 The beveling of the incision for the coronal approach parallels the hair follicles throughout the incision.

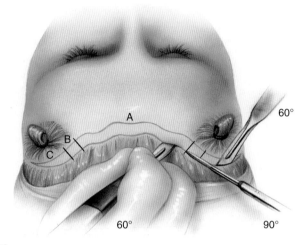

Figure 3-7 Varying angles of the blade are used during the trichophytic incision.

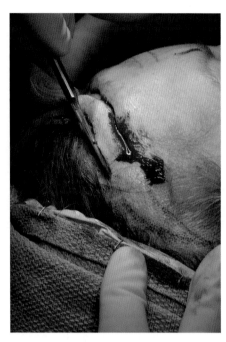

Figure 3-9 The angle of the blade transitions as the incision moves laterally.

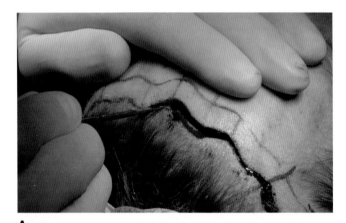

A

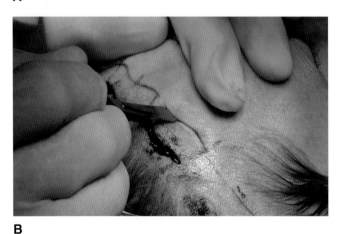

B

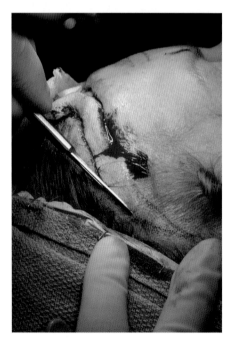

Figure 3-10 The lateral aspect of the trichophytic incision parallels the hair follicles as in the coronal incision.

Figure 3-8 The posterior aspect of the trichophytic incision is made through the first few anterior hairs (**A**). This incision transects the follicles so that they grow through, and thus mask, the healing wound. The anterior aspect of the trichophytic incision is performed; the angle of the bevel must be identical to that of the posterior portion of the incision to optimize wound healing (**B**).

regenerative properties. This bevel pattern is in opposition to the lateral, hair-bearing area of the incision. When the surgeon chooses this approach preoperatively, he or she should assess the growth pattern of these vital anterior hairs. If the hairs grow posteriorly, the patient may not be able to mask the incision by wearing the bangs forward, and this should be discussed with the patient. The second aspect of the incision is the interface of the anterior region of the incision with the hair-bearing areas laterally (see Figs. 3-7 and 3-9). At this juncture the beveling must be altered from transecting the follicles to running almost parallel to them. This is a brief transition and should quickly evolve into the standard follicle-sparing angle seen with the coronal lift as the surgeon goes deeper into the hair laterally (see Figs. 3-7 and 3-10). It should be noted that the surgeon must utilize the same angle of incision for both the posterior and anterior portions of the incision to ensure the best possible closure. The importance of proper beveling technique cannot be overemphasized. When done improperly, alopecia and noticeable—and thereby unattractive—scars result. Lack of attention to these details has produced results that give credence to the critics of these techniques. The hair is a great ally of the cosmetic surgeon as long as it is handled appropriately.

For the entire coronal incision and the lateral aspects of the pretrichial incision, the blade is advanced with a pushing motion, instead of the classical method of pulling the knife toward oneself. This technique allows better control of the knife through the thick skin of the forehead. It also enhances the surgeon's ability to follow the hair follicles correctly because the knife blade is visible. This is vital when considering the exacting manner in which the knife must be beveled for these procedures. Whether the coronal or trichophytic lift is performed, the incision must be beveled correctly throughout all aspects of the incision. The incision is carried down to the level of the subgaleal plane of dissection. After the incisions have been created the excess skin is removed. This is done one side at a time so that blood loss is kept to a minimum. As all surgeons who operate in this area know, the blood supply to the scalp is robust. Removing half of the excess skin and obtaining hemostasis will help to avoid untoward complications. Frequently, the superficial temporal vessels are transected laterally and this bleeding should be immediately addressed. We prefer bipolar cautery to reduce thermal damage to adjacent hair follicles. With this concept in mind, the surgeon should not pursue oozing vessels above the galea. There are no major vessels superficial to the galea and we will often attend to bleeding here with a cold compress in lieu of electrocautery. Cautery above this level places the hair follicles at undue risk. A complete examination of the incision should be performed prior to placing a cool, moist compress on the posterior portion of the incision. Bleeding can persist in the lateral aspects of the incisions and go unnoticed by the surgeon as he or she is focused elsewhere. The surgeon must check both lateral aspects of the incision periodically throughout the case to ensure adequate hemostasis. Large amounts of blood can be lost from scalp incisions. The contralateral skin is removed, hemostasis is obtained, and the anterior flap is then elevated.

A subgaleal dissection, with the No. 10 blade, is performed until slightly superior to the supraorbital rim (Fig. 3-11). This plane allows ease of dissection. With the excision of tissue in the open technique, we do not need to rely upon the periosteum readhering to the cranium to ensure that the lift holds. Although subperiosteal dissection is acceptable, this technique does not rely on

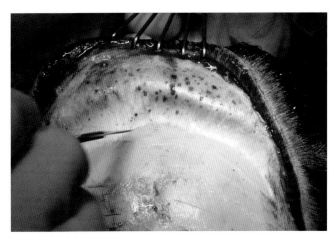

Figure 3-11 The subgaleal dissection is performed with the No. 10 blade.

periosteal refixation for its result and longevity; thus, it is easier and equally effective to dissect in the subgaleal plane.[55] We employ the term "sliding plane" because we feel it is descriptive of the dissection. The plane is elevated with a No. 10 blade and Anderson bear claw retractor in the original phase. When approaching neurovascular structures medially (supraorbital and supratrochlear nerves) and laterally (frontal branch of facial nerve), a nonpenetrating retractor is used (Fig. 3-12). The supraorbital and supratrochlear bundles are preserved at the orbital rim or notch, depending on the patient's anatomy. The frontal branch is also preserved by dissecting directly on the superficial layer of the deep temporalis fascia. When approaching the zygomatic arch we change dissecting instruments from a No. 10 blade to sharp, fine scissors and a cotton-tip applicator for blunt dissection (Fig. 3-13). The dissection is carried down to the arches bilaterally. We generally do not aggressively cauterize in this area secondary to potential thermal injury to the facial nerve; judicious bipolar cautery is advised if necessary.

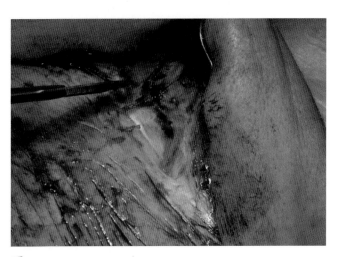

Figure 3-12 A nonpenetrating retractor is employed when approaching neurovascular structures.

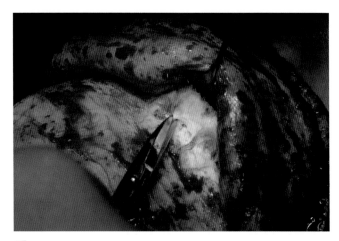

Figure 3-13 A sharp scissors and nonpenetrating retractor are used in the lateral component of the dissection.

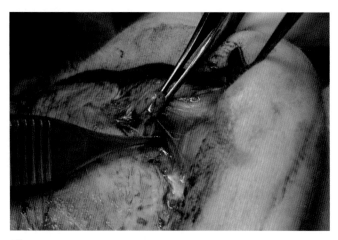

Figure 3-15 The corrugator excision is performed with bipolar cautery after transecting the muscle. This maneuver is aided by retraction in the vector of the muscle.

With the flap completely mobilized attention is then directed to the glabellar musculature (Fig. 3-14). The flap has been raised to the radix at this juncture, and using Adson forceps and sharp, fine dissecting scissors, the corrugators are dissected free and cauterized with bipolar cautery. This dissection is greatly aided by the assistant using a nonpenetrating retractor in the natural vector of the corrugator to help expose the muscle (Fig. 3-15). Care must be taken to avoid inadvertent trauma to the supratrochlear neurovascular bundle during this phase of the operation. Often, a supratrochlear vein is encountered in the region. It should be dealt with accordingly. The medial

2 to 3 cm is dissected free from the galea and the muscle is transected after bipolar cauterization at its medial attachment to the bone. The medial free edge of the muscle is grasped and pulled laterally until approximately 2 cm are freed for excision. Again the muscle is cauterized and resected with the sharp, fine scissors. This is a true advantage of the open technique. It allows for unparalleled exposure of this dense muscular complex.

With excision of this muscle the surgeon and patient can be assured of a long-term benefit unattainable with other methods such as botulinum toxin-A. The concern over muscle resection leading to a deficit of expression of the brow is understandable, but fortunately this consequence is exceedingly rare. Even with aggressive muscle resection the patient usually has adequate expression postoperatively.

The procerus is then addressed. With the flap elevated, the procerus is scored horizontally with a bovie (Fig. 3-16). This should be performed lightly through muscle alone. If done too deeply, the patient will be left with a

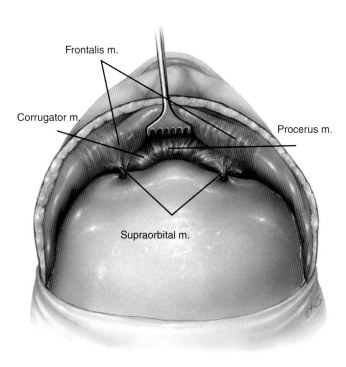

Frontalis m.

Corrugator m.

Procerus m.

Supraorbital m.

Figure 3-14 The anatomy of the everted forehead flap.

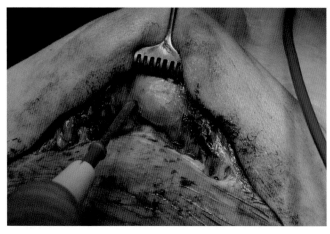

Figure 3-16 The procerus is scored horizontally with monopolar cautery.

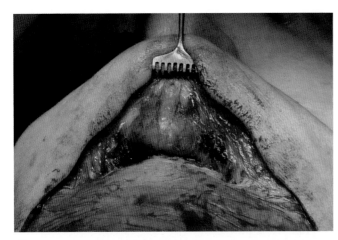

Figure 3-17 In select cases the glabellar region is scored vertically to alleviate excessively heavy brows.

soft tissue depression in the glabellar region. The scoring should center on the medial aspect of the muscle to ensure that the supratrochlear neurovascular bundles are left unperturbed. Occasionally, in the heavy brow we will also perform a vertical myotomy to allow for lateral spread of the glabella to address vertical rhytids (Fig. 3-17).

In most cases we will also perform a horizontal myotomy of the frontalis and a galeotomy (Fig. 3-18). We choose to perform this at the level of the most prominent midforehead rhytid. This is also performed with monopolar cautery in the midline. By performing this maneuver in the midline the surgeon allows the patient to retain muscle function laterally, permitting lateral brow elevation. The lateral borders of this incision are the medial aspects of the orbital rims. We are judicious in the use of this technique secondary to the concern of imparting a "surprised" look onto the patient.

A suction drain is then placed above the superior orbital rims and the field is copiously irrigated with an antibiotic solution. The drain is brought out through a puncture in the posterior, nonelevated flap. Care should be exercised not to traumatize the temporal vessel during placement of the drain, causing further significant bleeding. Both open techniques are closed in a two-layer fashion.

For the coronal incision, a galeal closure is performed with interrupted 2.0 Dexon (Fig. 3-19). This is followed by skin closure with wide staples (Fig. 3-20). The pretrichial lift closure is more detailed. The deep layer closure is done with 4.0 Maxon (Fig. 3-21). These deep sutures will cause a dimpling of the tissue immediately inferior to the incision in the midline. The patient should be informed of this preoperatively as this will resolve when the sutures dissolve. The skin in the visible region of the incision is then closed with interrupted 5.0 Prolene in a vertical mattress fashion (Fig. 3-22). Skin eversion is vital and must be attained with these sutures. Once complete with the vertical mattresses the suture line is further enhanced with the use of a running, locking 6.0 nylon suture to maximize the wound approximation (Fig. 3-23). The hair-bearing areas are closed with wide staples on the lateral components and standard staples as the surgeon

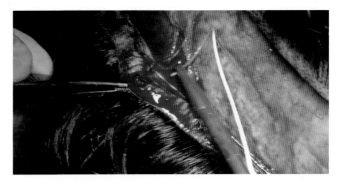

Figure 3-19 The galeal closure is performed with buried, absorbable sutures in the coronal technique.

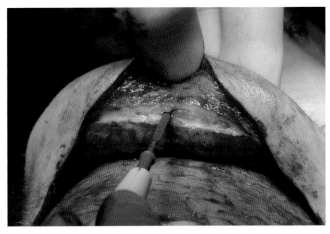

Figure 3-18 The frontalis is scored horizontally at the foremost forehead rhytid in most cases.

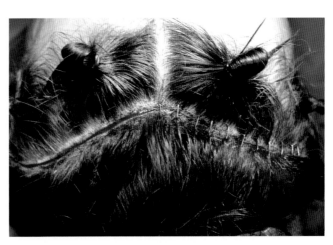

Figure 3-20 The coronal closure is completed with staples at the skin level. Please note the hair-to-hair apposition, a frequently misunderstood concept with this technique.

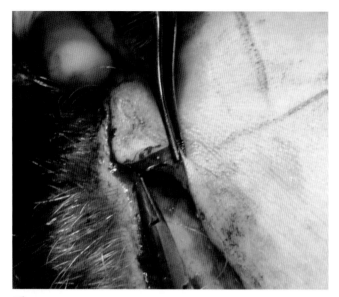

Figure 3-21 The trichophytic closure is begun with buried, absorbable sutures at the galeal level.

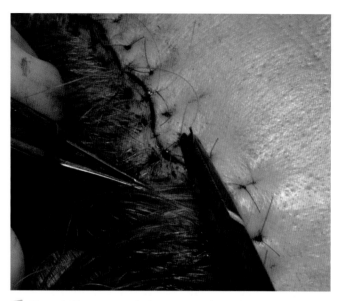

Figure 3-23 A running, locking 6.0 nonabsorbable suture is used to maximize wound closure and achieve the optimal postoperative result.

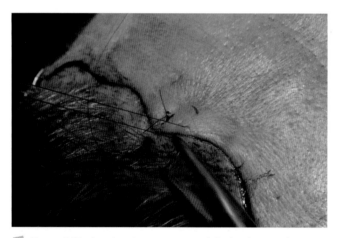

Figure 3-22 The skin closure is accomplished with vertical mattress sutures. We prefer nonabsorbable suture at the skin level to minimize the inflammatory response.

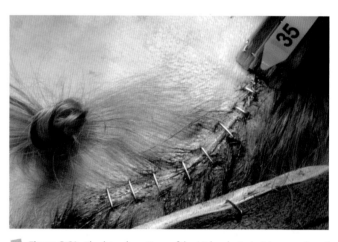

Figure 3-24 The lateral portions of the trichophytic incision are closed with large staples laterally and smaller ones medially.

nears the skin in the medial aspect of the incision (Fig. 3-24). Though somewhat more time consuming, this elaborate closure greatly enhances the patient's wound healing (Figs. 3-25 and 3-26).

The wound is then coated with antibiotic ointment and a nonadhesive piece of Telfa is placed over the incision. A light compressive dressing is then applied.

POSTOPERATIVE CARE

The drain is often removed in the recovery room on the evening of the procedure to decrease the headache and nausea that often accompany drains in this area.

Patient comfort dictates whether he or she may return home, go to a hotel, or spend a night in a medical facility. The dressing is removed on postoperative day 1 and no further dressing is necessary. The patient may immediately begin using hydrogen peroxide to keep the incision free of crusts. Showering with baby shampoo is allowed 48 hours after the procedure. The sutures for the pretrichial lift are removed on postoperative days 3 to 5, depending on the nature of the healing and logistics of removing sutures from other rejuvenation procedures that may have been performed. The staples are removed at 1 week after surgery. The pretrichial incision is immediately taped in the non–hair-bearing area after application of adhesive. The tape is worn continuously for 1 week after the removal of the sutures. After this point, the tape

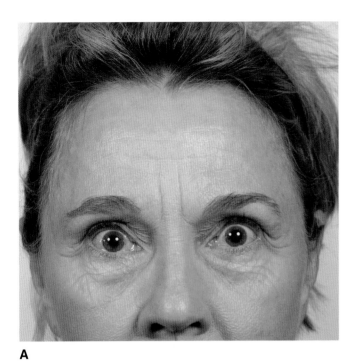

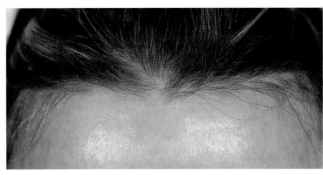

A

Figure 3-25 Preoperative frontal view of a 67-year-old woman (**A**). The tricophytic closure is barely visible when proper technique is used (**B**).

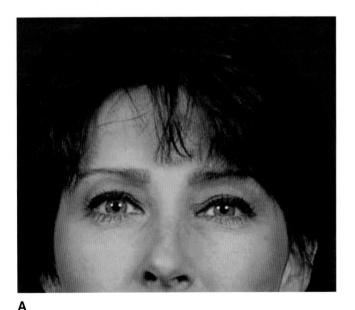

A

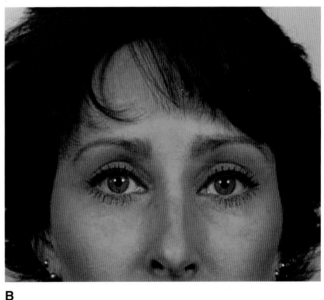

B

Figure 3-26 Preoperative (**A**) and postoperative (**B**) views of a 47-year-old patient who underwent a coronal browlift.

is kept on nightly for approximately 1 month. The tape minimizes tension on the skin, encouraging excellent camouflage of the healing wound. In the coronal approach all staples are removed 1 week after surgery, and there are no sutures to remove.

The patient is advised that the edema in the forehead will be most significant 2 to 3 days from the procedure. This edema can be quite uncomfortable for the patient. The patients are advised that this swelling will gradually resolve and they may commence mildly strenuous activity 3 to 4 weeks after the procedure. They are also advised to

avoid using a curling iron or a blow-dryer on a hot setting secondary to the changes in sensation in the first 6 weeks of the procedure. This parasthesia, a main issue with those who support the endoscopic techniques, is rarely an issue in our practice.

COMPLICATIONS

Despite the recent advances of endoscopic equipment and techniques, we prefer the open method because of its excellent result and patient acceptance. The highly publicized issues with the open approach—alopecia, numbness, scarring—have not been an issue in the senior author's practice for 25 years.[54,56,57] Although a logical argument can be made that these issues are serious, the theory and reality diverge (unpublished data). In addition, when one of the issues does arise, particularly numbness, the patient does not see it as a priority and is generally so pleased with the result that the issue fades. The patient is also counseled about this preoperatively so that it is not an unpleasant surprise if it does occur.

The most common troubling complication is that of parasthesia. The patient must be aware, preoperatively, that the forehead and scalp will be numb for several months, and possibly permanently. When discussed extensively in the preoperative phase this issue is managed adequately. In our experience, this is of marginal importance to the patient. It usually resolves in the appropriate time period and is almost always a nonissue when it has been addressed preoperatively.

Hematomas are also, fortunately, rare with the technique. Despite the copious blood supply to this region, hematomas are seldom seen. This is probably due to the tense nature of the closure, edema, and the unyielding cranium that tamponades any potential bleeding complications. The complication profile for the open browlift is excellent at 0.4% for hematoma formation, permanent alopecia, and "nerve damage."[58] Others have also found very acceptable complication rates.[15]

Alopecia is also a rare occurrence. In the coronal approach, the beveling of the incision and a hair-to-hair closure alleviate this concern. In the pretrichial lift, the hair will grow either through the healing incision or over it in the form of bangs. Rarely, a patient may not be a candidate if he or she has a high hairline and prefers to wear the hair back at all times or has hair growing in a vector unfavorable for masking the incision. Scar appearance is also greatly aided by meticulous attention to detail in the operating room, especially during the incision and closure.

One of the most noted complications of this procedure is the creation of a "surprised look," evidenced by a widened, elevated medial brow complex.[59] We minimize this issue by judicious removal of tissue and an appropriate resection of the glabellar musculature. Relieved of the need for overcorrection, as is needed in other techniques, we have not found this to be an issue in our practice.

An occasional issue that arises postoperatively is pruritus that occurs along the incision line. The patient may scratch and rub this area, causing a focal alopecia. This can be avoided with patient education. If the alopecia has already occurred, the patient is advised not to disturb the area further, and the hair often returns. Any undue scarring is very rare and can be treated with steroid injections of Kenalog-10.

Future Considerations

The continuing evolution of technology will undoubtedly benefit the patient in the long term. The surgeon must be careful, however, to adhere to proven surgical principles. We should expect that the patient's demands and desires will progress with these technologic advances, and we must stay at the vanguard to offer our patients the optimal care.

REFERENCES

1. Lexer E: Zur Geischsplastik. Arch Klin Chur 1910;92:749.
2. Passot R: La churugie esthetique des rides du visage. Presse Med 1919;27:258.
3. Hunt HL: Plastic Surgery of the Head, Face and Neck. Philadelphia: Lea & Febiger, 1926.
4. Noel A: La Chirurgie Esthetique et son Role Socia. Paris: Masson, 1926.
5. Joseph J: Nasenplastik und Sonstige Gesichtplastik Nebst Einen Anhang Uber Mammaplastik. Leipzig: Kabitzch, 1931.
6. Paul M: The evolution of the brow lift in aesthetic plastic surgery. Plast Reconstr Surg 2001;108:1409.
7. Brennan GH: The forehead lift. Otolaryngol Clin North Am 1980;13:209.
8. Connell BF: Eyebrow, face and necklifts for males. Clin Plast Surg 1978;5:15.
9. Kaye BL: The forehead lift: A useful adjunct to facelift and blepharoplasty. Plast Reconstr Surg 1977;60:161.
10. Core GB, Vasconez LO, Askren C, et al: Coronal facelift with endoscopic techniques. Plast Surg Forum 1992;15:227.
11. Liang M, Narayanan K: Endoscopic ablation of the frontalis and corrugator muscles: A clinical study. Plast Surg Forum 1992;15:58.
12. Vasconez LO, Gore GB, Gamboa-Bodadilla M, et al: Endoscopic techniques in coronal brow lifting. Plast Reconstr Surg 1994;94:788.
13. Isse NG: Endoscopic facial rejuvenation. Endoforehead, the functional lift: Case reports. Aesth Plast Surg 1994;18:21.
14. Ramirez OM: Endoscopic techniques in facial rejuvenation. An overview: Part I. Aesth Plast Surg 1994;18:141.
15. Wojtanowski MH: Bicoronal forehead lift. Aesth Plast Surg 1994;18:33.
16. Ramirez OM: Endoscopic full facelift. Aesth Plast Surg 1994;18:363.
17. Chasan PE, Kupfer DM: Direct K-wire fixation technique during endoscopic brow lifts. Aesth Plast Surg 1998;22:338.
18. Niazi ZBM, Salzberg CA: Endoscopic forehead lifts: The postoperatively adjustable technique. Plast Reconstr Surg 1998;101:2006.
19. Pozner JN: Simplified fixation for endoscopic brow lifts: Self-tapping, drill-free posts. Plast Reconstr Surg 1999;103:1326.
20. Loomis MG: Endoscopic brow fixation without bolsters or miniscrews. Plast Reconstr Surg 1996;98:373.
21. Marchac D, Ascherman J, Arnaud E: Fibrin glue fixation in forehead endoscopy: Evaluation of our experience with 206 cases. Plast Reconstr Surg 1997;100:704.
22. Mixter RC: Endoscopic forehead fixation with histocryl. Plast Reconstr Surg 1998;101:2006.

23. Newman JP, La Ferriere KA, Koch RJ, et al: Transcalvarial suture fixation for endoscopic brow and forehead lifts. Arch Otolaryngol Head Neck Surg 1997;123:313.

24. Landecker A, Buck JB, Grotting JC: A new resorable tack fixation technique for endoscopic browlifts. Plast Reconstr Surg 2003;111:880.

25. Schnur PL, Don SA: Forehead and brow lift. In Weinzweig J (ed): Plastic Surgery Secrets. Philadelphia: Hanley & Belfus, 1999.

26. Romo T III, Sclafani AP, Yung RT, et al: Endoscopic foreheadplasty: A histologic comparision of subperiosteal refixation after endoscopic versus bicoronal lift. Plast Reconstr Surg 2000;105:1111.

27. Chiu ES, Baker DC: Endoscopic browlift: A retrospective review of 628 consecutive cases over five years. Plast Reconstr Surg 2003;112:628

28. Swift RW, Nolan WB, Aston SJ, et al: Endoscopic brow lift: Objective result after one year. Aesth Surg J 1999;19:287

29. Troilus C: A comparison between subgaleal and subperiosteal brow lifts. Plast Reconstr Surg 1999;104:1079

30. Yarenchuk MJ: Subperiosteal and full-thickness skin rhytidectomy. Plast Reconstr Surg 2001;107:1045.

31. Hamra ST: A study of the long-term effect of malar fat repositioning in face lift surgery: Short term success but long-term failure. Plast Reconstr Surg 2002;110:940.

32. Elkwood A, Matarasso A, Rankin M, et al: National plastic surgery survey: Brow lifting techniques and complications. Plast Reconstr Surg 2001;108:2143.

33. Koch RJ: Endoscopic browlift is the preferred approach for rejuvenation of the upper third of the face. Arch Otolaryngol Head Neck Surg 2001;127:87

34. Murphy MR, Johnson CM: Unpublished data.

35. Godek CP, Buckey LP, Whitaker LA: Endoscopic versus open coronal forehead surgery: Surgeon preference and patient satisfaction. Plast Surg Forum 1999;22:182.

36. Guyuron B, Behmand RA, Green R: Shortening of the long forehead. Plast Reconstr Surg 1999;103:218.

37. Marten TJ: Hairline lowering during foreheadplasty. Plast Reconstr Surg 1999;103:224.

38. Michelow BJ, Guyuron B: Rejuvenation of the upper face: A logical gamut of surgical options. Clin Plast Surg 1997;24:199.

39. Marten TJ: Hairline lowering during foreheadplasty. Plast Reconstr Surg 1999;103:224.

40. McKinney P, Mossie RD, Zukowski ML: Criteria for the forehead lift. Aesth Plast Surg 1991;15:141.

41. Knize D: An anatomically based study of the mechanism of eyebrow ptosis. Plast Reconstr Surg 1996;97:1321.

42. Knize D: Limited-incision forehead lift for eyebrow elevation to enhance upper blepharoplasty. Plast Reconstr Surg 1996;97:1334.

43. Romo T III, Jacono AA, Sclafani AP: Endoscopic forehead lifting and countouring. Facial Plast Surg 2001;17:4.

44. Knize DM: A study of the supraorbital nerve. Plast Reconstr Surg 1995;96:564.

45. Gunter J, Antrobus SD: Aesthetic analysis of the eyebrows. Plast Reconstr Surg 1997;99:1808.

46. Whitaker LA, Morales L Jr, Farkas LG: Aesthetic surgery of the supraorbital ridge and forehead structure. Plast Reconstr Surg 1986;78:23.

47. Cook TA, Brownrigg AJ, Wang TD, et al: The versatile midforehead browlift. Arch Otolaryngol Head Neck Surg 1989;115:163.

48. Matarasso A, Terino EO: Forehead-brow rhytidoplasty: reassessing the goals. Plast Reconstr Surg 1994;93:1378.

49. McKinney P, Mossie RD, Zukowski ML: Criteria for the forehead lift. Aesth Plast Surg 1991;15:141.

50. Freund RM, Nolan WB III: Correlation between brow lift outcomes and aesthetic ideals for eyebrow height and shape in females. Plast Reconstr Surg 1996;97:1343.

51. Ellenbogen R: Transcoronal eyebrow lift with concomittant upper blepharoplasty. Plast Reconstr Surg 1983;71:490.

52. Roth JM, Metzinger SE: Quantifying the arch position of the female eyebrow. Arch Facial Plast Surg 2003;5:235.

53. Rafety FM, Brennana HG: Current concepts of browpexy. Arch Otolaryngol 1983;109:152.

54. Adamson PA, Johnson CM, Anderson JR, et al: The forehead lift: A review. Arch Otolaryngol Head Neck Surg. 1985;111:325.

55. Romo T III, Sclafani AP, Yung RT, et al: Endoscopic foreheadplasty: A histologic comparision of periosteal refixation after endoscopic versus bicoronal lift. Plast Reconstr Surg 2000;105:1111.

56. Adamson PA, Cormier R, McGraw BL: The coronal forehead lift: Modifications and results. J Otolaryngol 1992;21:1

57. Kerth JD, Torimui DM: Management of the aging forehead. Arch Otolaryngol Head Neck Surg 1990;116:1137.

58. Vinas JC, Caviglia C, Cortinas JL: Forehead rhytidoplasty and brow lifting. Plast Reconstr Surg 1976;57:445.

59. Freund RM, Nolan WB III: Correlation between brow lift outcomes and aesthetic ideals for eyebrow height and shape in females. Plast Reconstr Surg 1997;99:1808.

CHAPTER FOUR

Endoscopic Foreheadplasty

Nicanor Isse, MD

The aesthetic goal of foreheadplasty is to obtain a balanced brow position, preserving the natural relationship between the brow's head, body, and tail, and to improve wrinkles of the forehead and glabella. A minimally invasive technique for foreheadplasty was first introduced in 1992 and published in 1994.[1] The endoscopic foreheadplasty enables the correction of the brow position by modifying the depressor muscles of the brow and associated tissue while keeping the frontalis muscle intact so it can exert an upward force, thereby repositioning the brow. Since 1992, the technique has been enhanced by the adoption of more precise methods of patient selection; variations in tissue dissection, modification, and fixation; and the introduction of associated techniques such as chemical peeling, laser resurfacing, chemical denervation, and soft tissue fillers.

HISTORY

The history of foreheadplasty can be traced back for nearly 100 years. The very first description of foreheadplasty was done by Passot in 1919.[2] He described several horizontal skin excisions on the higher portion of the forehead to improve the horizontal wrinkles of the forehead. Skin excision on the temporal area reduced the crow's-feet and hood of the lateral brow. Passot later recommended direct skin excision above the brows with undermining.[3] In 1926, Hunt described the coronal, anterior hairline, and direct skin excisions on the forehead.[4] Claoue, in 1933, described undermining of the forehead.[5] In 1939, Fomon described a subcutaneous undermining with transection of the epicranium.[6] Castanares recommended modification of the frontalis muscle and transection of the frontal branch of the facial nerve, in addition to the forehead undermining and skin excision.[7] In 1964, Marino and Gandolfo started to modify the corrugator muscles in order to improve their results.[8]

In the 1960s and 1970s, Vinas described forehead lifts utilizing the bicoronal or pretrichial incision, depending on the patient's forehead height.[9,10] He also recommended the subgaleal dissection with detachment of the fascial adhesions to the glabella and supraorbital rim areas. He widely dissected the region under the superficial temporal

fascia. In 1972, Regnault described a biplanar approach on the temporal area to correct the crow's-feet.[11] Connell and associates, in the 1980s, published techniques that would modify the procerus and depressor supercilii muscles in order to improve the results of the bicoronal browlift.[12] Flowers, in 1991, emphasized the need for prioritizing the coronal browlift over the upper eyelids excision to obtain better aesthetic results in the periorbital area.[13] He also recommended corrugator muscle modification in the glabella and supraorbital rim area for sustained brow elevation, with minimal skin excision on the forehead area. In 1990, Tirkanis and Daniel introduced the biplanar approach to the forehead, using subcutaneous and subgaleal dissection.[14] In 1992, Isse introduced a minimally invasive technique for foreheadplasty using endoscopic techniques.[1] Since that time, the popularity of endoscopic browlift has continued to grow significantly.

PERSONAL PHILOSOPHY

As a person ages, the soft tissues of the face and forehead are drawn downward by a combination of static and dynamic forces. Gravity and depressor muscles oppose the elevators, leading to forehead wrinkles and malpositioning of the eyebrows and upper eyelids. Until the advent of minimally invasive surgical techniques, these conditions could be corrected only through direct incisions in the forehead or bicoronal incisions.

The technique for endoscopic rejuvenation of the forehead aesthetic unit was first introduced at the 1992 meeting of the Los Angeles Society of Plastic Surgery and published in 1994.[1,15] Alternative improvements in the technique have brought the procedure to the point at which excellent and sustainable results can be obtained with most patients. Moreover, advances in endoscopic instrumentation and imaging technologies have facilitated the adoption of this technique by a growing number of plastic surgeons. The basic concept of the procedure, however, remains unchanged: An endoscope is inserted through small incisions in the scalp, a wide area of the forehead is undermined, thereby releasing the soft tissue, depressor muscles are modified, and fixation is performed. The action of the frontalis muscle allows natural eyebrow elevation. Fixation is required to maintain the elevation on the lateral or temporal portion of the brow.

The endoscopic foreheadplasty offers several advantages over more invasive procedures. There is minimal hair loss, reduced scarring, decreased bleeding, a low incidence of prolonged or permanent numbness of the scalp, and most important, rapid recovery. There is a high rate of patient satisfaction for younger individuals, postmenopausal women with very thin hair, and individuals who object to a coronal incision.

This chapter presents a comprehensive review of the surgical technique for the endoscopic foreheadplasty. Factors that lend themselves toward successful outcome are presented. Some of the key technical improvements that have occurred as the procedure has evolved are examined, including the development of patient selection parameters and refinements in the techniques for dissection, tissue modification, and fixation.

ANATOMY

The muscles of facial expression in the forehead and their activity are described in Figure 4-1 and Table 4-1. From a dynamic viewpoint, the eyebrow can be divided into three parts: *medial*, *central*, and *lateral* (Fig. 4-2). The medial third of the brow (the head) lies medial to the supraorbital nerve in the glabella. This area is very rich in muscular activity and is controlled by the balance between the depressor and elevator muscles. The central third of the brow (the body) is an area limited medially by the supraorbital nerve and laterally by the superior temporal crest. It is balanced by the action of the frontalis muscle (elevator) and orbicularis oculi muscles (depressor). The lateral third of the brow (the tail) is located lateral to the superior temporal crest in the temporal region. This region is the thinnest portion of the brow and its dynamic activity is controlled mainly by depressor muscles (the orbital portion of the orbicularis oculi muscle). The frontalis muscle has little to no activity at this level and consequently suspension of the soft tissue is always necessary in the temporal area.

Three sets of muscles are involved in the mechanism of "human facial expression" around the brows, namely the *elevators*, *depressors*, and *corrugators* (see Table 4-1).[16,17]

The endoscopic foreheadplasty procedure has the ability to modify the frontalis, corrugator, orbicularis, procerus, and depressor supercilii muscles as needed.[18]

PREOPERATIVE ASSESSMENT

Endoscopic foreheadplasty is indicated when improvement of the brow position and shape is desired, or when the rhytids of the forehead, glabella, and periorbital areas need to be softened. These conditions may arise due to the following:

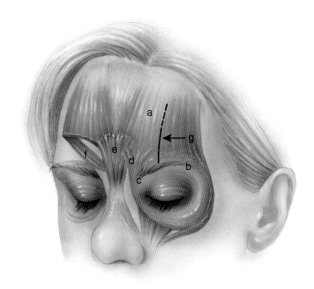

Figure 4-1 Muscles of the forehead. *a*, The frontalis muscle is the main elevator of the eyebrows. This muscle produces the horizontal rhytids on the forehead. *b*, The orbital portion of the orbicularis oculi muscle (OOM) is the main depressor muscle of the entire brow. Its activity forms the radial horizontal lines around the orbit. *c*, Deep head, the septal part of the OOM, produces further depression of the brow, resulting in forceful closure of the eyes and squinting. This muscle is generally mistaken for the corrugator muscle. *d*, The depressor supercilii muscle depresses the head of the brow and is responsible for the "reverse parenthesis line" around the medial head of the brow. Its action results in an "angry" facial expression. *e*, The procerus muscle depresses the head of the brow producing horizontal rhytids at the root of the nose. Its action is synergistic with the levator nasi. *f*, The corrugator supercilii muscle has a dual action of elevating the head of the brow (synergistic with the frontalis muscle at this level) and depressing the tail of the brow (synergistic with the OOM at this level). The corrugator produces flattening of the glabellar area, midforehead wrinkles, and notching of the brow at the level of the supraorbital nerve. *g*, The superficial or medial branch of the supraorbital nerve (SON) gives the sensory innervations of the forehead. The lateral branch of the SON innervates the scalp and is located under the periosteum in a more lateral position.

- Brow ptosis and malposition
- Glabellar rhytids (frown lines)
- Tissue sagging (root of nose)
- Pseudoptosis of upper eyelids
- Mild to moderate dermatochalasia (upper eyelids)
- Minimal ptosis of the upper eyelids
- Downward slanting of the lateral canthus
- Periorbital wrinkles (crow's-feet)

ENDOSCOPIC EQUIPMENT

Endoscopic browlift requires the use of a complete endoscopic unit: medical video camera, camera control unit, light source, monitor, and a fiberoptic cable.

DVD, VCR, or printer mounted on a movable stand may also be used. One-chip cameras are generally adequate for facial procedures. However, if crisp documentation of a specific case is required for publication or teaching purposes, the surgeon may wish to utilize a three-chip

Table 4-1 Muscles of Facial Expression in the Forehead and Their Activity

Muscle Movement	Muscle Name	Action	Facial Expression
Elevators	Frontalis	Elevation of brow	Attention
Depressors	Orbicularis oculi	Depresses entire brow	Reflection
	Procerus	Depresses medial brow	Aggression
	Depressor supercilii	Depresses head	Anger
Corrugators	Corrugator supercilii	Elevates and adducts head Depresses lateral brow	Pain

camera, which will provide superior resolution, detail, and definition.

An improved soft tissue endodissector/retractor with a downward curved tip can increase the visual field during the dissection. The retractor provides more control during tissue handling and avoids the creation of a false

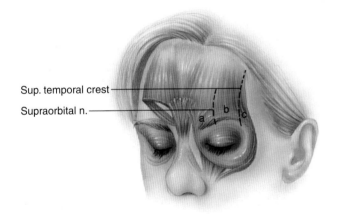

Figure 4-2 Segments of the brow. *a,* The head of the brow is located medial to the supraorbital nerve (SON) and contains most of the muscles of facial expression in the forehead (glabella). The repositioning of the brow in this area depends mainly on decreasing the muscle activity. "Tissue modification" is the best way to deal with the muscles via myotomy, myectomy, neurotomy "block," or chemical denervation. *b,* The body of the brow is limited medially by the SON and laterally by the superior temporal crest (STC). This region contains two muscles: frontalis as an elevator and orbicularis oculi muscle (OOM) as a depressor. Brow repositioning at this level occurs secondarily to the elevation of the medial and lateral brow. If the medial brow does not achieve the desired height, direct brow fixation is done at the paramedial location. Medial brow ptosis occurs secondary to OOM action and dermatochalasia (most commonly seen in older patients). *c,* The tail of the brow is located lateral to the STC in the temporal region. The pars orbitalis of the OOM produces an active depression of the tail of the brow, which could be exaggerated, depending on the degree of dermatochalasia. In this area, weakening pars orbitalis of OOM as well as fixation is necessary because the frontalis muscle does not exert any significant elevation of the brow at this level.

surgical plane, reducing surgical trauma and limiting tissue damage. Periosteal and soft tissue elevators are used, as well as a tissue "spreader" for the temporal and midface areas.

SURGICAL TECHNIQUE

A combination of intravenous sedation and local anesthesia is adequate, although general anesthesia can be used. Intravenous sedation is performed using 0.5% lidocaine (Xylocaine) with epinephrine (1:200,000) for the forehead, temporal area, eyelids, and scalp infiltration.

The following standard surgical steps are performed during an endoscopic foreheadplasty:
- Preoperative marking (Box 4-1)
- Incisions
- Creation of an optical cavity
- Dissection of the forehead and temporal areas
- Release of tissue attachment to bone and deep fascia
- Tissue modifications
- Fixation

THE INCISIONS

A central forehead incision and two paramedial incisions (right and left) approximately 4.5 to 5.0 cm lateral to the central incision are made behind the hairline (Fig. 4-3). These incisions measure about 1.2 to 1.5 cm in length. An incision is then made in the temporal region 2.0 cm behind the hairline and about 1.0 cm lateral to the temporal crest, measuring 1.5 to 2.0 cm in length.

CREATION OF AN OPTICAL CAVITY

A blind subperiosteal dissection is performed in the forehead area down to the midforehead line, and 1.2 to 2.4 cm posterior to the incisions, using a curved periosteal elevator (see Fig. 4-3). Using a blunt dissector, the temporal area is "blindly dissected" between the superficial (tempoparietalis fascia) and the deep temporal

Box 4-1 Preoperative Markings

1. Incisions (see description)
2. Temporal crest line
3. Posterior edge of lateral orbital rim
4. Superior edge of the zygomatic arch
5. Midforehead line: horizontal line marking the midpoint between the hairline and the brows
6. The trajectory of the temporofrontal branch of the facial nerve: a line drawn from the lowest portion of the tragus to an area about 1.5 cm cephalad to the superior edge of the brow at the level of the temporal crest

fascia for a distance of 2 cm anterior and posterior to the temporal incision.

DISSECTION OF THE FOREHEAD AND TEMPORAL AREA

"Blind dissection" is done initially to allow the instruments to be located under the periosteum in the frontal area (see Fig. 4-3). The endoscopic dissection is then performed in the forehead area. The endoscope is inserted through one of the forehead incisions while the periosteal elevator is inserted in another incision. The distal end of the endoscopic sheath has a curved elevator/dissector that creates an optical cavity when the very tip of the endoscope is tilted upward approximately 15 to 30 degrees. A magnified view of the regions is created.

In the temporal area, the dissection is initially performed using a blunt dissector and Metzenbaum scissors. "Vertical spreading" of the scissors maintains the correct plane of dissection. It is important to alternate the dissections between the frontal and temporal areas in order to avoid creating and working in a "tight tunnel." Working in a widely dissected area allows better visualization of the surrounding structures and better control of bleeding vessels.

RELEASE OF TISSUE ATTACHMENTS TO BONE AND DEEP FASCIA

Tissue attachments to bone and deep fascia are released in order to achieve mobilization and gliding of the superficial tissue over the deeper structures (Fig. 4-4). Several regions will require release, including both periosteal attachments and galea.

The periosteum is released at level of the glabella, supraorbital rim, and superior temporal crest. Horizontal and vertical periosteal release at the glabella improves the vertical wrinkles of the forehead. Horizontal release of the supraorbital rim will allow access to the deep galea of the orbicularis muscle and the suborbicularis planes. The vertical release of the periosteum will assist on the repositioning of the body and tail of the brow. Periosteal release of superior temporal crest together with the release of the temporal crest ligament and the superior orbicularis ligament will allow elevation of the body and tail of the brow, as well as improve the pseudoptosis of the upper eyelids.

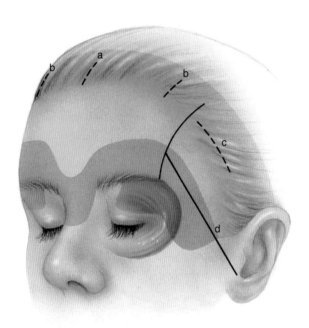

Figure 4-3 Incisions and dissection. *a*, The central incision is located at the center of the forehead, behind the hairline, measuring about 1.2 to 1.5 cm. *b*, Paramedial incisions are located 5 cm lateral to the central incision and are also about 1.2 to 1.5 cm. *c*, Temporal incisions are located in the temporal area, about 2 cm behind the hairline, and about 1.0 cm lateral to the temporal crest (TC). *d*, The trajectory of the frontal branch of the facial nerve is marked, starting at the level of the lower portion of the tragus heading toward a point 1.5 cm superior to the upper edge of the brow at the level of the TC. The light pink shaded area represents the initial nonendoscopic subperiosteal dissection, which extends down to the midportion of forehead laterally and close to the glabella medially. In the temporal area, the "blind" dissection is limited to the anterior hairline between the superficial and deep temporal fascia. The dark pink shaded area represents the "endoscopic dissection."

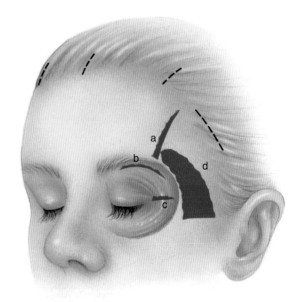

Figure 4-4 Release of tissue attachments. *a*, The temporal crest (TC) separates the frontal and temporal area during the subperiosteal or subgaleal dissection. The TC is thinner in the cephalad region near the scalp and thicker caudally toward the brow, where it is referred to as "superior orbital ligament." *b*, Superior palpebral ligament separates the pars orbitalis and preseptal regions of the orbicularis oculi muscle (OOM). *c*, The precanthal ligament is the thickening between the periosteum of the lateral orbital rim and the deep galea of the OOM. *d*, The orbicularis temporal ligament (temporal line of fusion) attaches directly onto the deep temporal fascia because the area does not have the superficial temporal fascia.

A sustained long-term elevation of the brow cannot been maintained without the release of the deep galeal ligaments and the myotomies of the lateral orbital pars of the orbicularis muscle. The deep galea is released at the level of glabella, superior palpebral ligament, superior orbital ligament (conjoined tendon), superior temporal crest ligament, orbicularis temporal ligament (temporal line of fusion), and precanthal ligament. Glabellar release (galea of procerus, depressors, and corrugators) stretches the soft tissue of the area, thereby smoothing out the glabellar wrinkles. The release of the superior palpebral ligament (deep galea of orbicularis oculi muscle attachment to the superior orbital rim) repositions the body and tail of the brow as well as improves the pseudoptosis of the upper eyelids by unfolding the preseptal orbicularis "festoon." Superior orbital ligament (conjoined tendon) is the most caudal portion of the temporal crest ligament at the junction of temporal crest and lateral orbital rim. Its release allows elevation of the body and tail of the brow. Superior temporal crest ligament (tempoparietalis fascia and deep galea of frontalis muscle attached to superior temporal crest) release allows elevation of the body and tail of the brow. The precanthal ligament is the attachment of the deep galea of the orbicularis muscle to the periosteum at the level of the lateral canthal raphe. Release of this ligament produces a tilt at the lateral canthal raphe as well as a more sustained elevation of the tail of the brow. The orbicularis temporal ligament (temporal line of fusion) is the attachment of the superficial fibroadipose tissue to the deep temporalis fascia. By releasing this ligament, the lateral brow is mobilized, adding to the long-term elevation of the tail of the brow.

An anatomically important area of concern is a series of vessels and sensory nerves that are present between the fibers of the orbicularis temporal ligament and are known as "the telephone formation" (Fig. 4-5). The medial zygomatic temporal vein (sentinel vein) is located lateral to the posterior edge of the lateral orbital rim and signals the trajectory of the temporal branch of the facial nerve. Transection of this vein further rotates the tail of the brow and lateral canthal region. This maneuver, however, might produce a long-standing or permanent postoperative venous congestion in the temporal area (varicosity). The lateral zygomatic temporal vein and artery, known as "the pointers," aim directly to the temporal branch of the facial nerve as it traverses the superior edge of the zygomatic arch. The medial and lateral zygomatic temporal nerves provide the sensory innervation to the temporal area (branches of the trigeminal nerve, V_2). These vessels and sensory nerves are aligned from the temporal crest to the superior edge of the zygomatic arch. The temporal branch of the facial nerve crosses superficial to this formation in the temporal area. This formation is also known as "the telephone pole."

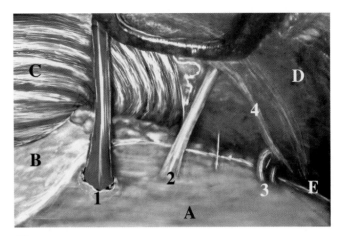

Figure 4-5 Endoscopic view of the temporal area. Deep temporal fascia (**A**). Lateral orbital rim (**B**). Orbicularis oculi muscle (**C**). Tempo-parietalis fascia (**D**). Zygomatic arch (**E**). Medial zygomatic temporal vein (sentinel vein) (**1**). Medial zygomatic temporal nerve (sensory branch of V2) (**2**). Lateral zygomatic temporal neurovascular bundle (**3**). Frontal branch of the facial nerve (**4**).

TISSUE MODIFICATIONS

"Tissue modification" refers to the weakening of the depressor muscles of the brow via myotomy and neurotomy. These maneuvers can be used to achieve specific aesthetic outcomes in all of the major area of the forehead (Fig. 4-6).[18,19] The glabella is the focus of the majority of the tissue modifications. Myotomy of the procerus produces elevation of the head of the brow and improvement of the horizontal rhytids at the root of the nose. The myotomy is

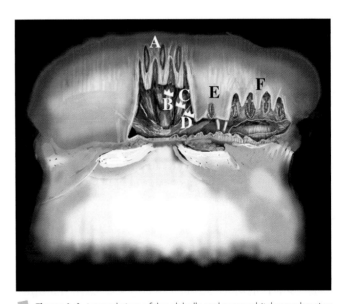

Figure 4-6 Internal view of the glabella and supraorbital area showing the periosteum release as well as myotomies. Periosteum release at the glabella (**A**). Myotomy of procerus muscle (**B**). Myotomy of depressor supercilii muscle (**C**). Myotomy of vertical-medial orbicularis oculi muscle (OOM) (**D**). Myotomy of corrugator/OOM decussation (**E**). Lateral myotomy of pars orbitalis OOM and neurotomy of the corrugator nerve (**F**).

carried out by incising the muscle transverse to its fibers using Metzenbaum scissors. Depressor supercilii myotomy produces elevation and slight separation of the head of the brow, reducing the "frown lines." This maneuver is done by avulsing the muscle with a tip of a closed Metzenbaum scissors. Myotomy of the corrugator supercilii muscle produces moderate separation of the head of the brow, correcting the vertical wrinkles of the glabella. This is accomplished by using electrofulguration to partially "coagulate" and remove the most superficial fibers of the muscle without transecting the muscle completely.

At the level of the supraorbital rim, the myotomy of the orbicularis oculi muscle (pars orbitalis) and neurotomy of the corrugator nerve provide further improvements in the aesthetic outcome of the endoscopic browlift. Medial to the supraorbital nerve, a single myotomy of the orbicularis oculi muscle is performed at the level of the decussating fibers of the corrugator and orbicularis muscle. This maneuver is carried out right under the eyebrow using a thin Metzenbaum scissors. The myotomy produces elevation and moderate separation of the head of brow. Lateral to the supraorbital nerve, multiple myotomies of orbicularis oculi muscle are performed, spanning a distance of approximately 2 cm. This elevates and rotates the body and tail of the brow. The pars orbitalis of the orbicularis oculi muscle is the strongest depressor of the brow, and its myotomy produces sustained and long-lasting elevation of the brow. Neurotomy of the nerve to the corrugator muscle is done incidentally at these two levels. This neurotomy produces mild separation of the head of brow.

FIXATION

Fixation is performed in order to "keep" the released tissue repositioned in the desired higher position (Fig. 4-7). Fixation should not be done forcefully to elevate the tissue without tissue release. In this situation, chronic action of the depressor muscle will drive the tissue downward, tearing the soft tissue and returning the brow to its original position. The three types of fixations are paramedian, bitemporal, and temporal.

Paramedian fixation is performed at the level of the paramedian incisions bilaterally. The periosteum and frontalis muscle are grasped at the caudal end of the incision with a 3-0 PDS and tunneled 10 cm posteriorly under the periosteum onto a "stab" incision. The periosteum and occipitalis tissue are then grasped with the suture (distance of 1 cm) and the suture is brought back anteriorly through the same tunnel. With the single skin hook the assistant will exert posterior tension as the surgeon ties a knot. This fixation is indicated for patients with severe brow ptosis and severe dermatochalasia. Fixation can also be utilized in patients who desire the

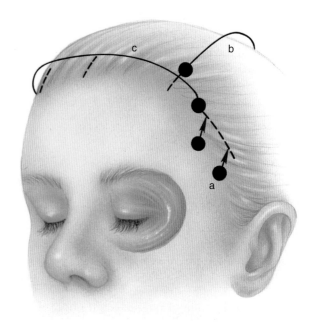

Figure 4-7 Fixation: temporal fixation (*a*), paramedial fixation (*b*), bitemporal fixation (*c*).

"arched brow" by producing maximum brow elevation at the level of the "midbrow."

Bitemporal fixation is routinely used for all cases. It produces an even elevation of the tail of the brows. The browlift is symmetrical because both lateral brows are elevated and suspended with the same suture (3-0 PDS). The suture is applied from the superficial temporal fascia at the medial end of the temporal incision, passing under the periosteum of the forehead to the opposite side, grasping the medial end of the contralateral superficial temporal fascia and temporal incision. This fixation method works well owing to the wide release of the temporal region and because the medial brow is elevated mainly by the action of the frontalis muscle after the depressor muscles are myotomized. The central brow (body of the brow) does not usually require fixation because it follows the new position of the medial and lateral brow.

Temporal fixation is performed to elevate and reposition the temporal area, as well as the lateral orbicularis muscle, producing slight slanting of the lateral canthal raphe. This maneuver is maximized when the medial zygomatic vein (sentinel vein) and precanthal ligaments are released. This fixation is done by suturing the temporoparietalis fascia (1.0 cm anterior to the temporal incision) to the deep temporal fascia as far posteriorly possible with a 3-0 or 4-0 nylon. Fixation sutures are utilized in the upper and lower part of the temporal incisions bilaterally. Figures 4-8 to 4-11 are preoperative and postoperative photographs of patients who have undergone endoscopic foreheadplasty.

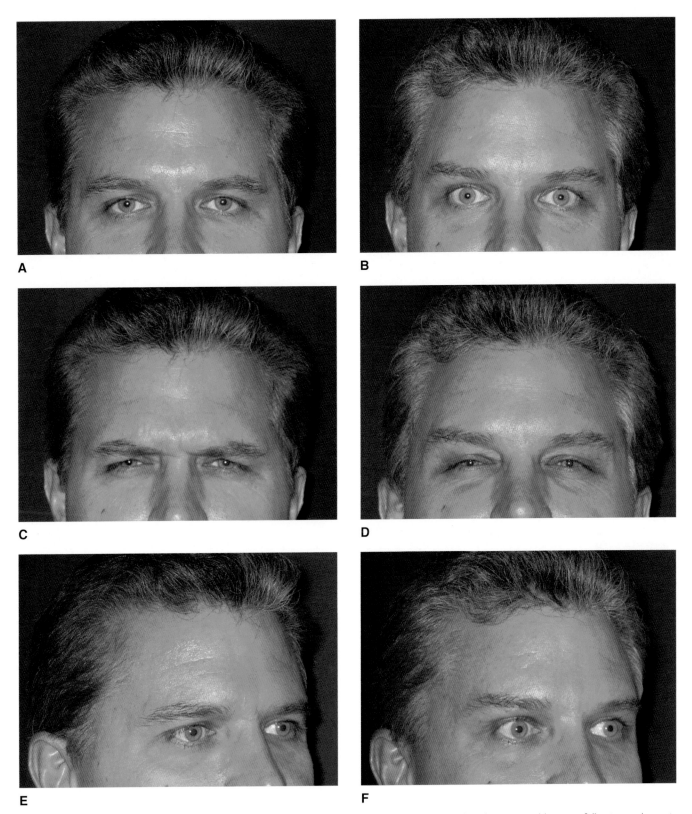

A

B

C

D

E

F

Figure 4-8 Preoperative (**A, C, E, G, I,** and **K**) and postoperative (**B, D, F, H, J,** and **L**) photographs of a 41-year-old patient following endoscopic foreheadplasty.

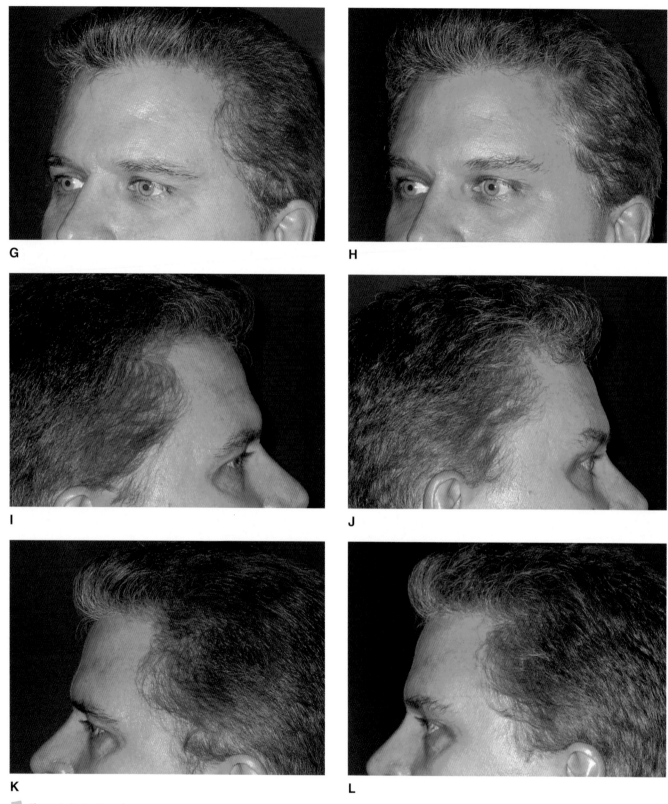

Figure 4-8 *Continued.*

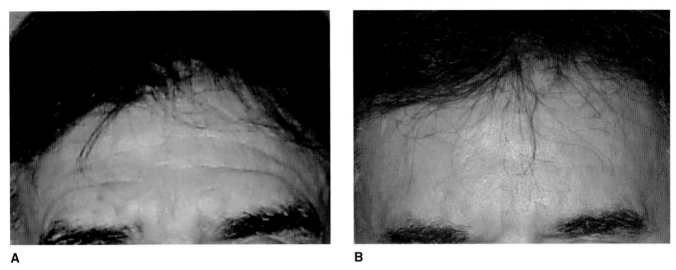

Figure 4-9 Preoperative photo showing wrinkles on the forehead secondary to frontalis muscle hyperactivity attempting to overcome the action of the depressors muscle (**A**). Postoperative view after endoscopic foreheadplasty (**B**). The horizontal wrinkles have almost disappeared. The tissue release plus the myotomies of the depressor muscles have diminished frontalis muscle activity.

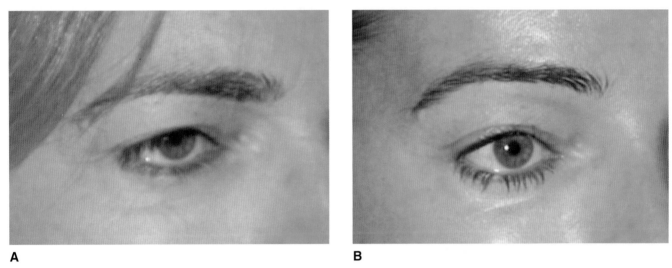

Figure 4-10 Preoperative view of a female patient with low positioning of the lateral brow as well as pseudoptosis of the upper eyelids (**A**). Postoperative photo after endoscopic foreheadplasty shows repositioning of the brow and improvement of the pseudoptosis of the upper eyelids without the need for "upper blepharoplasty" (**B**).

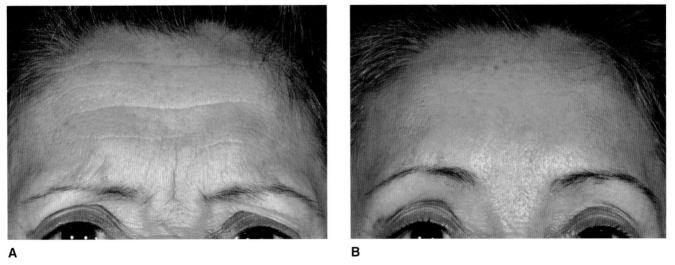

Figure 4-11 Preoperative photo of a patient with brow ptosis as well as rhytids in the forehead, glabella, and root of the nose (**A**). Postoperative photo following endoscopic foreheadplasty (**B**).

Special Considerations

Frontalis Plication

The endoscopic dissection is done routinely for all cases. Clinical circumstances will dictate additional maneuvers. If the patients have brow asymmetry, unilateral fixation is performed only on the ptotic brow, and unilateral myotomy of the orbicularis oculi muscle is performed on the lowermost brow. Furthermore, frontalis plication is applied to the more ptotic brow. Frontalis plication involves a horizontal incision behind the hairline measuring approximately 4 cm. Anteriorly and posteriorly, subcutaneous dissection is performed over the frontalis muscle for a distance of 2 cm. The frontalis muscle fibers are then split (1.5 cm) in the longitudinal fashion to allow subperiosteal undermining of the rest of the forehead as discussed previously. The frontalis muscle is then folded over and plicated with 4-0 vicryl (creating a fold of approximately 0.5 to 1.0 cm). Overlapping skin edges are trimmed and two-layered closure is performed (2 mm of skin overlapping is maintained to decrease scar widening postoperatively). Bilateral frontalis plication is performed in patients with severe bilateral brow ptosis, dermatochalasia, and horizontal rhytids of forehead.

Receding Hairlines and Baldness

Special attention to the incision must be made in patients who have receding hairlines or male-pattern baldness. The incisions are typically made about 7 cm superior to the brows and measure about 0.7 to 1.0 cm. The uppermost forehead rhytid can also be utilized. A small endoscopic elevator (sheath) is subsequently used. The forehead incisions are closed in multiple layers in order to minimize scarring.

Glabellar Endoscopic Foreheadplasty

Glabellar endoscopic foreheadplasty is recommended for the correction of the isolated ptotic medial brow and glabellar muscle hyperactivity. The dissection is limited to the glabellar area and may be performed through a frontal upper eyelid and nasal approach. The surgeon must take care not to break the balance of the brow; otherwise, the resulting medial brow will be in a higher position in comparison to the lateral brow.

Temporal/Lateral Frontal Endoscopic Foreheadplasty

Temporal/lateral frontal endoscopic foreheadplasty is recommended when the medial brow does not require improvement. This procedure allows for the elevation of the brow's tail, modification of the brow's contour, improvement of crow's-feet, or elevation of the lateral canthal raphe. Paramedian and temporal incisions are made. Subperiosteal dissection in the lateral portion of the forehead (lateral to the supraorbital nerve) is extended caudally down to the tarsal plate under the orbicularis muscle. Temporal dissection is done under the temporoparietalis fascia, down to the superior edge of the zygomatic arch, and medially over the periosteum of the lateral orbital rim.

POSTOPERATIVE CARE

Immediately after the operation the patient's forehead is taped and a head dressing (turban) is applied to decrease swelling. The drains and dressing are removed after 24 to 48 hours. The patients are encouraged to sleep with the head elevated for about a week. One week later the "tapes" and stitches are removed. Special attention is given to the hair around or inside the wound in order to prevent wound infection. Female patients can have their hair tinted after 2 weeks, assuming that all the wounds are completely closed.

COMPLICATIONS

The most common complications associated with endoscopic browlift are numbness of the scalp and temporary alopecia due to inflammation or edema. Paresis of the frontal branch of the facial nerve occurs less frequently (about 5%). These complications are all transient and none require additional surgery. Total recurrence of brow ptosis is rare, occurring in less than 2% of the cases. The usual cause of recurrent brow ptosis is severe bossing of the frontal bone (it is advisable to reshape the bony prominence during the procedure). Partial recurrence is about 1.2% in the author's experience.

REFERENCES

1. Isse NG: Endoscopic facial rejuvenation: Endoforehead, the functional lift. Case reports. Aesth Plast Surg 1994;18:21-29.
2. Passot R: La chururgie esthetique des rides du visage. Presse Med 1919;27: 258.
3. Passot R: Chirurgie Esthetique Pure: Techniques et Resultats. Paris: Gaston Doin & Cie, 1930.
4. Hunt HL: Plastic Surgery of the Head, Face, and Neck. Philadelphia: Lea & Febiger, 1926.
5. Claoue G: La ridectomie cervico-faciale par accrochage parieto-temporo-occipital et resection cutanée. Bull Acad Med (Paris) 1933;109:257.
6. Fomon S: Surgery of Injury and Plastic Repair. Baltimore: Williams & Wilkins, 1939.
7. Castanares S: Forehead wrinkles, glabellar frown and ptosis of eyebrow. Plast Reconstr Surg 1964;34:406.
8. Marino H, Gandolfo E: Treatment of forehead wrinkles. Prensa Med Argent 1964;51:1368.
9. Vinas JC: Plan general de la ritidoplastia y zona tabu. In Transactions of the 4th Brazilian Congress on Plastic Surgery, Porto Alegre, October 5-8, 1965, p 32.
10. Vinas JC, Caviglia C, Cortinas JL: Forehead rhytidoplasty and brow lifting. Plast Reconstr Surg 1976;57:445.
11. Regnault P: Complete face and forehead lifting, with double traction on "crow's feet." Plast Reconstr Surg 1972;49:123.
12. Connell BF, Lambros VS, Neurohr GH: The forehead lift: Techniques to avoid complications and produce optimal results. Aesth Plast Surg 1989;13:217.

13. Flowers RS: Periorbital aesthetic surgery for men: Eyelids and related structures. Clin Plast Surg 1991;18:689.

14. Tirkanis B, Daniel RK: The "biplanar" forehead lift. Aesth Plast Surg 1990;14:111.

15. Fodor PB: Editorial: Endoscopic plastic surgery, a new milestone in plastic surgery. Aesth Plast Surg 1994;18:31-32.

16. Sobotta J, Figge FHJ (eds): Atlas of Human Anatomy, 9th ed. Baltimore-Munich: Urban and Schwarzenberg, 1977, p 180.

17. Isse NG: The corrugator supercilii muscle revisited. Aesth Surg 2001;21:3, 293.

18. Isse NG: Endoforeheadplasty: The functional approach with emphasis on myotomies and myectomies. Fac Plast Surg Clin North Am 1997;4:2.

19. Isse NG: Endoscopic facial rejuvenation: Clin Plast Surg 1997;24:2.

CHAPTER FIVE

Blepharoplasty

Norman Pastorek MD, FACS • Andres Bustillo, MD

HISTORY

The history of eyelid surgery dates back to approximately AD 25, when Aulus Cornelius Celsus, a first century Roman philosopher, described the excision of upper eyelid skin for the "relaxed eyelid" in his *De re Medicina*. It is not known whether he was describing a true ptosis or an excess of skin. The first medical illustration of the aging eyelid was published in 1817 by Beer. A year later, Von Graefe first used the term "blepharoplasty" to describe a case of eyelid reconstruction following a cancer resection. It was during this period that many in Europe first began to advocate the removal of the upper eyelid skin to correct associated functional problems.

In 1844 Sichel described "ptosis adiposa" as a condition by which the excessive upper eyelid skinfold was filled with fat. He theorized that the disproportionate adipose tissue caused the skin to hang down over the lid. However, it was Fuchs who later correctly recognized the role of the fascial attachments between skin, orbicularis, tarsus, and the levator in the development of the supratarsal skinfold and the importance of its recreation in blepharoplasty.

In the early 1900s, many surgeons began to popularize the removal of upper eyelid skin for aesthetic enhancement. In 1907, an American surgeon named Conrad Miller wrote one of the first books on cosmetic surgery, entitled *Cosmetic Surgery in the Correction of Facial Imperfection*. His diagrams of blepharoplasty incisions are still similar to those used today. Kolle, in 1911, detailed the value and safety of preoperative marking of blepharoplasty incisions to avoid excessive skin removal. Adabert Bettman made important contributions with respect to postoperative scaring. He advocated precise apposition of wound edges with elimination of tension as well as early suture removal to avoid unsightly incisions.

In the early 1920s, Suzanne Noel, a Parisian surgeon, wrote a book on cosmetic eyelid surgery. Noel stressed the importance of preoperative planning using photographs. Noel is also credited with being among the first to recognize the psychological implications of cosmetic surgery. In 1924, Julian Bourguet was the first to describe the transconjunctival approach for the removal of orbital fat. Five years later, he described the removal of fat from the two separate compartments of the upper eyelid. He is also credited for being the first to publish "before and after" photographs of patients undergoing cosmetic eyelid surgery.

In the 1920s, Hunt described the coronal browlift, and shortly after Joseph popularized the trichophytic and midforehead browlifts. In the 1950s, Castanares precisely detailed the anatomy of the eyelids and made an important contribution by identifying the role of orbicularis resection in blepharoplasty. In the 1970s, Flowers introduced the supratarsal fixation for the low eyelid crease.

In the past two decades, the most notable advancements in blepharoplasty have been made in the avoidance of complications. The importance of preoperative evaluation for dry eye and other ocular diseases have been highlighted. Tenzel detailed the combination of horizontal lid shortening and lower lid blepharoplasty for lax lower lids. With this came the realization that such procedures should ultimately be performed at the lateral canthus to avoid lid margin incisions.

PERSONAL PHILOSOPHY

Blepharoplasty remains one of the most requested aesthetic facial procedures. Both heredity and aging can influence the appearance of the orbital area. The upper lid begins to show evidence of aging almost before any other facial feature. Familial fat pseudoherniation, though not a result of aging, can be seen to begin the early teen years. The eyes, more than any other facial feature, are a focus of attention to both the patient and observers. Eyelid changes, whether the result of heredity or the effects of aging, seem to take on a magnified importance in the orbital region. Because there is little room for error in blepharoplasty, both careful preoperative physical analysis and meticulous surgical execution are imperative for a successful outcome in blepharoplasty. In general, however, the benefits are much greater than the risks for these procedures. Both the surgeon and the patient universally find the results rewarding.

As in rhinoplasty or facelift surgery, each surgeon brings to the consultation and then to the operating room an artistic goal as to how the final result of blepharoplasty should appear. Although brow position is not part of blepharoplasty, brow position relative to the orbital rim is significant in the final appearance of blepharoplasty procedures. Some surgeons favor a very high brow position; others prefer a low brow. Many patients also have a personal bias in this regard. Patients will come to a surgeon often based on his or her personal philosophy relative to a "look" the surgeon is known for. This certainly is true in both rhinoplasty and blepharoplasty. As with most artistic vision, there is no absolute best, simply many individual sensitivities. There are certain goals, however, that every surgeon tries to achieve: (1) minimal scars in the upper and lower lids, (2) least possible redundant skin, (3) smoothest transition between bone and lid, (4) symmetry of the lid position, (5) symmetry of fat position, (6) maintenance of lid to limbus relationship, (7) durability of the procedure, (8) an overall unoperated appearance, (9) a nonfeminizing male upper lid, (10) rapid and uneventful postoperative course, and (11) absence of complications.

As is true for any surgical procedure, aesthetic or nonaesthetic, proper diagnosis and evaluation of the problem are of paramount importance. This process includes both physical and psychological assessment. Other factors of success in blepharoplasty include a complete explanation of the preoperative, intraoperative, and postoperative facets of the procedure to the patient. The surgeon must have a complete understanding of the technical aspects of upper and lower lid blepharoplasty and a complete grasp of how to manage minor and major complications that may occur. The information that follows is a compilation of a personal philosophy of upper lid and skin-muscle flap lower lid blepharoplasty.

The technique chosen for lower lid blepharoplasty merits special mention. Lower lid blepharoplasty can be performed through a skin flap, skin-muscle flap, a transconjunctival approach, or a combination of these approaches. Each has its advantages and enthusiasts. The author has used all of these approaches to the lower lid in various patients with varying lid problems. This chapter will discuss the skin-muscle flap, as it is the type of lower lid blepharoplasty most frequently used by the author. The advantage of the skin-muscle flap lies in versatility of being able to alter skin excess, skin tightness, muscle excess, muscle tension, fat volume, and fat repositioning. The use of suspension suturing, developed many years ago, allowed all the anatomic aberrations to be accommodated safely, without problems in lid margin positioning.

ANATOMY

EYELID ANATOMY

The lower lid margin has a tangential relationship to the lowest limit of the lower limbus. Seldom does the lower lid

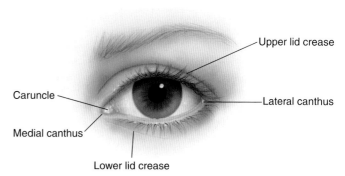

Figure 5-1 The eye is seen at rest with attention to the position of the upper lid over the upper cornea, midway between the upper edge and pupillary border.

cover the corneal margin by more than a millimeter. The upper lid margin is positioned over the upper cornea at midpoint between the upper edge and the pupillary border (Fig. 5-1). Occasionally in a normal eye there is visible sclera below the cornea. This variation may be aesthetically appealing in young woman, but more often its presence draws attention to the eyes and creates the illusion of prominence or exophthalmos. The lateral and medial angles of the palpebral aperture lie along a single horizontal plane.

The superior palpebral sulcus results from insertion of the levator aponeurosis into the lid skin (Fig. 5-2). This

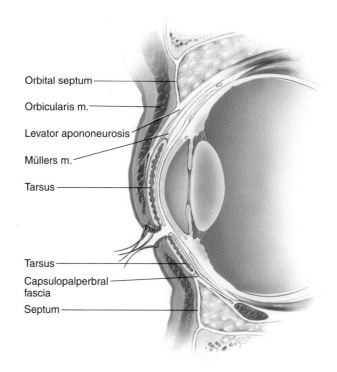

Figure 5-2 The upper eyelid and the relationship of the orbital septum, obicularis oculi, and orbital fat are illustrated. Note the tarsal plate and levator aponeurosis relationship with the levator attaching to the anterior surface of the tarsus and interdigitating with the skin at the lid crease.

insertion varies considerably in different persons. Measured from the lid margin, the fold or sulcus may be as high as 12 mm in eyes that have a high prominent, supraorbital rim and little fat in the superior compartment. Conversely, the lid fold may be as low as 5 to 6 mm above the lid margin in an eyelid that usually appears to be heavy and full. The inferior palpebral sulcus marks the lower margin of the inferior lid tarsus. The variable palpebral malar sulcus is formed by subcutaneous adherence of skin to deeper tissues.

EYELID SKIN

The average thickness of the eyelid skin is equal to that of a split-thickness skin graft. In no other area does the integument approach this fragile quality. The thinness and smooth texture of the lid skin transforms into a thicker, coarser, more sebaceous-type skin lateral to the bony orbital margins. The clinical significance of this transition of skin types is in the manner each recovers from surgical incision.

ORBICULARIS MUSCLE

Three distinct yet conjoined bands of striated muscle encircle the orbit just beneath the skin. These muscle bands act to close the eyes, protect the eyes, and through their pumping action medially aid expressing fluid into the lacrimal sacs.

The pretarsal muscle lies directly over the tarsal plates (Fig. 5-3). The preseptal muscle covers the more peripheral orbital septum, and the orbital muscle overlies the orbital bone margin, blending with the frontalis muscle over the eyebrow and the deeper corrugator supercilii muscle medially.

The medial canthal tendons are formed by the superficial heads of the pretarsal muscle. The tendon

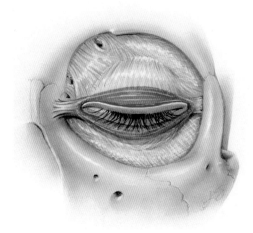

Figure 5-4 The upper and lower pretarsal muscles join laterally to form the lateral canthal tendon, which inserts on the lateral orbital tubercle.

attaches to the anterior lacrimal crest, and the superficial heads of the preseptal muscle attach to the medial canthal tendon. The deep heads of both the pretarsal and preseptal muscles attach to the posterior lacrimal crest posterior to the lacrimal sac.

The upper and lower pretarsal muscles join laterally to form the lateral canthal tendon, which inserts on the lateral orbital tubercle (Fig. 5-4). This tubercle is positioned just behind the orbital rim. The preseptal muscles join laterally to form the lateral palpebral raphe. The raphe is firmly attached to the skin in this area. There is a vascular space between the attachment of the lateral canthus and the more superficial raphe. Unlike the pretarsal and preseptal muscles, the orbital muscle has no firm lateral attachment except to the skin lateral to the lateral canthus. When the eye is firmly closed, the orbital muscle draws the lids medially, producing the crow's-feet wrinkling at the lateral angle.

ORBITAL SEPTUM

The orbital septum provides the skeletal framework of the eyelids (Fig. 5-5). Thin at its periphery, it attaches circumferentially to the bony orbital margin and is anatomically continuous with the orbital periosteum. Condensation and thickening of this septal layer gives origin to the wide, crescent-shaped superior tarsus and the small, bar-shaped inferior tarsus. The entire structure provides an effective diaphragm for the orbital contents and is an efficient barrier to inflammatory and neoplastic diseases that arise on either side of it.

Normally, the orbital septum supports the orbital contents, especially the orbital fat. The integrity of this membrane can be breached by trauma or weakened by hereditary predisposition. All the important intraorbital structures of surgical concern during blepharoplasty lie posterior to the orbital septum.

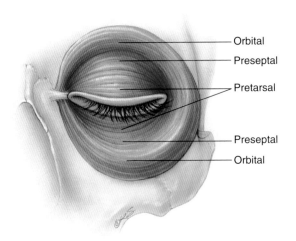

Orbital
Preseptal
Pretarsal
Preseptal
Orbital

Figure 5-3 The three aspects of the orbicularis muscle are depicted.

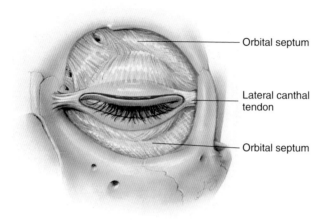

Figure 5-5 The orbital septum provides the skeletal framework of the eyelids.

ORBITAL FAT

Orbital fat provides a cushion and flotation to the intraorbital structures, both for stabilization and for frictionless movement. Intraorbital fat fills the posterior orbit, loosely separating the muscles, vessels, and nerves. The anterior compartmentalization of fat outlined by Castanares conceptualized the surgical anatomy, allowing for an orderly, thoughtful excision of pseudoherniated fat during blepharoplasty.

This anterior orbital fat is present just posterior to the orbital septum as three distinct compartments in the lower lid and two in the upper lid (Fig. 5-6). In the lower lid the medial and central compartments are separated by the inferior oblique muscle. This muscle lies diagonally from the globe above, downward, and medially toward the medial orbital wall. The lateral compartment is separated from the central space by facial extensions of the lateral and inferior rectus muscles. The medial fat compartment of the upper lid is isolated from the central

part by the superior oblique muscle. The quantity of fat in the upper compartment varies. It may stretch across the upper lid to the lacrimal gland or be present in a small pocket just lateral and adjacent to the medial compartment. In its appearance and consistency, the lacrimal gland in the most lateral position of the upper lid is entirely different from fat. A constant pattern of contrasts in texture and color is observed in the various pockets.

The fat of the medial lower compartment is always lighter yellow, or even white, when contrasted with the other compartments. It is also more firm and dense in comparison with the loose fluidity of the central and lateral divisions. The upper medial compartment may also share some of the pale and dense characteristics of the lower medial compartment, but the differences are not so striking. These color and texture differences allow for positive identification of the sometimes elusive medial pseudohernia during blepharoplasty.

Although it is generally true that these pockets of orbital fat are separate and distinct, surgical experience demonstrates that there may be interconnections rather than distinct boundaries, especially between the lower lateral and central compartments. Tension or traction in one area can often transmit reciprocal movement in an adjacent pocket that seems more than simple alteration in volume. During surgical excision, removal of one fat pseudohernia may cause an apparent lessening of the significance of the juxtaposed compartment. Surgical application of this observation is discussed later in the text.

TARSAL PLATES

The dense tarsal plates contribute rigidity and stability to the eyelids. The superior tarsal plate is 1 mm thick, with a horizontal width of 22 to 25 mm and a vertical dimension of 8 to 9 mm. The vertical dimension of the smaller inferior tarsus is 4 to 5 mm (Fig. 5-7A). Both tarsi merge with the lateral and medial lid ligaments at the canthi. The superior and inferior periphery of the tarsi are anatomically continuous with the orbital septum.

LEVATOR MUSCLE

The levator palpebral superioris muscle is the principal elevator of the upper lid. It spans 5.0 to 5.5 cm from its origin in the superior orbital apex to its insertion in the upper lid. As it passes over the superior rectus, it begins to thin and flatten. As the tendon emerges from beneath the bony superior orbital rim, it fans out into the levator aponeurosis. The aponeurosis extends across the full length of the superior tarsus. At the upper margin of the tarsus it fuses with the orbital septum (see Fig. 5-7B). Together they pass downward to attach firmly to the anterior surface of the tarsus and to the orbicularis muscle and the subcutaneous lid tissue. This attachment is responsible for the superior lid fold in the Caucasian eye. Above this fusion the orbital septum is separated from the

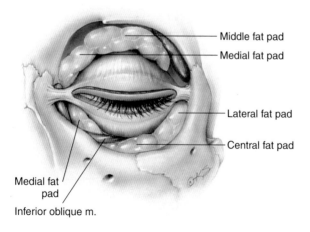

Figure 5-6 The fat compartments of the upper and lower lid are shown.

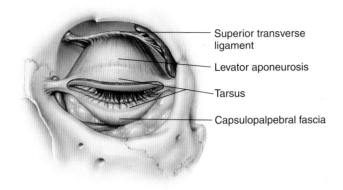

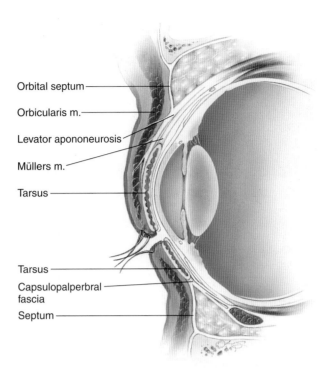

A

Figure 5-7 The tarsal plates provide stability to the lid (**A**). The upper plate is larger than the inferior plate. The levator aponeurosis extends across the full length of the superior tarsus (**B**). At the upper margin of the tarsus it fuses with the orbital septum.

B

aponeurosis by the preaponeurotic fat. The aponeurosis extends laterally into the lacrimal gland, separating it into two lobes and blending with the lateral canthal tendon; medially, it attaches to the posterior lacrimal crest.

Understanding and appreciation of the surgical relationship of the superficial orbital septum, the deeper orbital fat, and still deeper underlying levator aponeurosis are of extreme importance to the blepharoplasty surgeon.

PREOPERATIVE EVALUATION

PSYCHOLOGICAL EVALUATION

In blepharoplasty, as in all aesthetic surgery, it is important to establish that a reasonable and rational motivation exists for the procedure before any physical evaluation is begun. Those with sound motivations include (1) the patient who has considered blepharoplasty for some time, but because of other more pressing social, family, or financial considerations has had to postpone the consultation and surgery; (2) the patient whose livelihood depends on youthful appearance; (3) the patient with a significant aesthetic problem who has not focused on that problem as the source or cause of his or her life difficulties; and (4) the patient who verbalizes that the reason for the surgery is improved self-image and self-esteem.

Those with questionable motivations include (1) patients who present for blepharoplasty at the insistence of another person; (2) patients who have made a sudden decision about surgery; (3) patients who are overly focused on a barely perceptible eyelid irregularity; and (4)

patients whose demeanor, dress, or behavior are extreme or at odds with what is customarily expected in a person seeking aesthetic surgery.

Generally, the patient should not have unrealistic expectations of the aesthetic surgery. Patients who request eyelid rejuvenation surgery and have as their goal a return to an appearance of a younger age are usually good candidates and, fortunately, are in the great majority. Rarely, patients wanting blepharoplasty may seek a completely different look, that is, palpebral fissures that are bigger than natural or lateral canthal positions that are markedly elevated. These patients are pursuing a personal fantasy and may not ever be pleased with the results of aesthetic surgery. The patient who has a lifetime fullness of the upper lid (dermatochalasis) with minimal upper lid show is a special case. Upper lid blepharoplasty in these patients is not a rejuvenation procedure. The change that occurs with blepharoplasty is a completely different look. The newly defined look as demonstrated to the patient preoperatively is usually most welcomed, but a significant other may not welcome the new look. This is one of the few instances in aesthetic surgery in which someone other than the patient may be part of the decision-making process (Fig. 5-8).

MEDICAL EVALUATION

Medical conditions that would preclude any facial rejuvenation procedure should be elicited on the history form during history taking and elaborated on at the examination. Any systemic collagen disease, such as rheumatoid arthritis, systemic lupus erythematosus, and

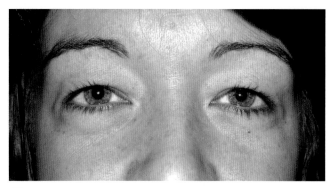

Figure 5-8 This 27-year-old patient presented for blepharoplasty with a history of "never having eyelids." These patients are among the very few for whom it may be prudent to involve a significant other in the consent for surgery. These patients will definitely look different following surgery. Both the surgeon and patient must preclude any misunderstanding with someone who was attracted to the original eyelid feature.

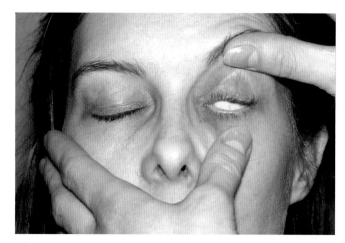

Figure 5-9 The rare patient who does not have a Bell's phenomenon must be identified preoperatively. The risk of exposure keratosis exists when the eyes do not roll upward upon closure of the eyelids.

periarteritis nodosa, carries with it a good possibility of associated dry eye syndrome.

Any of the medications (allopathic or herbal) that can interfere with the blood-clotting cascade should be eliminated at an appropriate time before surgery so that they are no longer a negative factor.

OPHTHALMOLOGIC HISTORY

The ophthalmologic history should include any vision problems, the need for corrective lenses, and any sign of actual or impending dry eye syndrome. Any history of conjunctivitis, styes, chalazion, or ocular herpes is significant. Recurrent chalazion is relatively common following blepharoplasty. It is also easily treated. It is considerably less alarming to patients if they are advised about the possibility before surgery. Lower lid edema, noted daily on awakening, may persist following blepharoplasty for several weeks. A history of previous blepharoplasty is significant, especially a history of multiple blepharoplasty. A history of upper lid injury in youth may be the cause of an unexpected lagophthalmos uncovered during an examination.

OPHTHALMOLOGIC EXAMINATION

The ophthalmologic examination must include a test of vision. Although a test of distance vision may not be suitable, a near vision test is easily performed using the text of the history form or a standard *near vision test card*. A vision test must be documented in the record. The upper lid protective mechanisms are evaluated by checking the following parameters: Bell's phenomenon (Fig. 5-9), lagophthalmos (Fig. 5-10), facial nerve function (Fig. 5-11), corneal sensitivity, and decreased blinking. The extraocular muscles should be evaluated and the results documented. The Schirmer test for dry eye syndrome is probably not indicated for every patient

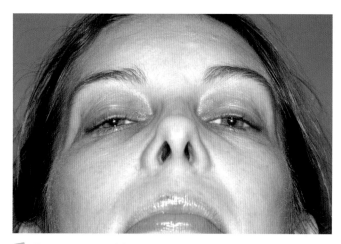

Figure 5-10 Lagophthalmos is determined by having the patient gaze downward while extending the neck. The upper lid is seen to be limited in its ability to cover the cornea and seem tethered. This can occur in any patient who has had previous upper lid blepharoplasty or an upper lid injury in youth

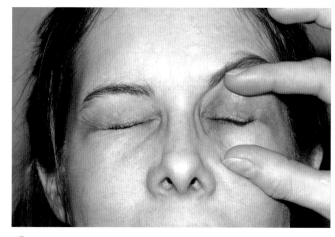

Figure 5-11 Minimal seventh cranial nerve weakness is determined by forcefully opening the eye against the patient's resistance.

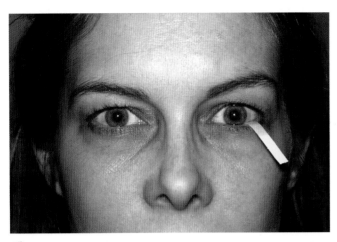

Figure 5-12 The Schirmer test will give a gross approximation of the lacrimal function. If the paper is minimally wet it indicates a major dry eye syndrome is present. It is probably more important to detect a minimal dry eye syndrome by history and then obtain an ophthalmologic examination when planning blepharoplasty.

undergoing blepharoplasty (Fig. 5-12). It is absolutely indicated for any patient who has a positive history of tearing, burning, or eye sensitivity. In these patients, an ophthalmologic consultation will be necessary prior to surgery to establish the level of the dry eye problem and to determine if the surgery is indicated. Patients with moderate to severe dry eye syndrome are probably not candidates for blepharoplasty. Patients with mild functional dry eye syndrome may be candidates for surgery. The upper lid visor function is responsible for corneal coverage, and upper lid blepharoplasty can precipitate dry eye syndrome more readily than lower lid blepharoplasty in a patient with functional dry eye syndrome. The blepharoplasty procedure in a patient with mild functional dry eye syndrome must be done with deliberate conservatism. Both the patient and the surgeon must recognize that a result on the undercorrected side of perfect is desirable. A visual field test is performed if there is a question of visual obstruction secondary to upper lid skin redundancy. A crude test can be performed with finger movement. However, if the procedure is being done specifically for visual field improvement it is probably best to have an independent examiner determine the extent of the problem.

EVALUATION OF EYELID AESTHETIC PROBLEM

The eyelid skin type should be noted. Is it dry, oily, thin, or thick? The type and extent of pigmentation is determined. Are the palpebral fissures symmetrical or asymmetrical? Most patients with asymmetrical palpebral fissures are unaware of the condition until it is pointed out to them. If it has always been present it is not seen as an abnormality. This condition is common. It is important that the condition be pointed out to the patient prior to

surgery. It may likely become a focus of attention following blepharoplasty as observers closely scrutinize the result and bring the asymmetry to the patient's attention. The relationship of the lid margin to the limbus should be recorded. Inequality of the upper lid relationship to the limbus may be secondary to a mild ptosis, may imply a unilateral exophthalmos, or can result from a unilateral lagophthalmos. Unilateral or bilateral mild exophthalmos is a common congenital variant. Asymmetrical positioning of the lower lid is less common, but can occur as a congenital condition. Any recent change needs evaluation. A static lifelong condition probably does not require further evaluation. However, an aggressive upper lid blepharoplasty can make an unnoticed palpebral fissure inequality very obvious.

The amount of upper lid skin redundancy is first estimated with the patient's eyes closed. The skin is gently grasped with a forceps from the medial to the lateral lid to give the surgeon an approximation of the amount of skin that can be safely removed at surgery. The extent of redundant skin lateral to the orbital rim is also evaluated. In this chapter the assumption is made that the brow position is adequate; that is, the brow is positioned above the orbital rim by observation and palpation. In this position, upper lid blepharoplasty can be done without brow lifting. If the procedure of upper lid skin excision ends at the orbital rim while redundant skin exists lateral to the rim, the resulting postoperative hooding will seriously mar the result. The skin lateral to the orbital rim should be incorporated in the upper lid procedure. The skin lateral to the orbital rim is thicker (it is facial skin) than the very thin eyelid skin. The scar will take longer to heal, will stay erythematous for a longer time, and will require the use of cover makeup. However, the end result is a much better looking upper lid. This needs to be explained to the patient. Though the medial and central upper lid is important, in modern upper lid blepharoplasty, the focus is on the elegant *lateral* upper lid.

The amount of medial and central fat pseudo-herniation in the upper lid is noted while gentle pressure is applied to the closed eyelids. Occasionally, a lateral upper lid fat compartment may be present. This almost always is associated with massive pseudoherniation of fat in the medial and central compartments. An apparent lateral fat compartment without large amounts of medial and central fat should make the examiner suspicious of ptosis of the lacrimal gland. If the lid skin is pulled tightly upward, lacrimal gland ptosis will present as a small nodule showing beneath the lateral orbital rim. If the gland is ptotic, the surgeon should plan to suspend it behind the orbital rim at the time of surgery.

Asymmetrical eyebrows must be evaluated in preparation for upper lid blepharoplasty. Asymmetry of the brows is common and hardly ever recognized by the patient until it is pointed out. The eyelid skin beneath the elevated brow usually is viewed by the patient as less redundant, while the skin beneath the lower lid is viewed as more redundant. If, in such patients, asymmetrical skin excisions are performed in the upper lid, the more dependent lid will be pulled even further downward. Unilateral brow elevation is highly recommended in these patients. Again, if the brow asymmetry has been present through out the patient's life the patient may not recognize this feature as abnormal. The patient must be educated about the consequences of performing the blepharoplasty without addressing the asymmetrical eyebrows. The asymmetry will always be more exaggerated following surgery. Some patients will elect not to address the brows despite the surgeon's best efforts to explain the less than ideal results. Brow asymmetry that exists only in animation is entirely different. This is a normal expressive variant. No attempt should be made to correct this type of animated brow asymmetry surgically. The animated asymmetry may respond to botulinum toxin treatment.

Occasionally, a prominent lateral bony rim may require reduction to complete an aesthetic effect. Though beyond the scope of this chapter, the procedure is performed via the upper lid incision with a bone burr. Fat excess may also be found in some patients to cause a heavy appearance in the area beneath the lateral upper brow. This fat may be removed by elevating the upper outer quadrant of orbicularis muscle and sculpting the fat over the upper outer orbital rim. The surgeon is cautioned to be sure homeostasis is complete because this fat is very vascular.

Testing the lower lid to determine tone will determine the vulnerability of the lower lid to postoperative scleral show, lateral "hound dogging," or ectropion. Simple observation of the lid can give the examiner an idea of the lid strength. If the patient has scleral show before surgery, the likelihood of this worsening with surgery must be considered and discussed with the patient, especially if this has been progressive. Some patients have had a small degree of scleral show for all their life. Not only may it be difficult to change this with surgery, but it may also not be desirable. These patients with lifelong scleral show may feel that their eyes are "smaller" without some white showing beneath the limbus. These cases make up a small percentage of the cases that present for surgery but are worth noting. The majority of patients will be distressed if there is an inferior repositioning of the lower lid. These patients and other observers will see a "rounded eye" postoperative result.

A simple snap test will reveal the lower eyelid tone (Fig. 5-13). The lower eyelid is grasped gently with the thumb and forefinger, pulled away from the globe and released. A normal lid will "snap" back to contact the globe with a spring-like action. Any degree of delay in this repositioning is indicative of poor lid tone. The slower the return, the more likely that some problem may occur if the blepharoplasty is not adjusted to account for this

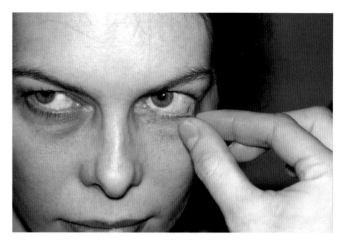

Figure 5-13 The snap test is important in determining the integrity of the lower lid. The normal lid will "snap" back against the globe when it is pulled away gently and then released. Any degree of slowing of the normal repositioning indicates the possibility of malposition of the lower lid margin following blepharoplasty.

laxity. The worse response is the lid that stays away from the globe until the patient blinks. The examiner must be careful to tell the patient to not blink during this test. Blinking as the lid is released will allow even the poorest toned lid to reapply itself to the globe, giving the examiner a false sense that the lid is normal. The surgeon must be alert to the patient with a negative vector. The negative vector is the anatomic observation, in a lateral position, of the globe being positioned more anteriorly than the orbital rim–malar bone complex. These patients are prone to lower lid malpostion following blepharoplasty. The most vulnerable case is the negative vector with an absent lid response to the snap test. A standard blepharoplasty procedure, in these patients, without specific attention to lid tightening will always result in some degree of unacceptable lid positioning. They are candidates for surgery in only the most experienced hands.

The lower lid orbital margin is palpated to determine if any of the baggy appearance of the lower lid is secondary to bony protrusion. Once the problem is ascertained to be fat pseudohernias, it is necessary to quantify the amount of fat. By having the patient gaze upward and then to the right and left the fat pseudo-herniation volume is amplified. This gives the observer an impression of the amounts and location of fat pseudoherniation—medial, central, and lateral—that will require treatment. The amount of skin redundancy is estimated by gently grasping the skin with a smooth forceps while the patient gazes forward. Orbicularis muscle hypertrophy is estimated by observing thickness just below the ciliary margin. Both skin and muscle may be responsible for any swag or festooning at the orbital rim. By having the patient squint the examiner can observe the orbicularis tighten and the subseptal orbital fat being pushed back into the orbit. It also gives the examiner an opportunity to show the patient what the lower

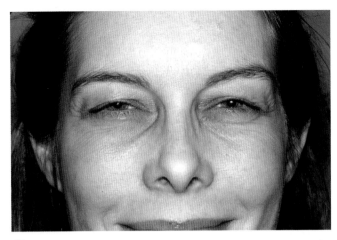

Figure 5-14 With the patient squinting the examiner can observe the subseptal orbital fat pushed back into the orbit. The fine wrinkles are readily apparent and not all of them will be alleviated by surgery. This should be explained to the patient.

lid will look like in terms of the absence of redundant fat and the amount of fine skin rhytids (Fig. 5-14). Not all these fine skin wrinkles will be alleviated by surgery. This should be explained to the patient.

It is important to discuss other anatomic features that will or cannot be changed during blepharoplasty. In darkly pigmented lids, the fine pale lid scar that is ideal may be more obvious. In patients with thin skin or a familial predisposition to a bluish hue from underlying vascular patterns the "dark circles" under the eyes probably will not change. The fine skin crepe patterns of the upper lid are more difficult to control than those of the lower lids. Lateral crow's-feet will not be eradicated by upper or lower lid blepharoplasty. Patients frequently expect periorbital skin problems will be eased at the time of the surgery. The limits of blepharoplasty must be explained before surgery. Any skin lesion such as keratosis, nevus, syringoma, trichoepithelioma, or xanthoma should be discussed as to the possibility of excision and the anticipated result.

As for all aesthetic surgery, photographic documentation is required preoperatively. Close-up 1:5 ratio photographs with frontal eyes open, frontal gaze upward, frontal eyes closed, oblique eyes open, and lateral eyes open should be obtained in addition to a 1:10 full-face view. Use of these photographs with a digital imaging system is the choice of the surgeon. It is not essential. The use of preoperative and postoperative photographs, at the conclusion of the consultation, as examples of possible outcomes is also the surgeon's choice.

SURGICAL TECHNIQUE

SKIN MARKING IN THE UPPER LID

The upper lid skin is cleaned with an alcohol pad to ensure that the marking will not spread. A surgical

marker of extreme thinness in selected to prevent a thick line. One millimeter of lid skin excision can make a difference in the surgical result. If the surgical mark on the lid skin is 2 mm thick on both the upper and lower limbs of the upper lid incision, it is possible to make a 4-mm error in the lid skin excision.

Two notations should be made before marking the skin. The relationship of the brow to the bony rim must be determined while the patient is in an upright position. The weight of the scalp will pull the brow upward when the patient is supine. This movement will carry some of the upper lid skin with it, giving an impression of less redundant skin than is actually present. Also, the amount of medial upper lid fat should be established while the patient is upright. The fat will fall back into the orbit in the supine position, giving a false sense of the amount of fat considered for removal.

The first skin marking is made just below the natural upper lid crease. The suture line will elevate slightly to settle at the natural lid level that is particular to each patient. The natural lid crease is usually apparent. If it is not, the patient is asked to open and close the eyes several times to make the crease appear. The average height of the crease is 8 to 10 mm above the palpebral margin at the center. This may vary between 6 and 12 mm. If the height at the lid center is lower than 8 mm, then the lid-crease marking is elevated to 8 mm to 10 mm. The marking parallels the natural curve of the lid. The medial mark terminates 1 to 2 mm medial to the puncta. The incision ends here. Incisions that continue into the concavity of the medial orbital rim may cause a webbed scar. If the incision is carried onto the nasal skin it is certain to cause an undesirable scar. Excess of creped skin in the medial portion of the eyelid present at the conclusion of the upper lid blepharoplasty can be removed with small vertical triangular skin excisions. These triangular excisions are positioned base down at the incision and rarely even require suturing. The lateral end of the upper lid incision continues along the natural lid crease to about five sixths of the lid. Here the incision should become more horizontal and then curve slightly upward. It is best to avoid the natural line that is seen as the lid crease extends into a lateral orbital skin rhytid. An incision in this area is often too low to cover with makeup. More important, however, a low incision may pull the tail of the brow downward to cause a persistent lateral hooding, thus countering the very purpose of the aesthetic procedure. Curving the incision upward to end between the lateral canthus and the lateral brow margin will reduce the lateral hooding by elevating the skin inferior to the incision upward. The incision ends in a position that is easily camouflaged by makeup (Fig. 5-15). Lateral extension beyond the orbital rim is not recommended in men.

The upper limb of the skin marking must be made to encompass all the redundant eyelid skin. The gravity effect of the scalp pulling the brows up must be countered

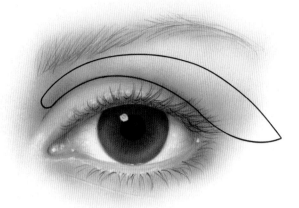 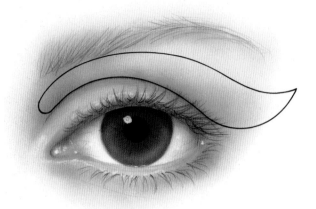

A   **B**

Figure 5-15 The diagram shows the classic position of the lateral upper lid incision falling into a natural lateral rhytid (**A**). Because of the downward thrust of the incision and the lack of any superior skin support in the lower lateral periorbital skin, the final result may be lateral lid hooding. The diagram indicates the upward sweep of the lateral upper lid incision that takes advantage of the natural lateral tether that is found in the temporal region (**B**). The tether becomes increasingly more significant in the skin lateral to the lateral brow. It becomes increasingly less significant in the skin adjacent to the lateral canthus and absent below this area. The authors have found an advantage in moving the lateral portion of the upper lid incision into this tethered area to elevate the skin in the lateral canthus.

by gently pushing the brow downward during the marking (Fig. 5-16). While the patient's eyes are closed the redundant skin is grasped with a forceps to estimate the amount to be removed. One blade of the forceps in placed at the lower lid mark while the other blade is used to gather as much skin as possible without elevating the upper lid margin away from the lower lid margin, so that the eye does not open (Fig. 5-17). The goal is to avoid opening the palpebral fissure and prevent lagophthalmos. Enough medial skin must remain to drape into the depression left by medial fat pocket excision. If the wound is closed by tenting the skin over the depression, a hypertrophic scar is almost certain to result. Both the

medial and the lateral ends of the marks must end in a 30-degree angle to avoid a "dog-ear" elevation (Fig. 5-18).

ANESTHESIA OF THE UPPER LID

If upper blepharoplasty is being done alone, it is easily performed as an ambulatory procedure under local anesthesia with a light premedication. A four-lid blepharoplasty may require a heavier premedication simply because the procedure is longer. If the blepharoplasty is being done as part of total facial rejuvenation, the surgeon will choose an intravenous analgesia or general anesthesia. The common requirement for blepharoplasty is the need

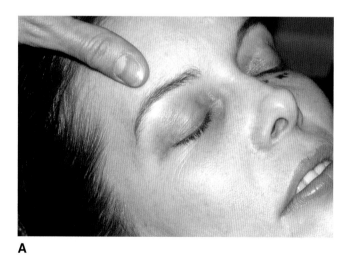 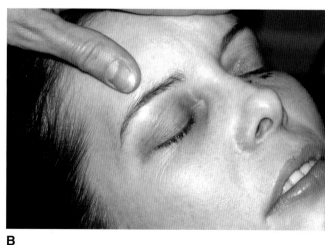

A   **B**

Figure 5-16 The brow-forehead complex is naturally elevated in the supine position (**A**). This elevation has a significant influence on the upper lid skin redundancy. The brow must be depressed to the normal upright brow position while calculating the amount of skin to be removed (**B**). The brow is depressed gently until a "stop" is felt. This is the normal position. The other alternative is to mark the upper lid skin while the patient is upright. The authors have found this latter method more difficult when measuring small or subtle skin excess.

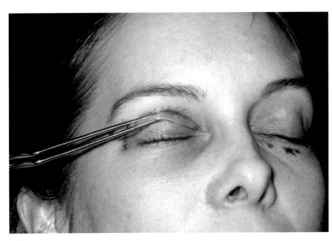

Figure 5-17 The amount of skin to be excised is the maximum that can be removed to leave no excess postoperatively, while complete eyelid closure remains intact. The authors find the small bayonet forceps to be easy to use for the measurement.

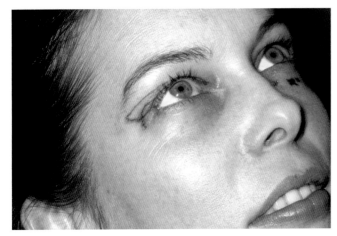

Figure 5-18 This view shows the marked upper lid with the eyes open. Note the amount of skin lateral to the lateral orbital rim. It is this lateral excision that gives beauty to the lateral lid and prevents lateral hooding.

for local infiltrative anesthesia. The author uses lidocaine (Xylocaine) 2% with epinephrine 1:100,000. Lesser concentrations seem to have a shorter effectiveness in the eyelid skin than in other areas of the face. Longer acting local anesthetics such as bupivacaine (Marcaine) may also be used. A mixture of these two anesthetics has been helpful in prolonging the pain-free period following surgery. This benefit must be weighed against the prolonged absence of eyelid closure function in the postoperative period. The total volume of infiltrative lidocaine 2% with epinephrine 1:100,000 should not exceed 1 to 2 mL per eyelid. Greater amounts will distort the eyelid and will not provide improved anesthesia. This amount of anesthetic will provide and sustain maximum anesthesia for 30 minutes and some anesthesia for 1 hour. Maximum epinephrine vasoconstriction occurs 10 to 15 minutes

following injection. The eyelids maintain anesthesia after infiltration for a shorter time than do other areas of facial skin. The addition of a small amount (1 to 10 mL of local anesthetic) of sodium bicarbonate to the local anesthetic may decrease the burning sensation of the local infiltration. The anesthetic is infiltrated with a 1.5-inch 27-gauge or 30-gauge needle from lateral to medial. The needle addresses the lid in a horizontal fashion, never vertically.

Sensory innervation of the upper lid comes from four branches of the ophthalmic nerve (cranial nerve V1). The lacrimal nerve supplies the lateral upper lid. The supraorbital nerve emerges through a groove or canal at the superior medial rim to supply the central and medial lid. Two smaller contributions, the supratrochlear and infratrochlear nerves, pierce the orbital septum above and below the trochlea of the superior oblique muscle. The maxillary nerve (cranial nerve V2) supplies the lower lid through a small zygomaticofacial twig and the superior branch of the infraorbital nerve. These nerves emerge via their respective lateral and medial foramen. There is little need for specific nerve blocks in blepharoplasty anesthesia. Nerve blocks for the upper lid require penetration of the orbital septum toward the orbital roof. It is also not advisable to attempt injection of the orbital fat in the upper or lower lids during initial injections. Penetration of vessels behind the orbital septum, with secondary bleeding and possible hematoma formation, is avoided if the anesthetic infiltration remains subcutaneous. The initial sensation for the patient is that the lids feel heavy and it is difficult to open the eyes. Once the anesthetic becomes effective the patient may have trouble closing the eyes because the orbicularis muscle is affected. The levator of the lid remains unopposed, opening the eye slightly. Any application of topical anesthetic solution to the conjunctiva or cornea should be avoided in standard blepharoplasty (nontransconjunctival approach) because there is no indication for interference with the protective corneal reflexes. Some surgeons prefer to use corneal shields for all blepharoplasty. The incidence of corneal injury without shields is extremely rare.

The timing of the injections depends on the speed and experience of the surgeon. The length of time needed for a four-lid blepharoplasty can vary from less than 1 hour (experienced surgeon) to 3 hours. Do not expect a lid to maintain anesthesia for much more than 1 hour. The lids should be infiltrated accordingly. The surgeon with modest experience may find it useful to anesthetize both upper lids initially; then, just before beginning the skin incision on the second upper lid, both lower lids are infiltrated. If all lids are anesthetized at the outset, the final or fourth lid may become sensitive just as the incision is made. The secondary infiltration could make precise skin and fat removal unnecessarily difficult. The average required times for completion of lid surgery should be recorded to allow a realistic schedule for anesthesia.

General anesthesia is rarely necessary for blepharoplasty. If general anesthesia is used, the surgeon and the anesthetist must be aware and sensitive to the problem of postintubation coughing and postanesthesia retching. These factors can add greatly to the postoperative edema and ecchymosis associated with blepharoplasty.

UPPER LID BLEPHAROPLASTY

The procedure begins with placing tension on the inferior limb upper lid marking, pulling it laterally to straighten the mark as much as possible (Fig. 5-19). The incision is made with a small blade (No. 15 Bard-Parker or No. 65 Beaver). The incision is made at a uniform depth through the skin beginning medially and continuing laterally in a single stroke. The incision is then made in the upper limb. The lateral angle must be very crisp at 30 degrees. This lateral angle can be made by turning the blade 180 degrees and stroking medially from the point of convergence. The lid skin is then removed with a curved Steven's scissors and a Brown-Adson forceps. Pushing the closed scissors in a medial direction in the subcutaneous space between the upper and lower limbs of the incision and spreading facilitate the removal. A decision is then made to remove or not remove orbicularis muscle (Fig. 5-20). Removal of orbicularis muscle allows for a greater definition of the upper lid cleft and a sculptured appearance of the upper lid. This advantage must be weighed against the fact that orbicularis function closes the eye and that the muscle is present in varying degrees in different individuals. Other considerations are that the deeply sculptured eyelid cleft can have an aging look (cadaveric) and the sculpted look in the male lid can appear feminine. Despite these considerations, some muscle excision is probably desirable in most cases except in older and thin-skinned patients in whom the muscle can be expected to be scant or thin. Point cautery is used to obtain absolute homeostasis.

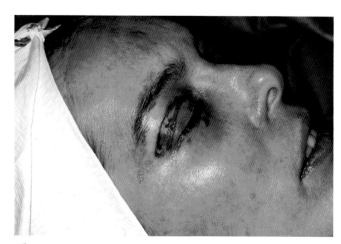

Figure 5-20 The thin upper lid skin redundancy has been excised with preservation of the underlying orbicularis muscle.

Following removal of the redundant skin and any indicated orbicularis muscle the medial fat pocket is exposed by gently spreading the medial orbital septum with a Steven's scissors or a fine hemostat. This can be facilitated by having the surgical assistant elevate the brow. The color of the medial fat is whiter than the yellow fat of the central compartment. The central fat can be close to the medial fat. The color difference can be helpful to avoid missing the medial fat pocket. The medial fat pocket can be visualized by observing the slight bulging while applying soft digital pressure to the closed eyelid. The medial fat is gently teased through the opening in the orbital septum (Fig. 5-21). A small amount of local anesthesia is injected into the fat. It is then clamped and excised. Enough fat is left at the point of excision to allow it to be cauterized. The local anesthesia is necessary to prevent pain with manipulation of the fat when this

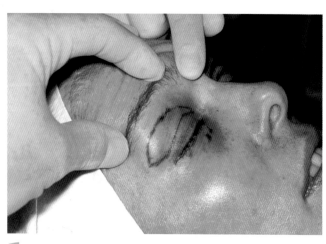

Figure 5-19 The skin is stretched taught to allow an easy sweep of the scalpel to incise the skin precisely along the surgical marking.

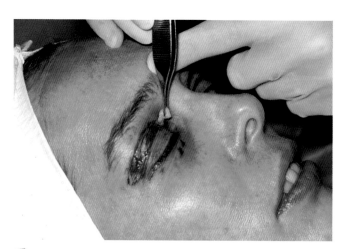

Figure 5-21 The medial fat pocket is exposed by applying a small amount of pressure to the globe and watching for slight bulging in the medial upper lid. The orbital septum is incised and the medial fat pocket is teased from the medial fat compartment.

procedure is done under local anesthesia. All the structures internal to the orbital septum maintain their sensitivity. The orbital septum is an effective barrier to the spread of local anesthetic. The upper medial fat pocket lies between the medial rectus muscle and the superior oblique muscle. The superior oblique muscle is at small risk of injury if too much tension is applied, drawing the fat up into the wound. The hemostat is applied only when it is clear that the muscle will not be clamped with the fat. The superior oblique muscle, however, is rarely seen. The fat is excised with a curved Steven's scissors. Enough fat is left to allow cautery with a hot tip cautery. The hot tip cautery is used because it allows pinpoint precision hemostasis. The use of electocautery will almost always cause pain in the posterior orbit even when the fat is totally anesthetized. It is not suitable for use under local anesthesia. After the medial fat is removed the central fat is located by applying gentle pressure to the globe. A small incision is made at the point where the orbital septum bulges. The fat is then gently teased into the wound. Only the fat that lies external to the septum without retracting back into the wound is removed. This will produce a smooth nonretracted central lid. Overexcision of fat in the central compartment is an error that often produces an A-shaped retraction that defeats the intended rejuvenation. The fat is clamped, cut, and cauterized in the same fashion as the medial fat. The levator aponeurosis is superficial and clearly visible beneath the central compartment fat.

Rarely, in extremely heavy lids, there is a lateral fat compartment over the position of the lacrimal gland. If the lacrimal gland is seen to be ptotic preoperatively, it is easily repositioned by using a 6-0 polypropylene suture to secure the gland capsule to the orbital roof just internal to the orbital rim. The gland color is pink and the consistency is lobular, which differentiates it from orbital fat. Occasionally, a broad heavy bony orbital rim will require reduction with a bone burr. Also, in particularly heavy lateral lids a separate fattiness can be found deep to the upper outer orbitalis muscle (ROOF, or retro-obicularis orbital fat). Removal of this fat gives a refinement to the heavy outer orbital rim. This retro-orbicularis fat is extremely vascular, and complete homeostasis is important.

Repair of the wound can be accomplished with several varied sutures. However, the author finds polypropylene the most nonreactive, resulting in the finest scars. Nylon is somewhat more reactive and is more difficult to remove because its friction quotient grips the tissue when it is used as a continuous suture. Absorbable sutures are the most reactive in the skin, producing redness that is not seen with polypropylene. Braided or multifilament sutures are the worst sutures to use for eyelid incision closure. They are notorious for leaving suture tunnels and skin suture marks.

The upper eyelid skin wound is closed beginning with simple 6-0 polypropylene (Prolene) sutures from lateral

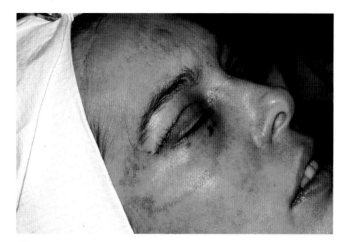

Figure 5-22 The upper lid wound is closed initially with several 6-0 Prolene simple sutures laterally. The wound tension is highest laterally. The remainder of the wound is closed with a single subcuticular 6-0 Prolene suture. The ends are left free and are not tied.

to medial to close the lateral one fourth of the wound. The orbital septal incisions are not repaired. The lateral or facial skin part of the wound is under the most tension and is the most likely to separate if closed with a running suture. The remaining wound is closed with a running subcuticular suture beginning medially and continuing to the simple interrupted suture closure (Fig. 5-22). The ends of the sutures are left untied and long and are taped to the skin above the eyebrows. The surgeon must handle the eyelid skin very gently. If a forceps is used, only the subcutaneous tissue is grasped. If any area of the closure seems to need support, individual simple sutures are placed using only a surgical twist instead of a knot. Any skin redundancy noted at the medial end of the wound in handled by removing small triangles of skin (base down at the wound edge) both above and below the wound edge.

Skin glue alone has not been found satisfactory as a primary closure following upper lid blepharoplasty. The authors find the suture closure technique to produce consistently finer scars. Skin glue is used in selected cases as a supplemental closure following suturing. It is also useful for closing wounds that have separated because of trauma in the immediate postoperative period. The use of $\frac{1}{8}$-inch sterile surgical tape to cover the sutured wound gives additional support and security in the immediate postoperative period.

Figure 5-23 presents one case of upper lid blepharoplasty. Figure 5-24 presents a more extensive case. Figures 5-25 to 5-27 show pre- and postoperative views of individuals who have undergone upper blepharoplasty.

LOWER LID SKIN MUSCLE FLAP BLEPHAROPLASTY

The lower lid incision should be made parallel to a line 2 to 3 mm below the cilia of the lower palpebral margin. It

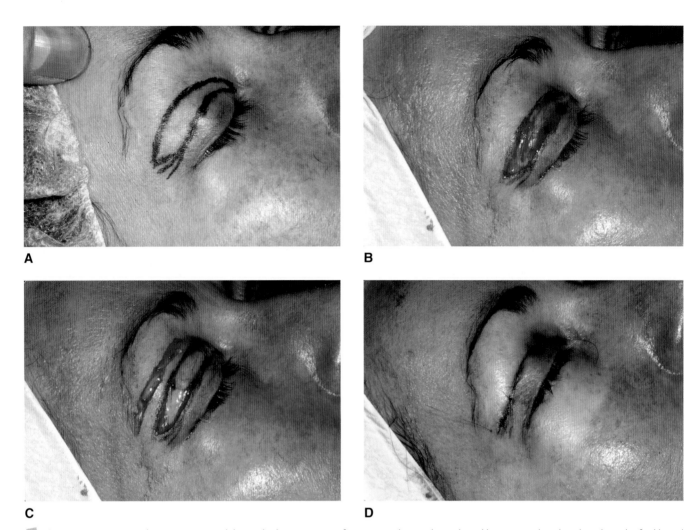

Figure 5-23 In part **A**, this patient's upper lid is marked in preparation for surgery. The two lower lateral lines were placed to show how the final lateral skin marking configuration is chosen to elevate the lateral "crow's-foot "area rather than pull the skin lateral to the orbital rim downward. In part **B**, the redundant skin has been removed. Patients, such as this one, with moderate orbicularis muscle hypertrophy can benefit from an excision of muscle from the central aspect of the wound. The muscle excision will provide a more attractive lid cleft definition. In part **C**, the orbicularis muscle has been excised and placed on the upper lid to display the amount and extent of the muscle excision. The cuff of muscle is always removed centrally with some muscle remaining at the wound edges. Part **D** shows wound closure with multiple simple sutures laterally and a single subcuticular suture medially and centrally. The sutures are removed at 4 days.

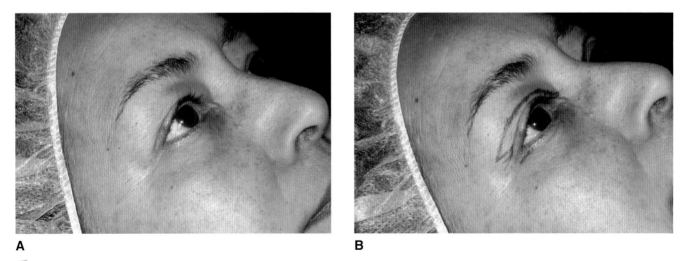

Figure 5-24 This patient has significant skin excess, muscle hypertrophy, and fat pseudoherniation (**A**). Skin marking of the upper lid shows the amount of redundant skin beyond the lateral orbital rim (**B**).

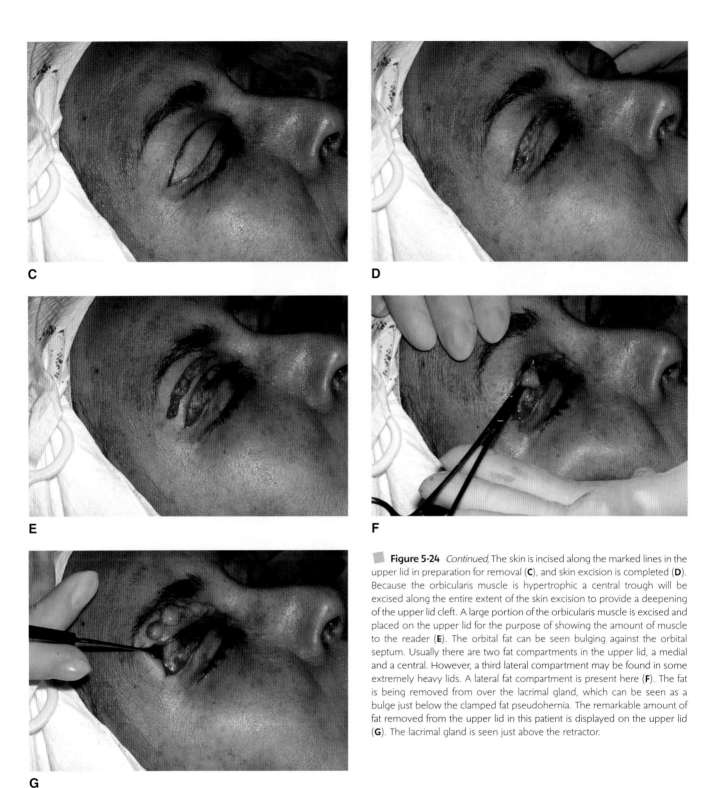

C

D

E

F

G

Figure 5-24 *Continued,* The skin is incised along the marked lines in the upper lid in preparation for removal (**C**), and skin excision is completed (**D**). Because the orbicularis muscle is hypertrophic a central trough will be excised along the entire extent of the skin excision to provide a deepening of the upper lid cleft. A large portion of the orbicularis muscle is excised and placed on the upper lid for the purpose of showing the amount of muscle to the reader (**E**). The orbital fat can be seen bulging against the orbital septum. Usually there are two fat compartments in the upper lid, a medial and a central. However, a third lateral compartment may be found in some extremely heavy lids. A lateral fat compartment is present here (**F**). The fat is being removed from over the lacrimal gland, which can be seen as a bulge just below the clamped fat pseudohernia. The remarkable amount of fat removed from the upper lid in this patient is displayed on the upper lid (**G**). The lacrimal gland is seen just above the retractor.

extends medially along this line no farther than the inferior lid puncta. Laterally, the incision curves upward as it maintains the 2- to 3-mm distance parallel to the ciliary margin. It then breaks at the lateral canthus into a more horizontal position and a lateral skin crease. Older methods required that this lateral portion of the incision angle downward and that the skin be advanced laterally to excise a triangle at the lateral lid. The resultant scars were obvious, uncorrectable, and a permanent reminder of the blepharoplasty surgery. The method described here involves a superior elevation. It is usually necessary to mark only the lateral limb of the incision because the infraciliary incision is always the same position. It is actually easier to observe the infraciliary crease without

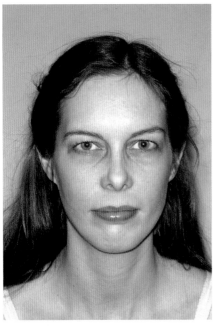

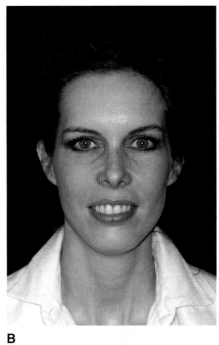

A

B

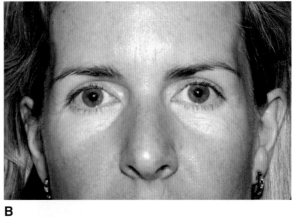

Figure 5-25 Preoperative (**A**) and 6-month postoperative (**B**) frontal views of a 34-year-old woman who underwent upper lid blepharoplasty.

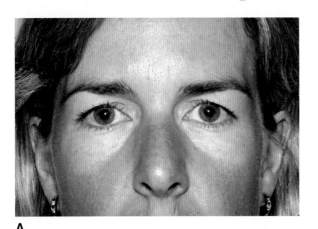

A

B

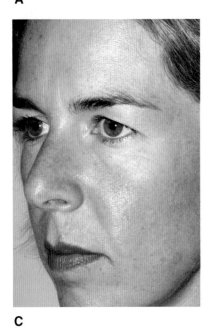

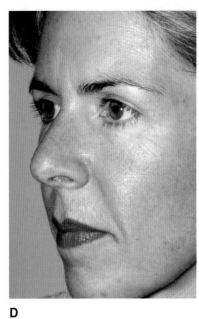

C

D

Figure 5-26 Preoperative (**A**) and 6-month postoperative (**B**) frontal views of a 32-year-old woman who underwent upper lid blepharoplasty. Preoperative (**C**) and 6-month postoperative (**D**) oblique views of upper lid blepharoplasty.

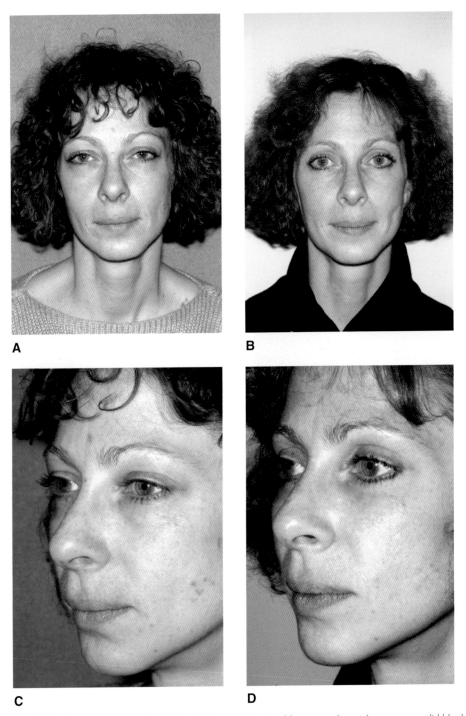

Figure 5-27 Preoperative (**A**) and 1-year postoperative (**B**) frontal views a 34-year-old woman who underwent upper lid blepharoplasty. Preoperative (**C**) and 1-year postoperative (**D**) oblique views.

the marking. Again, it is important to use the finest point marker on the skin.

The marked skin is incised with a No. 15 Bard Parker blade or a No. 67 Beaver blade down to the orbicularis muscle while the upper lid is opened slightly to observe and assure that the incision in no lower than 2 to 3 mm from the lash line (Fig. 5-28). The remainder of the incision is made with a small, sharp, straight scissors. The

lower blade of the scissors is used as a pushing dissector subcutaneously as the upper blade cuts through the skin in a straight line in the natural crease 2 to 3 mm below the lash line (Fig. 5-29). No cilia are cut. The incision ends medially at the lower lid puncta, never beyond. Any medial extension of the incision invites postoperative problems with tear drainage. A small skin flap is then developed for approximately 3 mm to expose and preserve

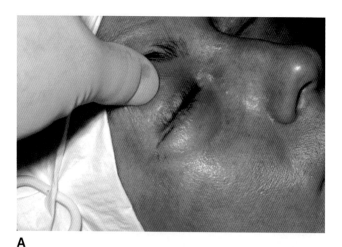

A

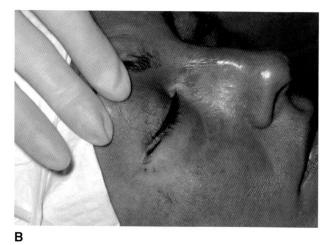

B

Figure 5-28 The lateral lower lid wound site is marked 2 to 3 mm below the lash line only in the lateral 6 to 7 mm of the lid (**A**). The lateral lower lid wound is incised with a scalpel (**B**).

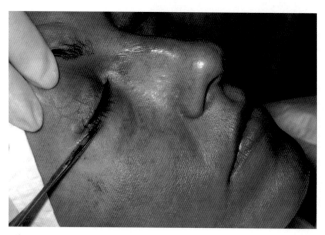

Figure 5-29 Following a blade incision of the lateral lid at 2 to 3 mm below the lash line, the remaining incision is made at the same distance below the lash line with a small sharp scissors.

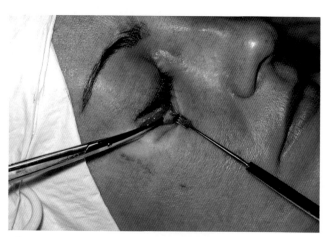

Figure 5-30 The skin flap is developed for approximately 3 mm to expose and preserve the pretarsal fibers of the orbicularis oculi muscle.

the pretarsal fibers of the orbicularis oculi muscle (Fig. 5-30). By preserving this pretarsal muscle sling, the lower lid can be expected to have a more immediate tension response after surgery, reducing the possibility of scleral show or ectropion. A curved Steven's scissors is the used to separate the pretarsal and preseptal muscle to the puncta (Figs. 5-31 and 5-32). Blunt dissection with a cotton-tipped applicator sweeps and separates the orbicularis muscle from the orbital septum down to the bony inferior orbital rim exposing the lateral, central, medial orbital rims.

A decision is made at this point to excise, preserve, or reposition the orbital fat. When abundant fat is present in all compartments, some fat must be removed. The author has found that fat preservation with repositioning can be valuable when a deep tear-trough deformity exists. In the central lid precise fat excision will create a smoothness at the bony rim–central orbital septum junction. In the lateral and central compartments the fat is removed to a level 1 mm below the bony rim. The fat is removed by

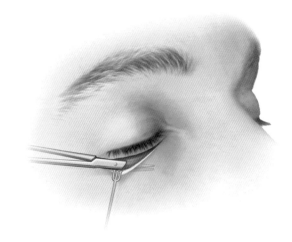

Figure 5-31 The diagram shows the path of the scissors separating the pretarsal and the preseptal muscles. The pretarsal muscle is left intact to act as an active muscle sling in the immediate postoperative course. The lower lid function is realized more quickly to help prevent any of the sequelae of a lax lower lid.

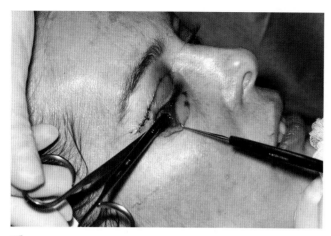

Figure 5-32 The surgical photograph shows the same orientation as in the previous figure. The small Steven's scissors is used to tunnel between the orbicularis muscle above and the orbital septum below. The scissors is then turned 90 degrees and the muscle is transected.

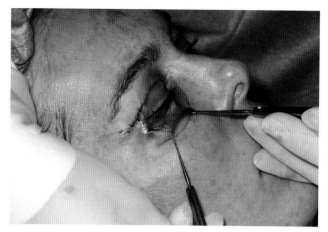

Figure 5-33 The medial fat compartment is handled differently depending on whether a tear-trough deformity is present. If a tear-trough depression could benefit from elevation, a pocket is developed by elevating the medial orbicularis muscle from its attachment to the maxilla. This attachment is tenacious. The orbital septum is incised at the orbital rim (arcus marginalis) and the fat is spilled into the wound. The medial orbital fat is then tucked beneath the muscle. It does not need to be sutured in this position to be effective, although it can be sutured to the periosteum.

first incising the orbital septum and then teasing the fat into the wound. If this is done under local anesthesia it must be done with gentleness. Aggressive traction will cause pain. The fat redundancy is then infiltrated with local anesthesia, clamped, excised, and cauterized. (The same procedure is followed as in the upper lid described previously.) The central compartment fat is always the most obvious. The lateral compartment orbital septum is the thickest. The medial fat compartment is usually the most elusive. Identification and notation of this compartment preoperatively is important. At times, it may by necessary to apply gentle pressure to the closed eye and watch for the location of orbital septum bulging to locate the medial fat compartment. Once identified, the orbital septum is incised with the scissors and the fat is teased into the wound. Before infiltrating and clamping the fat, the inferior oblique muscle should be observed. In contrast to the upper lid, this muscular structure is almost always visible and should be found before clamping to avoid injury to the muscle. The fat in this medial location is also more dense and vascular than the other compartments of the lower lid (Figs. 5-33 to 5-35). Homeostasis must be absolute to avoid a bleeding medial fat stump that could retract back into the orbit.

When a preoperative tear trough problem is in need of correction, the medial fat is handled differently. There have been many papers and presentations on this subject. Most authors have recommended that the fat or the orbital septum be sutured into the tear-trough depression. At times, especially when this technique is first used by the surgeon, the lid margin can be pulled downward or worse, everted when the orbital septum is sutured to the periosteum. The tarsal plate and the orbital septum are a single continuous structure. The author has found the following technique useful. In those individuals who require filling of the tear trough, the medial orbitalis

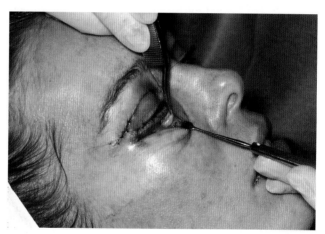

Figure 5-34 If no tear-trough deformity exists and the medial fat compartment is seen as a medial fat pocket, then the fat is excised. The fat is teased into the wound. The amount of fat that lies on the opened orbital septum is usually the correct amount to be removed. The goal is to have the level of the fat at 1 mm below the orbital rim.

muscle (the portion of the orbicularis muscle extending over the orbital rim) is elevated with a small short dissector for a distance of approximately 1 cm. This area must be thoroughly infiltrated with local anesthetic if the procedure is done under local anesthesia. Once the muscle is elevated, the surgeon should observe if the elevation is completely under the tear trough. Incising the orbital septum along the orbital rim opens the fat compartment. The fat is then allowed to spill into the wound. It is pushed gently into the space beneath the elevated muscle. It has not seemed necessary to secure the fat in the new position. Whether the fat is secured with sutures or not the results have effaced the depth of the tear trough.

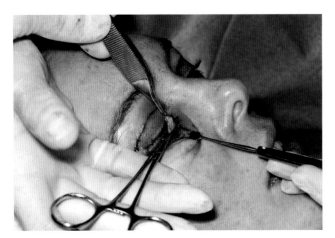

Figure 5-35 When the patient is under local anesthesia, the fat is infiltrated with a small amount of local anesthetic; it is clamped and excised. Enough fat is left remaining to allow cautery of the fat stump without touching the forceps. The authors use a hot tip cautery for hemostasis. Under local anesthesia, electocautery applied to the clamp itself will cause pain in the posterior orbit no matter how effectively the fat has been infiltrated with local anesthetic.

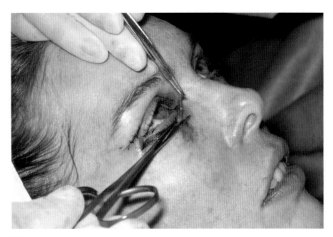

Figure 5-36 Skin removal is of critical importance in lower lid blepharoplasty. Even 1 mm too much can result in a scleral show, yet 1 mm less can result in a perceived persistent redundancy. With the patient in upward gaze an amount of skin is removed so that it appears that 1 to 2 mm *too much* has been removed. Experience has shown that the lateral suspension suture will close this gap. The result will be an attractively tight appearing lower lid without scleral show. Both skin and the attached preseptal orbicularis muscle are removed. If only skin is removed, a slight elevated roll will result just beneath the lash line.

Once the medial fat has been dealt with, the surgeon should go back to the lateral compartment to be sure that the proper amount of fat has been removed. One of the most common complaints following lower lid blepharoplasty is the presence of persistent bulging in the area of the lateral fat compartment. If more fat can be teased into the wound, it should be removed.

Once homeostasis is obtained, the skin-muscle flap is redraped superiorly. Under local anesthesia, the redundant skin is removed while the patient is looking upward, with a straight Steven's scissors (Fig. 5-36). The amount removed should leave a small gap between the upper and lower limbs of the lower lid incision. The suspension suture will close this gap. If the patient is under general anesthesia, the lower lid is positioned so that the lid margin is crossing the limbus at an appropriate position. At this point, the decision about how much lower lid skin is to be removed during blepharoplasty should be made. If the lower lid falls inferiorly and redundant skin and muscle are removed to accommodate this inferiorly positioned lid, a rounded palpebral fissure, scleral show, or ectropion becomes a definite possibility. After the redundant lid is excised, the surgeon should observe the field to see if any thickness of muscle is present along the inferior limb of the wound. As the skin-muscle flap is draped superiorly it is not uncommon to see the preseptal muscle overlie the pretarsal muscle, causing an elevation or ridge below the subciliary incision. Women always want this subciliary area smooth. Any redundant muscle is removed. Homeostasis is again established. At this point, the suspension suture is then placed (Figs. 5-37 to 5-50). The suspension is always a vertical vector elevation. The suture found to be most effective is the 5-0 clear Prolene. The suture

placement is between the deep preseptal orbicularis muscle and the lateral orbital rim periosteum at the region of the lateral orbital tubercle. The knot should be buried. If any tethering is noted in the skin of the lower lid, the suture should be placed at a deeper level. It is also important not to place the suture so tightly that the lower lid skin gathers at the lateral rim. The skin at the lateral extreme of the wound should be smooth. The suture must be cut on the knot.

Once the suspension suture has been placed, the wound is closed with a running 6-0 Prolene suture from

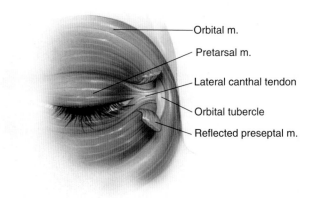

Figure 5-37 The diagram indicates the two position points of the suspension suture for lower lateral support. The superior position is through the periosteum at the orbital tubercle. The lower position is through the preseptal orbicularis muscle in direct vertical line from the superior position. The muscle in the diagram shows the muscle reflected for the purpose of anatomic demonstration.

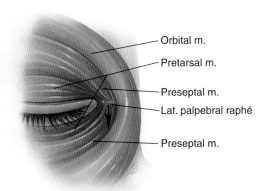

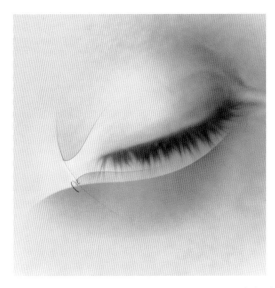

- Orbital m.
- Pretarsal m.
- Preseptal m.
- Lat. palpebral raphé
- Preseptal m.

Figure 5-38 The vertical arrow shows the position of the suture placement in relationship to the lateral palpebral raphe and the preseptal muscle.

Figure 5-41 The illustration shows transparent view of the lateral suspension suture placement. The suture is tight and the knot is buried.

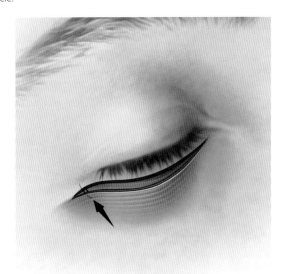

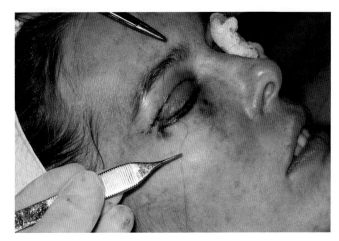

Figure 5-39 The illustration shows the position of the lateral suspension suture with the small wound gap in the lower lid.

Figure 5-42 The suspension suture being used here is a blue polypropylene 5-0 suture for demonstration purpose. The actual suture used is a clear polypropylene suture. Note that the suture is at the lateralmost extent of the lower lid incision.

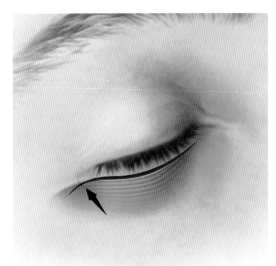

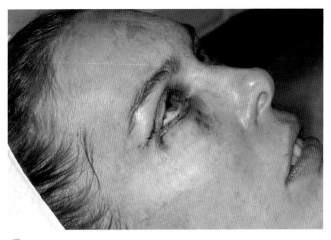

Figure 5-40 The illustration shows the upper movement of the lower lid with tightening of the suspension suture. All tension is removed as the two wound edges become apposed. The wound is then closed under no tension.

Figure 5-43 The patient with the lateral suture in place is asked to look upward to demonstrate the maximum tension on the lower lid incision. Note that without the placement of lower lid sutures there is no separation of the wound. The suspension suture is relieving all tension.

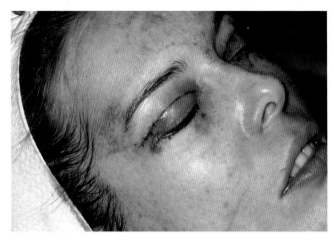

Figure 5-44 A few simple sutures have been used to close the lower lid wound. The alternative closure would be a running cutaneous 6-0 polyropylene suture. The authors find it difficult to use a subcuticular suture in the lower lid.

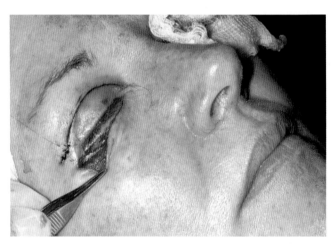

Figure 5-45 In this patient the orbital fat has been dealt with by excision and repositioning. The decision is now made about the amount of redundant skin and the lateral suspension suture. Note that the incision in the lower lid extends slightly beyond the lateral canthus margin.

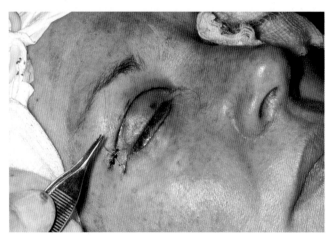

Figure 5-46 The lower lid skin-muscle flap has been elevated and draped over the superior margin of the incision. With the patient's eyes closed there is no tension on the skin-muscle flap.

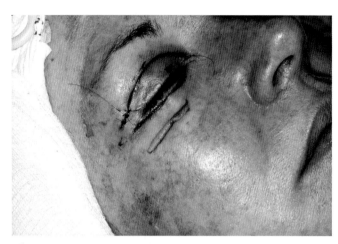

Figure 5-47 The amount of skin removed here with the patient's eyes closed seems appropriate. But, without the suspension suture the patient will develop a scleral show as healing occurs. The lid must be supported when this amount of skin is removed using the skin-muscle flap approach.

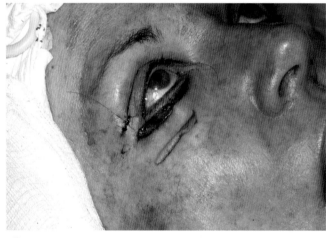

Figure 5-48 With gazing upward and opening the mouth a remarkable separation of the wound occurs. Without the assistance of the suspension suture the downward traction would most likely result in scleral show, lateral "hound dogging,' or the round eye presentation.

lateral to medial. The medial ends of the suture are left long and taped to the cheek skin. Short suture ends can turn back toward the globe to irritate the cornea. Three $\frac{1}{4}$-inch sterile surgical tape strips are place laterally to provide an upward pull on the cheek skin to decrease any downward pressure on the wound. Figures 5-51 to 5-54 show pre- and postoperative views of patients after lower blepharoplasty.

POSTOPERATIVE CARE

No bandages are used on the lids, but the eyes are covered by cold compresses as continuously as possible until bedtime the day of the surgery. The wounds are lubricated with a steroid-antibiotic ophthalmic ointment. If the upper lid wounds have been covered with $\frac{1}{8}$-inch sterile surgical

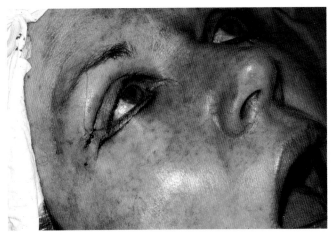

Figure 5-49 The lateral suspension suture has been placed between the lateral orbital tubercle periosteum and the exact vertical pretarsal orbicularis muscle on the skin-muscle flap. Note that the suture has been placed deeply in the muscle. No puckering or tethering is seen in the lower lid skin. Also observe that the orbicularis muscle has been draped over the malar bone to create a smooth transition between the orbital margin and the lower lid. It is this smoothing effect of the suspension suture that has eliminated the need for fat repositioning in the lateral half of the lower lid.

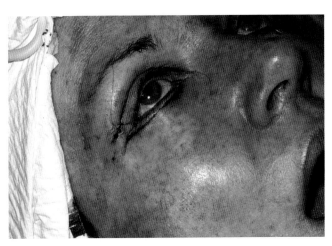

Figure 5-50 The strength of the suspension suture can be seen as the patient gazes upward with her mouth wide open. With this maximum tension on the wound there is no separation at the wound. The final skin sutures can be placed gently with enough force to simply bring the edges together.

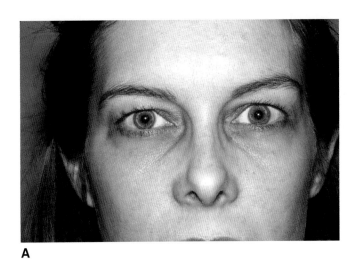

A

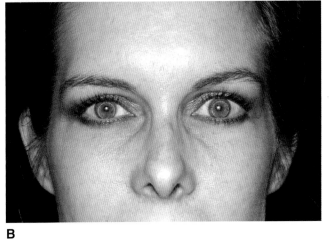

B

Figure 5-51 Preoperative (**A**) and 1-year postoperative (**B**) frontal views of a 34-year-old blepharoplasty patient.

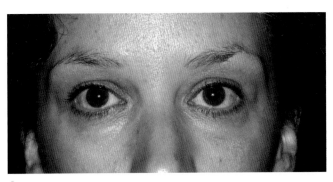

A

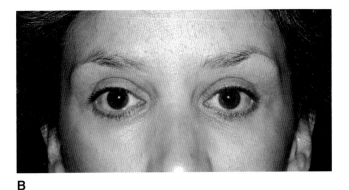

B

Figure 5-52 Preoperative (**A**) and 1-year postoperative (**B**) frontal views of 42-year-old blepharoplasty patient.

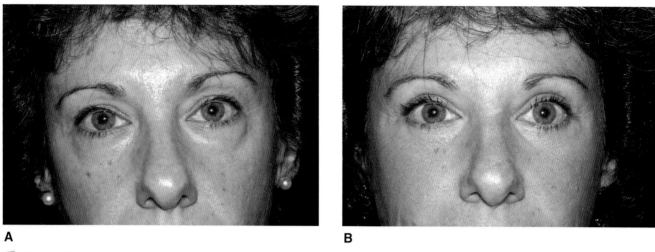

A   B

Figure 5-53 Preoperative (**A**) and 9-month postoperative (**B**) frontal views of a 43-year-old blepharoplasty patient.

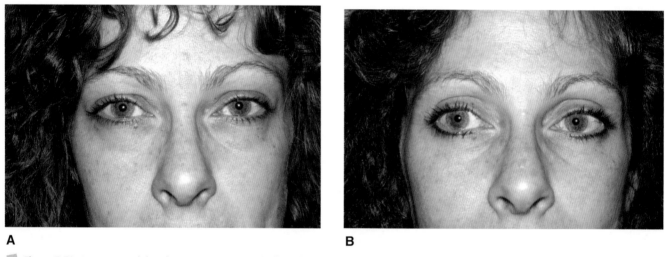

A   B

Figure 5-54 Preoperative (**A**) and 1-year postoperative (**B**) frontal views of a 33-year-old blepharoplasty patient.

tapes, then the ointment is not used. Some bloody spotting will be noted and should not cause alarm. Pain is not a major problem. A burning sensation for 1 to 1.5 hours after surgery is not unusual. This discomfort can almost always be relieved with minor analgesics such as acetaminophen with or without codeine. Anything that would produce vasodilatation should be avoided. The patient is instructed not to consume coffee, alcohol, or highly spiced foods and to keep exertion limited to activities of daily living. On the second postoperative day, compresses are used 20 minutes per hour. Maximum postoperative edema is usually seen on the morning of the second postoperative day. Sutures are removed on the fourth postoperative day. Makeup can be applied on the fourth postoperative day to the lid skin and to the wound itself on the sixth postoperative day. Contact lens use may begin on the fourth postoperative day. Most patients feel comfortable returning to work or normal activities on the seventh postoperative day. Partial exercise can begin at

2 weeks and full exercise at 4 weeks. One or 2 weeks before the operation, the patient is given preoperative and postoperative instructions and an accounting of the expected events following surgery. This material is best prepared from the surgeon's own experience.

Serious complications of blepharoplasty are, fortunately, uncommon. There are many frequent minor or lesser complications and sequelae that occur following blepharoplasty. These lesser sequelae are complex and related to subjective aesthetic judgments as well as to specific objective observations. Many of these sequelae are temporary and are related to variations in the healing process.

Most texts on blepharoplasty list the complications of blepharoplasty and the management of these problems. Although a complete understanding of these more specific complications is imperative, each surgeon must develop a much broader perception of the postoperative blepharoplasty course to include all gradations of normal

Box 5-1   Problems Seen Shortly After Surgery

These problems can be expected to resolve quickly, in 1 or 2 weeks:

- Chemosis, especially of the lower lateral lid (1 week)
- Subconjunctival hemorrhage (3 weeks)
- Separation of the lateral lower lid from the bulbar conjunctiva (may be helped by surgical tape support in the immediate postoperative period)
- Tearing
- Burning sensation
- Visual blurring secondary to ointment
- Edema of the lids
- Pain (unusual beyond the first few postoperative hours, may be felt with coughing or sneezing if a suspension suture has been used)
- Asymmetry secondary to swelling
- Insensitivity of the upper lids noted when applying makeup

postoperative healing, postoperative problems, and true complications that deviate from the ideal result. *When this more graduated approach is related to the postoperative course chronologically in days and weeks, it becomes a valuable informational source to the patient.*

SLOWLY RESOLVING PROBLEMS

These postoperative problems generally resolve after the second postoperative week.

Eyelid Ecchymosis

The usual progression of ecchymosis is from blue-black through magenta to yellow and on to normal skin color within 1 to 2 weeks. An occasional patient may retain a uniform or patchy subcutaneous hemosiderin deposit for a considerable time. This most commonly occurs along the palpebral malar sulcus following a particularly dense ecchymosis in the darkly pigmented patient. It is totally unpredictable in patients with no previous history of bruising. Permanent pigmentation is very rare. Particularly stubborn problems may take up to 18 months of continuous reassurance. No particular treatment seems to hurry the resolution process. However, some patients seem to benefit from the application of *Arnica montana*. Camouflage makeup is an appropriate recommendation.

Tearing

Tearing and burning may persist as a mild annoyance beyond the immediate postoperative period without any visual disturbance. This is secondary to the minimal palpebral margin separation, which allows some drying of the conjunctiva. These symptoms are almost always self-limiting, but the use of artificial tears *before retiring* may be advisable. Continued follow-up is necessary until the symptoms abate.

Contact Lens Difficulties

Some difficulty with the insertion of contact lens may be anticipated. The alteration of the lid tension may change the clarity of vision. A change in lens prescription should wait several months of healing. Some patients who maintain the use of hard contact lenses may discover difficulty in removing the lens. The lens issuer can provide a small suction cup device specifically designed to assist removal. The problem should be anticipated prior to the surgery.

Recurrence of Dormant Inflammatory Lesions of the Upper Lid

Long-dormant chalazions can be reactivated in the first few weeks following surgery. A preoperative questionnaire is helpful in alerting the surgeon to anticipate this problem. This relatively painless swelling of the upper lid results from the obstruction of the opening of a meibomian gland. The swelling is localized between the upper lid margin and the incision. The problem is not an infection, but an inflammation related to the inspissated accumulation of glandular secretion. Surgery is not indicated. The problem responds to warm compresses and possibly prophylactic antibiotics.

Hyposensitivity of the Lids

The hyposensitivity of the upper lids may persist beyond the immediate postoperative period. It is most likely secondary to persistent mild lid edema. It always resolves.

Wound Problems at the Time of Suture Removal

The lateral extension of the upper lid incision may be subject to overlapping during the postoperative edema phase of healing. If this is found, the wound should be teased open and the wound resutured. If healing is allowed without addressing the overlap, an unattractive scar will result.

Changes in Texture and Appearance of Lower Lid Skin

Noticeable laxity, fine creping, and slight shine can be expected to persist in the lower lid skin for 10 days or more when postoperative edema is pronounced. This appearance can be most upsetting to the unprepared patient. Calm reassurance is helpful.

Persistent Sensation of Tightness

A sensation of tightness or resistance to opening or closing the eyes without any evidence of a functional problem may persist for several weeks. Explaining that this is a self-limiting condition will relieve anxiety.

Contact Dermatitis

Antibiotic ointments, especially those containing neomycin, are a common source of contact dermatitis. In patients not previously sensitized, a recurrence of lid edema associated with itching may develop after several days of ointment usage. It is common for patients to continue to use the ointment on the lids beyond the immediate postoperative period for which it was intended. Discontinuing the ointment and the use of cold compresses usually will reverse the problem. Oral corticosteroids are used for the most severe cases.

OTHER POSTOPERATIVE PROBLEMS

It is important that patients fully understand all of the problems that will or will not be resolved with blepharoplasty. Nonresolvable problems in the periorbital area are the most frequent source of alienation between the patient and surgeon. Although these problems are not seen as complications from the surgeon's viewpoint, they may be considered a complication by the patient.

Malar Bags

The persistence of malar bags probably evokes the most persistent postoperative complaints. Uninformed patients always expect their removal as part of blepharoplasty or find their relatively increased prominence following removal of lid fat intolerable. The malar bag is always seen as a stigma of aging and the patient is not easily swayed from this conclusion. Preoperative discussion of the problem is obviously imperative.

Animated Lateral Wrinkling

Lateral temporal and upper malar wrinkling that occurs when the patient smiles is not changed by blepharoplasty. It may become relatively more conspicuous. The patient may have not had a preoperative awareness of the problem or may be disappointed that the blepharoplasty did not eradicate them. The patient will hold a mock smiling appearance to demonstrate to the surgeon how unhappy he or she is with the results of the procedure. This condition must be evaluated and carefully discussed with the patient before surgery. Botox treatment following the surgery will definitely help the appearance.

Other preoperative sources of postoperative dissatisfaction are persistent fine wrinkling, asymmetrical palpebral fissures, asymmetrical brow position, persistent scleral show, and persistent lid pigmentation.

AESTHETIC PROBLEMS FOLLOWING BLEPHAROPLASTY

Persistence of Fat Pseudohernias

Persistent fat pseudohernias most commonly occur in the lateral compartment. The compartment should be evaluated preoperatively with the patient in extreme superolateral gaze to determine the extent of the fat problem. This fat compartment can be elusive. The author always deals with this compartment first and goes back at the

conclusion of the procedure to check that more fat is not present. Additional fat can be removed after a minimum of 3 months of postoperative healing. It can be removed via a transconjunctival approach or via a subciliary approach. The thickness of scar tissue in the area and the thickness of orbicularis muscle make the dissection deceptively deep to remove the redundant fat.

Persistent fat in the medial and the central compartments of the lower lid can usually be removed via a transconjunctival approach.

Persistence of fat in the medial upper lid is also common when there is an extraordinary amount of fat preoperatively. The fat is removed via an incision in the upper medial lid incorporating the original scar. Again, subcutaneous scar tissue may make the excision more difficult than the surgeon anticipates from the appearance of the problem. Additional skin is excised only if there is overlap of the skin edges following removal of the fat.

Persistence of Redundant Skin in the Lower Lid

The surgeon with limited experience should view this problem not as a complication but as an acceptable conservative consequence and an easily corrected alternative to a complication. It is difficult for even the most experienced surgeon to attain consistent perfection in the amount of skin removal. The surgeon should acknowledge the problem when the patient inquires. Denying or minimizing the significance of the redundancy could be particularly upsetting to the patient in the short-term postoperative period. Once the patient hears that the redundancy is a minimal problem to "fine tune" once healing has occurred, anxiety abates. The skin excess can be dealt with by skin flap or minimal skin-muscle flap excision.

Persistent Redundant Skin of the Upper Lid

Most cases of minimal upper lid skin persistency are secondary to a miscalculation of the brow position while the patient was supine. The upward displacement of the brow gives an erroneous measure of the amount of upper lid that will require removal. This is especially true of the lateral brow and skin. Persistent medial skin is more common in the aged eye. The apparent skin excess seen in the patient following secondary upper lid blepharoplasty is noted only with eyes open. The patient and surgeon may estimate the excess at 2 to 3 mm. However, with eyes closed there is no excess and no skin can be grasped with a forceps. These patients should not have additional skin removed. It will lead to a lagophthalmos and may cause the brows to descend.

Prominent Orbicularis Ridge Beneath the Lower Lid Incision

This problem results when the preseptal orbicularis muscle in the skin-muscle flap is elevated and overlaps the pretarsal muscle. At the time of wound closure this muscle overlap and consequent ridging should be obvious and its presence anticipated. This problem can be addressed following complete healing of the wound. A small skin flap is elevated, the muscle is excised, homeostasis is established, and the wound closed.

Scar Problems

Asymmetrical scars of the upper lid can be avoided if the lid skin is marked under magnification with a very fine pen. A wide pen mark can lead to a difference of 2 mm between eyes in the final scar. It is important to remember that the lower limb of the upper lid incision will always elevate as the wound is closed. Also, if the natural lid crease is at different positions when comparing the two lids an adjustment must be made to bring the two upper lid scars into symmetry.

Webbed Scars

A webbed scar can result from carrying the medial upper lid incision beyond the medial canthal sulcus and onto the nasal skin. Healing of this scar will elevate into a web. By using the web as the central limb of a Z-plasty, the problem can be eliminated.

Vertical Scars in the Lateral Lower Lid

Early texts on blepharoplasty advocated a subciliary incision ending with an incision angled downward at the canthus that allowed for the lid skin to be pulled laterally. The skin laterally was excised as a Burrow's triangle. This always resulted in an obvious scar, which is almost impossible to camouflage. This technique is not advised. The lower lid incision should always be horizontal. The direction of lid pull should always be vertical.

Scars in Mid Upper and Lower Lid

Scars in this area usually result from overlapping the skin edges or wound separation during the initial healing stage. The wound edges should be adjusted at the time of suture removal and resutured.

Suture Marks

Suture marks occur when undue tension is placed on the wound edges or when the sutures are allowed to remain long enough to produce inflammation at the suture placement sites. Monofilament sutures always cause less inflammation than braided or absorbable sutures. Removal of sutures by the third or fourth day is essential in preventing suture marks.

Suture Tunnels and Incisional Milia

The use of any braided suture material encourages epithelial growth along the path of the suture. The resultant tunnel will trap epithelial debris. The solution is to connect the two openings with a tiny blade incision. Milia or small sebaceous cysts may result from blockage of many eyelid sebaceous gland ducts along the suture line or trapping of epithelial debris in the wound. Milia appear as extremely superficial white skin inclusions; sebaceous cysts are deeper. Either is easily resolved by a minute pointed blade incision and expression of the sebaceous material.

PROBLEMS OF LOWER LID POSITION

Scleral Show

Ideally, the lower lid margin contacts the corneal limbus. Postoperatively the lid margin may be displaced 1 mm inferiorly following conservative skin-muscle excision. It can be seen following a skin-muscle blepharoplasty in which no skin was removed, even when the preoperative muscle tone was normal. This minimal scleral show or almost scleral show is an equivocal complication, especially since it is frequently seen as a normal variant. Usually, this minute scleral show is considered as complementary to the "wide-eyed" or "bright-eyed" youthful appearance following blepharoplasty. The surgeon may notice the minimal displacement of the lid, but is wise to allow the patient to initiate and reference to it.

Moderate Scleral Show, Inferior Rotation of the Lid Margin, and Ectropion

These complications may result from unrecognized lid laxity preoperatively, excessive removal of lid skin, or both. Indication for surgical intervention to reverse a minimal scleral show is determined by the patient's perception of the problem. An optimistic approach to some resolution of the problem over time is warranted. Upward massage and closed-eye squints (to strengthen the orbicularis) will produce some reversal of minor lower lid displacement. If the visible sclera remains a focus of dissatisfaction over a period of months, an additional procedure, such as lateral orbicularis muscle suspension following minimal elevation of skin and muscle, usually produces a satisfactory elevation of the lid margin.

Moderate to severe scleral show, lateral lower lid rotation (hound dogging), or ectropion following blepharoplasty will require either horizontal lid shortening alone when the complication is related solely to poor lid tension or a horizontal lid shortening in combination with skin grafting (and possible mucosal grafting) when the skin deficit has caused a vertical shortening and tethering of the lid. Certainly, prevention by careful preoperative assessment and conservative surgery is preferable to producing these complications.

PROBLEMS OF UPPER LID POSITION

Blepharoptosis

Postoperative lid ptosis either existed preoperatively and was not recognized or is secondary to some interference with the levator mechanism. The levator can be injured if the fat dissection is carried deep in the central compartment or laterally where it becomes more superficial and divides the lacrimal gland. Mild ptosis can persist for several months following a blepharoplasty procedure that includes fixing the lid skin to the levator just above the tarsal border (supratarsal fixation). This procedure has been fostered as a way to obtain a deep upper lid sulcus but is not recommended by the authors.

Correction of a persistent ptosis should await resolution of the healing process following blepharoplasty.

Lagophthalmos

The inability to completely close the palpebral fissure following blepharoplasty is usually temporary. With normal lacrimal function and a normal Bell's phenomenon, it is usually noticed when the patient sleeps and causes no discomfort. It also may be seen as a slight tethering when the patient's head is back and looking downward. This minimal lagophthalmos is most commonly seen following secondary or tertiary blepharoplasty or when a primary blepharoplasty is done in conjunction with a browlift or foreheadlift. The constant tendency for the upper lid skin to stretch as an accommodation to tension usually prevents functional problems following generous excisions of upper lid skin. However, there are limits to the ability of the upper lid to accommodate. The cases most prone to functional lagophthalmos problems are aggressive secondary or tertiary blepharoplasty, aggressive forehead-brow elevation in conjunction with upper lid blepharoplasty, and cases in which an earlier eyelid trauma had produced a lagophthalmos but went undetected before surgery.

At the completion of the upper lid wound closure in primary blepharoplasty it is common to see a palpebral fissure separation of up to 4 mm. Much of this observation is due to activity of the levator while the orbicularis is anesthetized. If the palpebral fissure separation is 5 to 6 mm, the possibility of lagophthalmos is real. Overestimation of skin excision can occur when the thin lid marking is spread widely during four-point skin fixation at the time of the skin incision. It is not difficult to replace a strip of upper lid skin if over-resection is suspected at the conclusion of the procedure. A strip of replaced skin will be totally viable without the need for a pressure bandage. The replaced skin will be totally unnoticeable in several weeks.

HEMATOMA OF THE LIDS

Careful homeostasis at every point of the blepharoplasty procedure has been persistently emphasized in this chapter. Development of a hematoma in the immediate postoperative period requires reopening the wound and establishing homeostasis. In the first few hours following surgery, hematoma must be differentiated from edema and ecchymosis. These problems usually involve the lower lid. Progressive enlargement, elevation of the lower lid

margin, a deep purple discoloration, and firmness to touch are indications of the need for prompt exploration. When the bleeding involves a vessel associated with fat resection the vessel can be hard to find because of extravasation and the fat stump retracting back into the orbit. The time to control these vessels is at the moment any bleeding is detected following release of the fat stump. Slow development of ecchymosis and a pitting edema just above the orbital rim is more likely edema than a hematoma. Pitting edema is unlike the tense fullness found with hematomas. This ecchymosis and edema can be treated expectantly.

Lid hematoma discovered after the immediate postoperative period should be allowed to liquefy (7 to 9 days) and be removed by needle aspiration and gentle pressure expression. This may require several daily visits for repeated treatments. Failure to remove the clot will result in a firm nodular scar that may persist for many months.

OVERCORRECTION OF FAT POCKETS

Excessive removal of fat from the lower lid can give a cadaveric appearance as the concave effect of the lower lid brings the bony rim into relief. In this chapter, the authors have addressed repositioning of the medial fat in those patients in whom a tear-trough deformity exists medially. Certainly, in these cases, fat removal will worsen the appearance. In the central and lateral lid the fat removal is carefully executed so that the level is no more than 1 mm below the bony margin. In the upright position this will translate to a smooth transition between the bony rim and the remaining central and lateral orbital fat.

If over-resection of fat is recognized intraoperatively, orbital fat can be replaced in small amounts as needed. These grafts of orbital fat have a high success rate. If the over-resection is noted in the postoperative period, injected fat from donor submental or abdominal regions may be used in small amounts to elevate the depressed area. Some experience is needed to produce a perfect result. Fat injected in this area can move to an adjacent area of the lid.

FUNCTIONAL PROBLEMS ASSOCIATED WITH BLEPHAROPLASTY

Dry Eye Syndrome

Dry eye syndrome is the most common functional problem following blepharoplasty. In most cases this is related to exposure of the cornea in patients with a subclinical dry eye syndrome. In patients with minimal dry eye problems that have only a functional and no anatomic component preoperatively, a perfectly performed blepharoplasty should have little negative effect on increasing the problem. But the surgeon can never know if the dry eye syndrome might progress coincidentally with the blepharoplasty. In patients with an anatomic cause for the dry eye syndrome, if the anatomic component can be corrected with the blepharoplasty, they may experience an improved quality of life. If the anatomic cause of the dry eye syndrome were worsened, then the dry eye syndrome would become more severe. In these patients, the easiest solution is not to operate. If the patient is accepted as a surgical candidate, the most conservative approach and procedure is indicated. Patients with certain systemic diseases are known to be prone to postoperative blepharoplasty dry eye syndrome; these diseases include systemic lupus erythematosus, scleroderma, Wegener's granulomatosis, ocular pemphigoid, Stevens-Johnson syndrome, ocular rosacea associated with acne rosacea, and paresis or paralysis of the seventh cranial nerve.

A history of any ocular symptom of itching, foreign body sensation, burning, or mucoid secretion should alert the examiner to a potential problem. Surgery in these patients is performed only after ophthalmologic consultation.

Once a patient presents with dry eye syndrome following blepharoplasty the use of artificial tears, nocturnal lubricants, and lid taping to ensure corneal protection and the participation of an interested ophthalmologic colleague are all necessary over an extended period.

Epiphora

Tearing following blepharoplasty is common in the immediate postoperative course. Persistence of tearing may indicate interference with the lacrimal canaliculi by mechanical obstruction, distortion secondary to lateral tension, or external rotation of the puncta out of the normal tear collection pathway.

Examination of the outflow tract by an ophthalmologist experienced in this testing may be necessary to evaluate obstruction and to assure an anxious patient that there has been no injury to the duct system.

Surgery on the lacrimal system for epiphora should follow only after 6 months of hopeful spontaneous resolution.

ORBITAL HEMATOMA

In addition to the cessation of medication known to cause operative bleeding, preoperative laboratory evaluation is indicated with any history of easy bruising, previous surgical bleeding, or a suspicious family history.

Intraoperative orbital bleeding is rare during blepharoplasty. The method of lid anesthesia advised in this chapter specifically avoids penetration of the orbital septum with a needle to prevent intraorbital vessel injury. Cautious intraoperative attention to homeostasis, especially when fat is being excised, has been stressed.

Any recurrence of bleeding following cautery homeostasis requires immediate attention before visualization of the bleeding vessel is obscured by extravasation.

Orbital hematoma in the immediate postoperative period is also a rare complication. The sudden intense pain associated with lid swelling and proptosis is a surgical emergency. Bleeding is usually arterial and associated with lower lid blepharoplasty. Increasing pressure within the orbit can damage the optic nerve and lead to blindness. Any sudden increase in pain in the immediate postoperative period must call attention to the possibility of orbital hematoma. The wound should be opened, clots expressed, and the vessel controlled. If the orbital pressure causes any decrease in vision or if the intraocular pressure approaches 80 mm Hg, a lateral canthotomy and inferior cantholysis should be performed. These procedures release the diaphragmatic confining effect of the orbital septum and inferior lateral canthal tendon and thus decompress the orbit, relieving pressure on the central retinal artery and optic nerve. The wound should be left open and small drains should remain in place for 24 to 48 hours.

DIPLOPIA

The extraocular muscles are always at risk in blepharoplasty. The superior oblique, inferior oblique, and the medial rectus muscles can be damaged if medial compartment fat is clamped without first specifically observing that the fat is free of any muscle. Extraocular muscles may be traumatized by cautery, by blind clamping for homeostasis, or during direct cautery dissection of fat. Fortunately, most visual disturbances from muscle imbalances secondary to surgical trauma show progressive improvement with eventual return to normal. Secondary surgery to restore continuity of transected muscle or balance by muscle resection may be required when the injury is severe, but usually such surgery is recommended only after several months of observation.

BLINDNESS

Blindness following blepharoplasty is an extremely rare occurrence. In most cases other than orbital hematoma, there has been no specific causal relationship between the blepharoplasty and the loss of vision. The suspected cause of the blindness—toxic amblyopia, idiopathic optic nerve atrophy, retrobulbar optic neuritis, or optic nerve changes secondary to systemic disease—seems beyond preventability. Still, the possibility of blindness following blepharoplasty does exist. To the author's knowledge, all reported cases thus far have followed surgery on the lower lids, and all have been unilateral. The moral issue of performing blepharoplasty on a patient with one seeing eye must be resolved by the individual surgeon and the patient's informed consent.

Future Considerations

Though the current surgical treatment of eyelid to reverse the effects of aging and correct the effects of heredity will continue to be important in the future, newer procedures may be expected to either augment or replace what we now see as state of the art. Many modalities may augment or even replace surgical treatment of the aging eyelid. Many light therapies of various wavelengths have been available in the recent past, and the progress in this area of medical skin rejuvenation has been most remarkable. A steady progression of lasers has proved effective in the treatment of the eyelids. Intensive pulsed light, intensive fluorescent pulsed light, LED (light-emitting diode) therapy, and photodynamic therapies all have had some recent profound effect on eyelid skin. Newer variations and advances are inevitable. Treatment for collagen induction by surgical needling, radiofrequency treatment, and fine point laser penetration for collagen stimulation all have had some positive effect on the eyelid skin. The future for this type of treatment looks very positive. The rapid development of dermatologic treatment by topical application will undoubtedly continue to be of great value in the treatment of the aging eye. There is no limit to the possibilities. There exists the possible breakthrough in gene therapy or hormonal therapy that may applicable in this area of interest. The progressive surgeon must be acutely aware of all that is new in this area of expertise, but also must be aware of which new modalities and products are of proven use and which are being popularized by medical suppliers and manufacturers creating public interest in the media before the modalities are clinically validated.

SUGGESTED READING

1. Baker SR: Orbital fat preservation in lower lid blepharoplasty. Arch Facial Plast Surg 1999;1:33-37.
2. Castanares S: Blepharoplasty for herniated infraorbital fat: Anatomical basis for a new approach. Plast Reconstr Surg 1951;8:46.
3. Castanares S: Anatomy for a blepharoplasty. Plast Reconstr Surg 1974;53:587.
4. Fagien S: Reducing the incidence of dry eye symptoms after blepharoplasty. Aesthet Surg J 2004;24:464-468.
5. Honrado CP, Pastorek N: Longterm results of lower-lid suspension blepharoplasty: A 30-year experience. Arch Facial Plast Surg 2004;6:150-154.
6. Katzen LB: The history of cosmetic blepharoplasty. Adv Ophthal Reconstr Surg 1986;5:89-96.
7. Jelks GW, Jelks EB: Preoperative evaluation of the blepharoplasty patient: Bypassing the pitfalls. Clin Plastic Surg 1993;20:213-223.
8. McCord CD, Boswell CB, Hest TR: Lateral canthal tightening. Plast Reconstr Surg 2003;112:222-237.
9. Pastorek N: Upper lid blepharoplasty. Facial Plast Surg 1996;12:157-169.
10. Patipa M: The evaluation and management of lower eyelid retraction following cosmetic surgery. Plast Reconstr Surg 2000;106:438-453 (discussion, 454-459).
11. Zide BM, Jelks GW: Surgical Anatomy of the Orbit. New York: Raven Press, 1985.

CHAPTER SIX

Transconjunctival Lower Blepharoplasty

Harry Marshak, MD • *Steven C. Dresner, MD*

HISTORY

Even though the history of upper eyelid cosmetic blepharoplasty dates back 2000 years, cosmetic blepharoplasty of the lower eyelids was not described until the early 20th century.[1] Julian Bourguet first described the transconjunctival approach to excising herniated orbital fat from the lower eyelid in 1924.[2] Castanares made significant contributions to the field by describing the fat compartments of the upper and lower eyelids.[3] In 1960, Reidy described the skin-muscle flap approach, which became the accepted lower blepharoplasty technique for over 20 years.[4] Although it still is one of the most commonly performed techniques, the skin-muscle flap procedure has a high rate of postoperative complications such as lid retraction and ectropion.[5] During the 1970s, Parkes described the pinch technique for the treatment of excess skin of the eyelid.[6] He advocated excising excess fat, when indicated, from an anterior approach, after the pinch of skin was removed. In 1978, Furnas described the use of the skin-muscle flap for lower eyelid festoons.[7] In the 1980s, Tenzel and McCord described performing lateral eyelid tightening procedures at the time of lower lid blepharoplasty in patients with preoperative eyelid laxity.[8,9]

The transconjunctival blepharoplasty (TCB) became popular and accepted when Baylis reintroduced the technique in 1989 as a safe lower blepharoplasty approach with minimal risk and complications.[10] He advocated the use of the pinch skin excision technique in conjunction with TCB, when indicated. In 1992, Hamra repopularized the skin-muscle flap approach.[11] The TCB, however, continues to be the preferred lower blepharoplasty technique for most ophthalmic plastic surgeons and many plastic surgeons owing to its reduced incidence of complications.

PERSONAL PHILOSOPHY

There are many advantages of TCB over traditional subciliary skin-muscle flap blepharoplasty. It is the primary procedure we perform in our practice for fat prolapse in the lower eyelid. The transconjunctival approach avoids the need to incise the orbicularis oculi muscle or the orbital septum, thus dramatically reducing the risk of postoperative lid retraction and ectropion. By not cutting the muscle, there is also much less bleeding associated with the surgery. TCB also allows for a much shorter surgical time. This lower blepharoplasty technique, when performed properly, is quick, easy, and gives a natural, nonsurgical postoperative appearance.[12]

We believe that most lower blepharoplasty procedures could be performed with some variation of the TCB. The primary indication for TCB is blepharochalasis with prolapse of the orbital fat pads anteriorly, causing an unacceptable cosmetic appearance. This is generally secondary to atrophy or loss of elasticity of the orbital septum due to aging changes or chronic inflammation. Also, certain patients genetically have fat prolapse and will seek correction at a younger age.

A skin pinch blepharoplasty is performed in 50% of the patients when excess skin is noted following fat removal or at the preoperative examination. Failure to perform a skin pinch when indicated will lead to further pronouncement of the excess skin in the lower eyelid. Fat repositioning can be performed in conjunction with TCB in patients with significant tear-trough deformity. Lateral canthopexy is indicated in the presence of a moderate amount of laxity of the lower eyelid. Lateral canthoplasty is required when patients present with severe lower eyelid laxity or ectropion. Failure to address these conditions at the time of TCB can result in iatrogenic postoperative eyelid malposition.

Chemical peel or laser skin resurfacing can be performed at the same time as TCB, but it is not our preferred method. CO_2 laser blepharoplasty is more time consuming and has the potential risks of operating room fires and damage to the globe and surrounding structures. Furthermore, because some form of cautery is required on the field to control bleeding anyway, we find it easier to use cutting cautery for the entire procedure.

TCB is contraindicated in patients with "festoons" of the lower eyelid or individuals with midfacial ptosis from facial nerve paralysis. These patients are better treated with a traditional subciliary skin-muscle flap approach to the orbital fat, with excision of excess skin and muscle, along with canthoplasty to prevent eyelid retraction. They may also require midface elevation.

ANATOMY

The lower eyelid can be divided into an anterior, middle, and posterior lamella (Fig. 6-1). The anterior lamella consists of skin and orbicularis oculi muscle. The orbital septum comprises the middle lamella, while the posterior lamella consists of the tarsal plate, lower lid retractors, and conjunctiva. It is the tarsal plate that gives the eyelid its strength and structure. Its height is approximately 4 to 5 mm and its thickness is about 1 mm. The lower lid retractors, also known as the capsulopalpebral fascia, originate from the tendon of the inferior rectus muscle and insert on the inferior border of the tarsal plate. The orbital septum originates at the inferior orbital rim as the arcus marginalis and fuses with the capsulopalpebral fascia just before its insertion on the tarsus. The orbital septum serves as the anterior boundary for the orbital fat. It is the weakening of the septum with age or recurrent

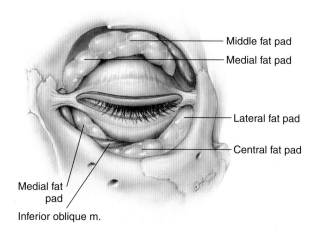

Middle fat pad
Medial fat pad
Lateral fat pad
Central fat pad
Medial fat pad
Inferior oblique m.

Figure 6-2 Preaponeurotic orbital fat pads. There are three fat pads in the lower eyelid: medial, central, and lateral. The medial and central pads are divided by the inferior oblique muscle. The central and lateral pads are divided by the inferior arcuate ligament. The inferior oblique muscle is almost always encountered as it divides the medial and central fat pads.

inflammation that allows for the anterior herniation of the orbital fat.[11,13]

There are three fat pads in the lower eyelid: medial, central, and lateral (Fig. 6-2). These fat pads are surrounded and divided by fine septae. The medial and central pads are divided by the inferior oblique muscle. The central and lateral pads are divided by the inferior arcuate ligament. The inferior oblique muscle originates from the inferior medial orbital wall and traverses through the lower eyelid to insert on the posterior lateral aspect of the globe. Its anterior course divides the medial and central fat pads of the lower eyelid. Extreme care must be taken to avoid damage to this muscle during blepharoplasty.

The caruncle is located next to the medial canthus and represents the transition zone between the nonkeratinized epithelium of the conjunctiva and the keratinized epithelium of the skin. Incision of the caruncle should be avoided during surgery because scarring in this area can occur and can be unsightly and uncomfortable for the patient. The canaliculus extends medially from the punctum and carries tears into the lacrimal sac. The vertical portion extends 2 mm inferior to the punctum. The horizontal portion then extends 8 mm medially to the lacrimal sac, running 1.5 to 2 mm inferior to the lid margin. It is critical not to cut the canaliculus during surgery as severe tearing problems will result. TCB incisions should never extend medial to the punctum.

PREOPERATIVE ANALYSIS

A complete history and physical examination are performed in the blepharoplasty consultation (see

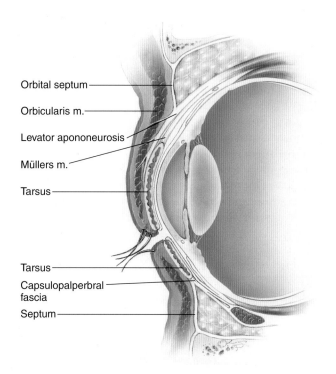

Orbital septum
Orbicularis m.
Levator apononeurosis
Müllers m.
Tarsus
Tarsus
Capsulopalperbral fascia
Septum

Figure 6-1 Eyelid cross-sectional anatomy. The lower eyelid can be divided into an anterior, middle, and posterior lamella. The anterior lamella consists of skin and orbicularis oculi muscle. The orbital septum forms the middle lamella and the posterior lamella consists of the tarsal plate, lower lid retractors, and conjunctiva. The lower lid retractors, also known as the capsulopalpebral fascia, originate from the tendon of the inferior rectus muscle and insert on the inferior border of the tarsal plate. The orbital septum originates at the inferior orbital rim as the arcus marginalis and fuses with the capsulopalpebral fascia just before its insertion on the tarsus

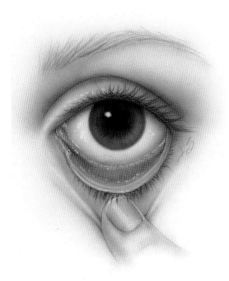

Figure 6-3 Snap test. The lower eyelid is pulled downward and outward. The rate of return of the eyelid is measured before the patient blinks. The lid laxity is directly related to the length of time it takes for the lower eyelid to return to its normal position. The patient has severe laxity if the lower eyelid does not return to normal position prior to the patient blinking.

Chapter 1). It is important to evaluate the degree of fat prolapse in each of the three fat compartments of the lower eyelid to determine a plan for appropriate surgical excision. The patient can be laid back in the examination chair, allowing gravity to retract the prolapsed fat pads posteriorly. The patient can be given a mirror to show how he or she might look if the fat pads are recontoured. An assessment should then be made as to the presence and degree of excess skin of the lower eyelid. This assessment is best performed with the patient looking up, to give the surgeon an idea of how much skin can be safely removed. A snap test is also performed to evaluate lid laxity (Fig. 6-3). The surgeon must determine all the pertinent preoperative factors that can lead to postoperative lower eyelid malposition at the time of the consultation.

With this information in hand, a surgical plan can then be created. This would entail one of the following: skin-muscle flap; TCB; TCB and skin pinch technique; TCB and canthopexy; or TCB and canthoplasty.

SURGICAL TECHNIQUE

TCB can be performed under local anesthesia, monitored anesthesia, or general anesthesia. The advent of laryngeal mask airway (LMA) has made general anesthesia much easier. The LMA avoids the need for endotracheal intubation and muscle relaxants. It can be used in conjunction with a propofol drip allowing for quick awakening and recovery after the procedure. We believe LMA in conjunction with a propofol drip provides the safest method of anesthesia in most patients because it allows the anesthesiologist to have control of the airway without the need for muscle paralysis as required with an endotracheal tube. Furthermore, because oxygen is being delivered to the patient through the LMA and not via mask or nasal cannula, the risk of operating room fire from electrocautery or laser is greatly reduced.

The preferred local anesthetic is 1% lidocaine with epinephrine mixed equally with 0.50% bupivacaine with epinephrine and a 1/10 mixture of hyaluronidase. The lidocaine and bupivacaine provide early and late local anesthesia. The epinephrine provides hemostasis. Hyaluronidase causes lysis of intercellular bonds, allowing for better dispersion of the injection. This reduces the amount of postinjection edema, allowing for better manipulation of the tissue during TCB and skin pinch procedures. Approximately 5 mL of the local anesthetic mixture is injected into each lower eyelid transconjunctivally via the eyelid fornix. Only one injection site is required. Gentle pressure is applied to facilitate spreading of the solution and to prevent hematoma formation.

The surgery starts with the retraction of the lower lid using a rubber-coated Desmarres retractor by the assistant (Figs. 6-4 and 6-5). The globe is protected and retracted posteriorly with the Jaeger lid plate. The coating of Desmarres and Jaeger lid plate prevent possible conduction of the electrocautery to the eyelid and globe. The conjunctiva and lower eyelid retractors are then incised 3 mm below the inferior border of the tarsal plate with a Colorado tip electrocautery, which provides precise cutting and coagulation. The incision should begin lateral to the level of the punctum and extend the full length of the lid.

The dissection is begun centrally, to avoid the inferior oblique muscle, and performed in layered fashion through the conjunctiva and lower eyelid retractors (Fig. 6-6). Care is taken to avoid cutting too deep until the inferior oblique muscle can be identified. A cotton-tip applicator is used to ballot the conjunctiva and lid retractors inferiorly and allow the fat pads to reposition anteriorly. During incision and dissection of the lower eyelid, care must be taken to avoid perforation of the skin anteriorly. Perforation usually occurs when the surgeon is unclear as to the level of dissection.

Once the fat pads are identified, gentle posterior pressure on the globe is applied to allow the fat pads to prolapse forward. Each fat pad is gently teased anteriorly with forceps. The base of the fat pad is cauterized to contract the fat posteriorly and to provide hemostasis. The amount of fat to be debulked is then excised with cutting cautery. Only a moderate amount of fat should be excised from each fat pad to prevent a skeletonized appearance of the orbit postoperatively. The excised segment of each fat pad is set aside so that an equal amount of fat can be taken from the corresponding area on the contralateral eyelid. If an asymmetry was noticed

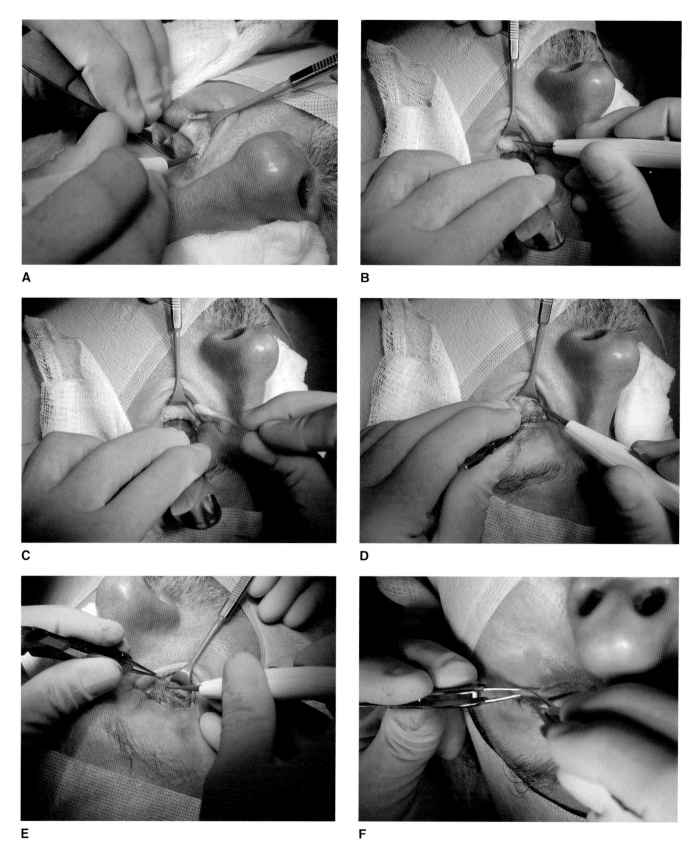

Figure 6-4 Intraoperative photos of transconjunctival lower blepharoplasty. The conjunctival fornix is exposed and the initial transconjunctival incision is made (**A**). The lid is retracted with a coated Desmarres retractor and the eye is protected with a lid plate. The incision is made with the Colorado tip bovie. The fat pad is exposed as the conjunctiva and lower lid retractors are incised (**B**). A cotton-tip applicator is used to ballot the tissue and expose the fat (**C**). The lateral, central and medial fat pads are exposed (**D**). The fat is excised with cutting electrocautery (**E**). Skin is grasped between two forceps during the pinch blepharoplasty (**F**).

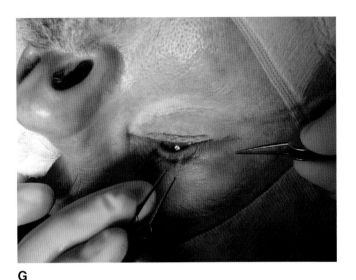

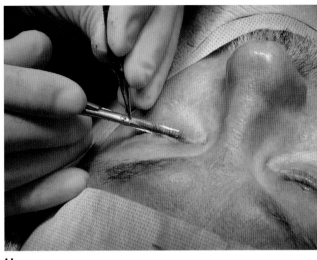

G   **H**

Figure 6-4 *Continued.* The skin stands up by itself after pinching (**G**). The skin is then excised with scissors (**H**).

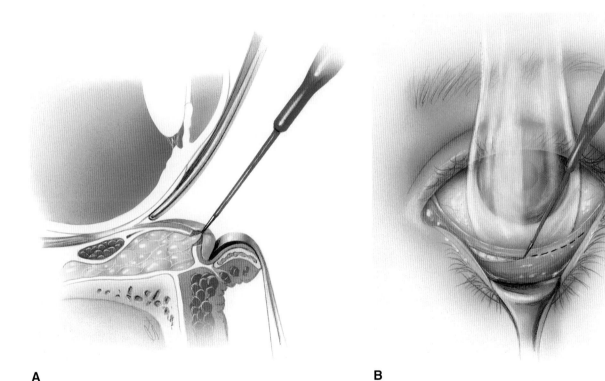

A   **B**

Figure 6-5 View of the transconjunctival incision. Desmarres and Jaeger lid retractors are used to expose the conjunctiva of the lower eyelid (**A** and **B**). The conjunctiva and lower eyelid retractors are then incised 3 mm inferior to the inferior border of the tarsal plate with Colorado tip electrocautery. The incision should begin lateral to the level of the punctum and extend the full length of the lid.

during the preoperative evaluation, a disproportionate amount of fat should be excised. At the end of the case, the conjunctiva and lower lid retractor flap is draped superiorly into its anatomic position, covering the wound. Suturing of the wound is not necessary.

Fat transposition can be performed in conjunction with TCB in patients with tear-trough deformity (Fig. 6-7). TCB is performed normally, with debulking of the central and lateral fat pads. A pocket is dissected at the medial orbital rim, either in the subperiosteal or suborbicularis plane. The medial fat pad is then placed into the pocket as a pedicle flap. It is positioned over the rim to correct the tear-trough deformity. Transcutaneous sutures are used to hold the pedicle in position.[14]

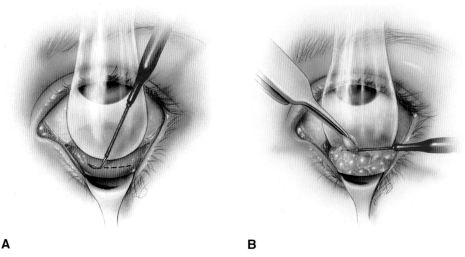

A   **B**

Figure 6-6 Lower eyelid dissection. The dissection is begun centrally, to avoid the inferior oblique muscle, and performed in layered fashion through the conjunctiva and lower eyelid retractors (**A**). A cotton-tip applicator is used to ballot the conjunctiva and lid retractors inferiorly and allow the fat pads to reposition anteriorly (**B**). Once the fat pads are identified, gentle posterior pressure on the globe with the Jaeger retractor is applied to allow the fat pads to prolapse forward. Each fat pad is gently teased anteriorly with forceps. Only a moderate amount of fat should be excised from each fat pad.

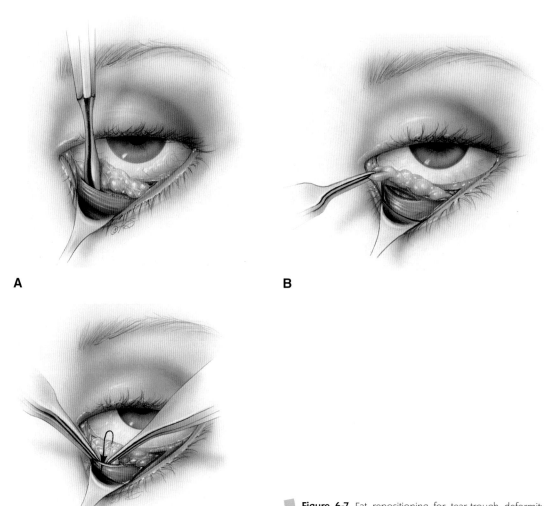

Figure 6-7 Fat repositioning for tear-trough deformity. Tear-trough deformity is an indentation in the nasojugal fold. This area can be partially improved with fat repositioning during the transconjunctival lower blepharoplasty. A pocket is dissected at the medial orbital rim, usually in the subperiosteal plane (**A**). The medial fat pad is then placed into the pocket over the orbital rim as a pedicled vascularized flap (**B** and **C**).

Lower lid pinch blepharoplasty is performed if excess skin is noted (Fig. 6-8). The anesthetic solution is injected subcutaneously along the subciliary line. The local anesthetic with hyaluronidase provides excellent hydrodissection of the skin from the underlying orbicularis muscle. The excess skin is then pinched upward along the subciliary plane with two forceps. The pinched skin is then excised with scissors. After hemostasis is obtained with cautery, the skin is closed with a 7-0 Prolene running suture.

When excess skin is noted in association with moderate lid laxity, a pinch blepharoplasty is combined with a lateral canthopexy (Fig. 6-9). After the pinched skin is excised, a button-hole is made in the orbicularis muscle at the lateral aspect of the wound to expose the lateral orbital rim. The retinaculum of the anterior crus of the lateral canthal tendon is identified. A 5-0 Vicryl suture on a P-2 needle is passed through the retinaculum and the periosteum of the lateral orbital rim. This suture is tied temporarily. The tightness and contour of the lower lid are examined. After the canthopexy is performed on the contralateral lid, the contours of both lower lids are compared for symmetry. The sutures are tied permanently. A 6-0 Vicryl suture is used to close the orbicularis. The skin is then closed with a 7-0 Prolene running suture. Figures 6-10 to 6-12 show results of patients who have undergone TCB.

POSTOPERATIVE CARE

Postoperatively, the patients are prescribed tobramycin eye drops, cephalexin, and analgesics. Head elevation and cold compresses are recommended for the first 72 hours, followed by warm compresses for the next 72 hours. Sutures, when present, are removed at 5 to 7 days after the surgery.

COMPLICATIONS

Postoperative hemorrhage is the most feared complication of blepharoplasty. Because the fat pads retract into the orbit, bleeding from the area can get trapped in the orbit. This can lead to retrobulbar hemorrhage and compression of the optic nerve. Meticulous hemostasis at the end of the procedure, with particular attention to the fat pads, is required to prevent this potentially sight threatening complication.

Because the lower lid retractors are incised at the beginning of the procedure and generally not sutured at the end, the potential for developing postoperative entropion exists. This can usually be prevented by ensuring that the conjunctival lid retractor flap is draped upward and left apposing the lower border of the tarsus at the end of the procedure. If postoperative entropion develops, it is treated with lateral canthoplasty. The lower lid retractors may need to be reattached to the inferior border of the tarsus if the entropion is severe.

Care must be taken not to cause a skeletonized appearance by excising an excessive amount of fat. Removing too little fat will also lead to patient dissatisfaction, especially in the lateral fat pad region. This is in contrast to the upper eyelid, where the most common cause of undercorrection is failure to locate and adequately excise the medial fat pad. To avoid this undercorrection, the trans-

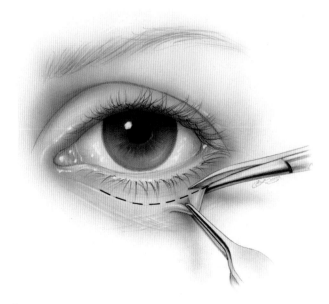

A

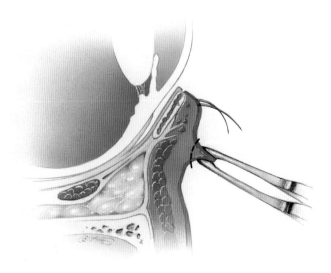

B

Figure 6-8 Lower eyelid pinch blepharoplasty. Excess skin is pinched upward along the subciliary plane with Brown-Adson and small forceps. The upper level of the incision is below the lash line. The pinched skin is excised with scissors.

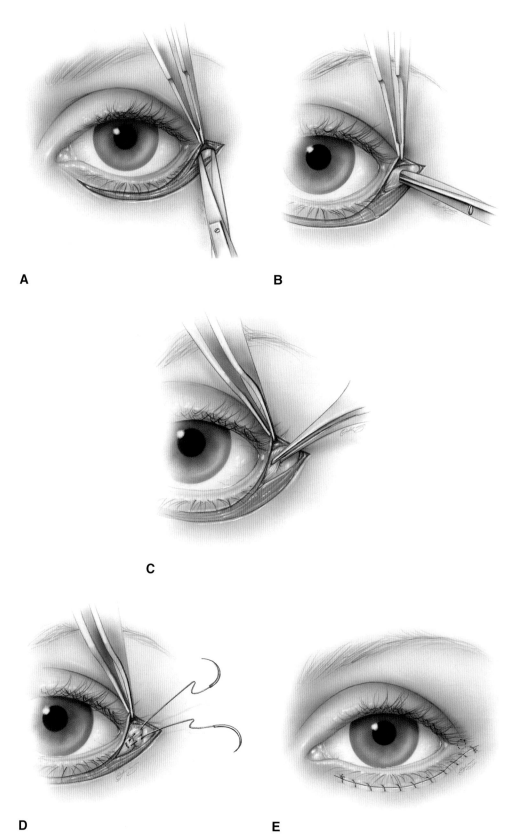

A

B

C

D

E

Figure 6-9 Lateral canthopexy. After the pinched skin is excised, a button-hole is made in the orbicularis muscle at the lateral aspect of the wound to expose the lateral orbital rim (**A**). The retinaculum of the anterior crus of the lateral canthal tendon is identified (**B** and **C**). A 5-0 Vicryl suture (P-2 needle) is passed through the retinaculum and the periosteum of the lateral orbital rim (**D**). This suture is tied temporarily while the tightness and contour of the lower lid is examined. The extended skin incision is then closed (**E**).

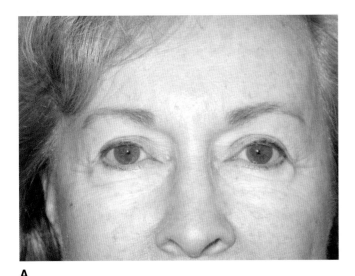

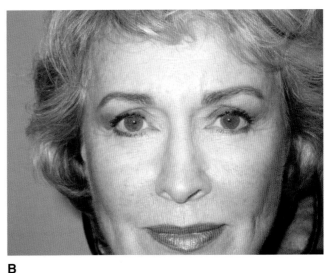

Figure 6-10 Preoperative (**A**) and postoperative (**B**) views of a 58-year-old woman with dermatochalasis who underwent transconjunctival lower blepharoplasty.

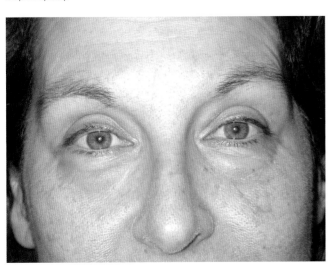

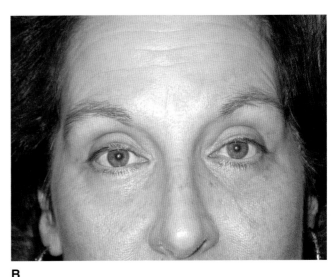

Figure 6-11 Preoperative (**A**) and postoperative (**B**) views of a 60-year-old woman with dermatochalasis and excess skin who underwent transconjunctival and pinch lower blepharoplasty.

conjunctival incision must be carried out lateral enough to identify the lateral fat pad. After excising a moderate amount of fat from the three pockets, the lower lid should be examined from the skin side to ensure that there are no bulges of fat remaining.

Damage to the inferior oblique muscle during the dissection will generally lead to postoperative diplopia. Mild trauma to the muscle often causes reversible symptoms, but transection of the muscle will lead to a permanent ocular motility disorder. The eye can sustain injury during any eyelid procedure, but transconjunctival surgery presents a larger risk. Trauma, including penetration, can occur from ill-placed cautery, sutures, or excessive pressure. Corneal abrasion can occur during any manipulation of the eye, especially from the lid plate.

Corneal abrasions are extremely painful and can lead to corneal ulcers. They must be treated with ophthalmic antibiotic drops or ointment. If they persist more than 24 hours, ophthalmologic consultation is recommended. Full-thickness globe penetration can occur from needles, sutures, or cautery. This is a sight-threatening condition that also requires immediate evaluation by an ophthalmologist.

The TCB must be performed in a precise manner. Several pitfalls can occur during the surgical dissection. An incision that is too low in the fornix will lead to poor wound closure and scarring of the inferior cul-de-sac. If the incision is extended too far medially and into the caruncle, scarring can lead to entropion. A common error involves carrying the dissection into the deep posterior plane. A deep dissection can lead to retained anterior fat

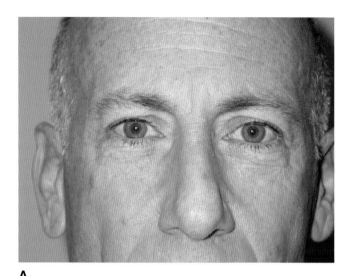

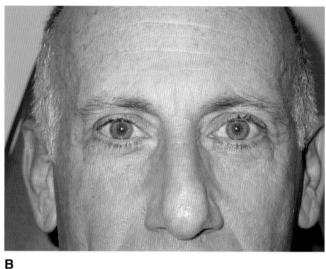

A

B

Figure 6-12 Preoperative (**A**) and postoperative (**B**) views of a 53-year-old man with dermatochalasis, excess skin, and lower lid laxity who underwent lateral canthopexy, transconjunctival and pinch lower blepharoplasty.

pockets in addition to risking trauma to the globe, inferior oblique, and inferior rectus. Fat pads are in a sense pyramids, and therefore, dissection and excision of fat too close to the base of the pyramid may allow excess fat to remain at the apex of the pyramid.

Future Considerations

The trend for conservative lower eyelid rejuvenation will continue well into the future. TCB will continue to serve as the workhorse of lower eyelid surgery as patients and surgeons become more aware of poor aesthetic results and postblepharoplasty eyelid malposition. The role of midface rejuvenation and volume restoration will also continue to gain acceptance as important adjunctive procedure to enhance the overall results of lower blepharoplasty. Noninvasive procedures may some day replace the need for lower eyelid skin excision as newer technologies provide safer results in all skin types.

REFERENCES

1. Katzen LB: The history of cosmetic blepharoplasty. Adv Ophthalmic Plast Reconstr Surg 1986;5:89.
2. Bourguet J: Les hernies graisseuses de l'orbite. Notre treitement chirugical. Bull Acad Med (Paris) 1924;92 (3 ser):1270.
3. Castanares S: Blepharoplasty for herniated intraorbital fat; anatomical basis for a new approach. Plast Reconstr Surg 1951; 8(1):46.
4. Reidy JP: Swellings of eyelids. Br J Plast Surg 1960;13:256.
5. Edgerton MT Jr: Causes and prevention of lower lid ectropion following blepharoplasty. Plast Reconstr Surg 1972;49(4):367.
6. Parkes M, Fein W, Brennan HG: Pinch technique for repair of cosmetic eyelid deformities. Arch Ophthalmol 1973; 89(4):324.
7. Furnas DW: Festoons of orbicularis muscle as a cause of baggy eyelids. Plast Reconstr Surg 1978; 61(4):540.
8. Tenzel RR: Complications of blepharoplasty. Orbital hematoma, ectropion and scleral show. Clin Plast Surg 1981; 84(4):797–802.
9. McCord CD Jr, Shore JW: Avoidance of complications in lower lid blepharoplasty. Ophthalmology 1983;90(9):1039.
10. Baylis HI, Long JA, Groth MJ: Transconjunctival lower eyelid blepharoplasty. Technique and complications. Ophthalmology 1989;96(7):1027.
11. Hamra ST: Repositioning the orbicularis oculi muscle in the composite rhytidectomy. Plast Reconstr Surg 1992; 90(1):14.
12. Zarem HA, Resnick JL: Expanded applications for transconjunctival lower lid blepharoplasty. Plast Reconstr Surg 1999;103(3):1041.
13. Doxanas MT: Minimally invasive lower eyelid blepharoplasty. Ophthalmology 1994;101(8):1327.
14. Goldberg RA, Edelstein C, Balch K, et al: Fat repositioning in lower eyelid blepharoplasty. Semin Ophthalmol 1998;13(3):103.

CHAPTER SEVEN

Asian Blepharoplasty

Samuel M. Lam, MD • Young-Kyoon Kim, MD, PhD

Asian blepharoplasty represents a unique topic in aesthetic surgery. Successful surgery of the Asian upper eyelid mandates a thorough knowledge of the divergent anatomy, peculiar cultural predilections, aesthetic interests, and precise operative techniques. Failure to understand all of these important dimensions will undermine a surgical endeavor. This chapter will help instruct novices to experienced facial cosmetic surgeons on all of these fundamental considerations to ensure uniform, consistent surgeon and patient satisfaction. The discussion of operative technique focuses on the limited, or partial-incision, as well as the full-incision method of "double-eyelid" crease formation that has served as the major methods on which the authors have relied in several thousand clinical cases.

HISTORY

The first creation of a supratarsal crease can be traced back to the late 19th century, when a Japanese surgeon named Mikamo performed a suture-based procedure in three reported clinical cases.[1–3] Viewed within the cultural context of the Meiji restoration, Mikamo's seminal work may be deemed simply as an expression of westernization that was in vogue during that epoch of rapid assimilation of Western ideals. However, Mikamo's writings show that his aesthetic references were for the most part internally derived, that is, he claimed that 80% of the indigenous Japanese people already had a double eyelid crease naturally and that a single eyelid configuration imparted a "monotonous and impassive" countenance that ran counter to what "writers and painters have regarded as an indicator of beauty."[2,3] He also commented on the functional impairment that a single lid could impose by way of "narrowed vision."

After Mikamo, almost 30 years of silence passed before another Japanese surgeon documented his experience with the "double-eyelid" procedure. After World War II, a burgeoning interest in Asian eyelid surgery arose owing to the rise of intermarriage according to the Hawaiian surgeon Leabert Fernandez in 1959.[4] The Malayan surgeon Khoo Boo-Chai popularized the suture technique for Asian blepharoplasty in 1963 and claimed that the motivating factors for surgery included the desire for socioeconomic

advancement by emulating a Western societal norm, removing the stigma of distrustful-looking "beady" eyes, and enhancing the prospect for marriage.[5] Millard also pioneered techniques in Asian blepharoplasty, advocating orbital lipectomy to achieve the desired objective.[6] Since the 1980s, McCurdy has observed an undeniable trend away from true "westernization" procedures in which high Caucasian-looking folds and hollowed out eyelids from overzealous lipectomy have given way toward conservative, more natural-looking results that retain ethnicity.[7] Asian blepharoplasty remains the most popular cosmetic surgery for Asian patients today with a wide range of surgical options available to attain a supratarsal fold as well as to modulate related structures such as the epicanthus.

PERSONAL PHILOSOPHY

AESTHETICS AND CULTURAL CONSIDERATIONS

An ongoing debate that will not abate any time soon concerns whether Asian eyelid surgery constitutes a betrayal of native ethnicity in favor of Western ideals or in fact represents a simple expression of Asian beauty without external, Western references. Clearly, this chapter does not seek to answer this very difficult question definitively because the answer lies in subjectivity, bias, and opinion. Nevertheless, as stated, true "westernization" procedures that involved creation of a very high supratarsal crease and hollowed eye appearance that closely approximated a Western countenance have not been in vogue for the past decade or more. Today, Asians who live both abroad and in East Asia favor a natural-appearing crease and eyelid shape that matches that of their native peers and that can be found on their peers who never have had surgery (i.e., that occurs as a natural trait). However, the influence of Western media images and Caucasian beauty on Asians living in the Occident or Orient alike is undeniable. Globalization of a defined standard for beauty has emerged in which racial boundaries have been partly effaced by interracial marriage and increased use of non-Caucasian models.

Understanding the cultural biases that influence a decision for Asian eyelid surgery involves more than commentary about aesthetic ideals. Asians, particularly those who live abroad in Asia or who have recently emigrated to the West, often have very different, and what may be construed as peculiar, attitudes and motivating factors for cosmetic surgery that a Western surgeon should consider during the consultation process. For instance, beyond aesthetic interests, an Asian patient may be seeking a change in his or her fortune, as dictated by cultural folklore. A higher nose bridge, wider eyes, and longer ear lobes are all associated with bringing a person good luck and fortune. If the patient desires a cosmetic procedure to ward off evil spirits and gain fortune, the surgeon should be wary about pursuing surgery for the obvious reason that the patient may be quite unsatisfied afterward if the expected newfound luck does not materialize.

Further, in the postoperative setting, Asian patients can be highly critical of their cosmetic results and may be susceptible to judgmental and negative commentary of their family and friends regarding their decision to have cosmetic surgery or the outcome. A supportive and nurturing approach to the patient will help the surgeon to satisfy and to cope with the demanding nature of many Asian patients. Different ethnicities also tend to react differently postoperatively, with Koreans who fall on one extreme in their potential for vociferous and repeated chimes of dissatisfaction compared to the reticent Japanese who remain silent about what may trouble them and instead decide to voice their discontent to another surgical colleague. These broad generalizations are not intended to denigrate any particular ethnicity but to provide the Western surgeon unaccustomed to the behavior and biases of Asian patients a framework with which to address the patient in a constructive manner.[7]

TECHNIQUES FOR UPPER BLEPHAROPLASTY IN ASIANS

Many surgical techniques exist for management of the Asian upper eyelid, but for sake of academic clarity, they can be classified into three main headings: full-incision,[8] partial-incision,[9] and suture-based methods.[10] The variations and modifications of techniques for Asian blepharoplasty closely approximate the number of practitioners of the art, as every surgeon performs a slightly different technique based on experience and preference. Nevertheless, this proposed classification scheme provides an insightful method to view the unique advantages and disadvantages of each type of surgery so that the thoughtful surgeon can find his or her own chosen method or choose the right method for a particular patient.

The full-incision method provides the surgeon with the ability to remove redundant skin and excess muscle as well as fine tune the shape of the eyelid crease. Continuing the full incision into the epicanthal region (or making a separate incision in the epicanthus) permits modulation of

the epicanthus as part of the surgery. However, the full-incision method is more labor intensive and may require longer operative time. In addition, the chance for scarring, especially medially near the epicanthus where there is a biologic propensity toward cicatrix formation, is increased. The recovery period during which time the height and fullness of the created crease appears unnatural is also the longest of all three major methods and can last from several months to a full year. Revision surgery can be the most demanding, as exploration and correction at the level of the levator requires extreme care and attention to prevent complication arising from inadvertent levator injury. Despite these limitations, the full-incision method remains the most ideal for the more mature Asian patient who has concomitant dermatochalasis and who wants a double-eyelid created.

The suture-based method offers the benefits of quick operative as well as recovery time. The patient will most likely have a natural-looking lid-crease height in a matter of days to weeks instead of months. Also, the surgeon does not truly need to understand the intricacies of surgical anatomy, as the suture is simply passed through from skin to conjunctiva and back again. However, the suture method also does not permit any removal of fat, which can be problematic for two reasons. The fullness of the upper eyelid is not truly addressed, and the adipose tissue that becomes sandwiched between the levator and skin may serve as a barrier for permanent adhesion that would lead to early fold loss.[11] Owing to these limitations, the authors rarely rely on suture-based surgery, especially in the older patient who may require some skin removal along with double-eyelid creation.

The partial-incision method offers a balance between the full-incision and suture-based methods. Through a limited, 1.5-cm incision, the only adipose compartment that contributes significantly to eyelid fullness can be easily reduced and a significant levator-skin adhesion established. The shorter incision minimizes the risk of epicanthal webbing or scarring that may arise with the full-incision method. Further, the recovery time falls somewhat in between that of the suture-based and the full-incision methods: approximately 3 to 4 months until the lid-crease height should appear completely natural in most cases. The fact that no skin is removed also permits the overlying skin to redrape over the incision, thereby camouflaging it during the healing process. The authors argue that no skin needs to be removed (in the younger age group), as the aesthetic deficit of the creaseless Asian eyelid concerns the relatively low position of the central adipose tissue and the lack of a supratarsal crease, both conditions of which are addressed with the partial-incision method. Revision surgery for the patient with a partial incision is also considerably easier than with the full incision. However, the more abbreviated incision may be associated with a greater chance of eventual fold loss than the full-incision method; but measures can be taken to minimize this chance, as will be explained in the forthcoming section on surgical technique. The authors reserve the full-incision method for those individuals over 40 years of age whose dermatochalasis would justify some concomitant skin removal. If epicanthal advancement is favored, a separate, limited incision can also be made medially to address this area with the flexibility of undertaking the epicanthoplasty at the same setting as double-eyelid creation or at an earlier or later date given the fact that the two incisions remain separate and distinct.

TECHNIQUES FOR LOWER BLEPHAROPLASTY IN ASIANS

Blepharoplasty of the lower eyelid differs little from that of the Caucasian: a transcutaneous or transconjunctival approach may be used with good success. Accordingly, a detailed step-by-step description of lower-lid blepharoplasty will not be described in this chapter. A transconjunctival approach may be preferable in the Asian patient for several reasons. Lower-eyelid dermatochalasis is much less prevalent in the Asian patient; therefore, skin removal is often unnecessary. Even if removal of skin redundancy is required, a skin pinch technique can be safely combined with the transconjunctival method. Also, the predilection of the Asian skin toward hypertrophic scarring and prolonged erythema may make a transconjunctival approach better suited. Experience and judgment will be important when deciding which method to use. Lower-eyelid rhytidosis would typically be easily treated in the fairer skin of Caucasians with 35% trichloroacetic acid peel or ablative laser rejuvenation but should be cautiously approached in Asians owing to the risk of a protracted healing phase, including hyperpigmentation, hypopigmentation, prolonged erythema, and scarring.

SUMMARY OF APPROACH: EVALUATION OF THE YOUNGER VERSUS THE OLDER ASIAN PATIENT

For Asian upper blepharoplasty, the younger patient may be easily addressed with the partial-incision method. This relatively quick and straightforward method permits the surgeon to address the aesthetic concerns of the majority of younger patients. As the preponderance of double-eyelid blepharoplasty procedures are performed in the younger age group (teenage years through the 30s), the partial-incision technique has remained the principal method for Asian upper blepharoplasty in the authors' practices.

Conversely, older patients (late 30s and beyond) may have either already had a double eyelid created in the past or do not desire this alteration in their appearance. For older patients who request formation of a supratarsal crease, the surgeon must exercise judgment as to which method may be the most suitable for the patient. For early

brow descent/dermatochalasis, the partial incision may still be used but with the incision placed slightly higher to accommodate for the skin redundancy that will fall over the incision. Because patients beyond the teenage years and early 20s may not tolerate the lengthy time that the full-incision method will render their appearance unnatural, the partial-incision method may be favored for the shorter healing time.

For the more mature patient with greater brow descent/dermatochalasis, the full-incision method is preferred so that skin redundancy can be addressed at the same time. Preferably, a browlift should be performed first at a minimum of 6 weeks antecedent to the double-lid blepharoplasty, as almost every mature patient has some degree of brow descent that would warrant correction. However, many Asian patients may resist undergoing a staged procedure because of the lengthened recovery time, associated cost, and possible unfamiliarity with browlifting. If a browlift is declined, the surgeon should be careful not to remove so much upper-lid skin, as to exacerbate brow ptosis or prevent a future browlift. If an older patient requests upper facial rejuvenation and *would like to retain a single-eyelid configuration*, the surgeon can remove upper-eyelid skin by measuring an arbitrary height (e.g., 5 to 7 mm above the ciliary margin) on both upper eyelids using Castroviejo calipers. During the blepharoplasty, the surgeon should avoid entry into the postseptal fat in the central compartment, as fixation of the skin to the underlying structures arising from surgical dissection may result in unwanted crease formation. Medial fat removal alone, however, rarely leads to any measurable degree of crease fixation.

ANATOMY

The Asian upper eyelid has been characterized and caricatured as uniquely different from that of other races, specifically in the fullness of the lid appearance, absence of a discernible supratarsal crease, a narrowed palpebral fissure, webbing or downturn of a skinfold medially (known as the epicanthus), and superior obliquity of the eye at the lateral canthus. These characteristics are present to a large extent in the Asian races, but by no means should these anatomic traits be considered monolithically universal in scope. Subtle and distinct variations exist among the ethnic races (Koreans, Japanese, Chinese, etc.) and differ markedly even within a particular ethnicity. For instance, there is a higher observed frequency of a single eyelid configuration in the Korean race, whereas 70% of southern Chinese possess a well-delineated supratarsal fold. Overall, approximately 50% of East Asians have a single, noncreased eyelid.[12]

The classification of the Asian upper eyelid into creased and creaseless is not entirely accurate. In fact, three morphologies of the Asian upper eyelid are present:

a defined supratarsal crease, a low eyelid fold, and a complete absence of any fold (Figs. 7-1 and 7-2).[13] The type of eyelid crease is determined by the height at which the levator aponeurosis inserts into the dermis. Many investigative techniques—including magnetic resonance imaging (MRI), scanning electron micrography, cadaveric histologic analysis, and intraoperative surgical evaluation—have explored the anatomic nature of levator insertion in the Occidental versus the Oriental eyelid.[14-16] The levator has been found to insert into the dermis at variable distances above the ciliary margin (or not at all) in the Asian but overall at a lower height than in the Caucasian (Fig. 7-3). It has also been reported that the levator aponeurosis itself does not insert into the dermis, but instead fine fibrous septae that extend from the tarsus toward the dermis account for the formation of the palpebral fold.

The puffiness of the Asian upper eyelid has been attributed to an excess of preaponeurotic adipose tissue in the single-eyelid configuration. Alternatively, it has been proposed that the patient with a low or absent levator-to-

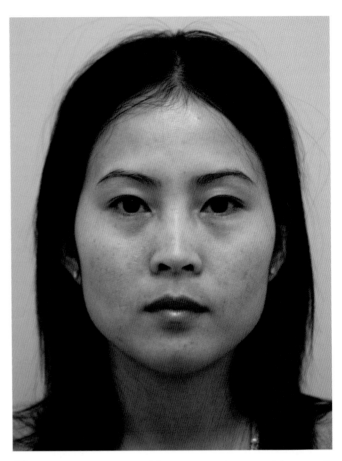

Figure 7-2 This 32-year-old Vietnamese woman exhibits a well-defined, but relatively low, supratarsal crease naturally. She did not have eyelid surgery.

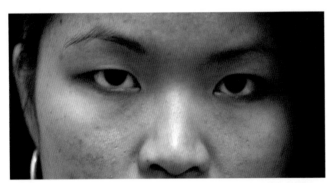

A

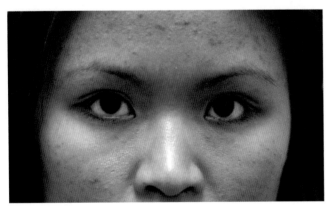

B

Figure 7-1 This 23-year-old Chinese woman exhibits a rudimentary supratarsal fold on her left side and an absence of a fold on her right side (**A**). As evident, her right eyelid is fuller and lower than the left, because the small, rudimentary left crease has retained her postseptal orbital fat in a relatively higher position on the left side. A partial-incision technique was performed at 8 mm above the ciliary margin to impart a more symmetrical and defined supratarsal crease bilaterally (**B**).

skin insertion also has a relatively low fusion of the orbital septum with the levator aponeurosis (the so-called septo-aponeurotic sling), allowing the fat to descend further downward and thereby yield a fuller eyelid appearance. Therefore, the Asian may in fact have the same amount of preaponeurotic adipose tissue but exhibit greater fullness only because of the relative lower descent of fat. Because Asians tend to have lower eyelid creases than their Western counterparts, even individuals with well-defined creases still may have some greater degree of fullness relative to Caucasians. Accordingly, this feature should be surgically preserved, as a hollowed eyelid looks particularly unnatural on an Asian compared with on a Caucasian. The unrestricted descent of preaponeurotic fat over the pretarsal region also contributes to a narrower palpebral fissure, which may yield a ptotic appearance of the upper eyelid (known as pseudoptosis orientalis).

The epicanthal fold that is present in 40% to 90% of Asians may further narrow the palpebral aperture. The epicanthal fold of skin curves downward along the medial extent of the eyelid and can partially or completely obscure the caruncle, or lacrimal lake. This anatomic feature has been attributed to the vertical shortage and

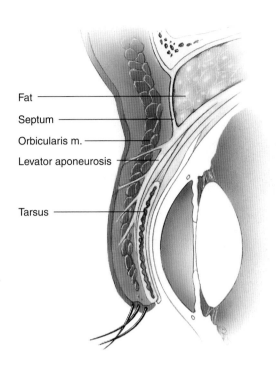

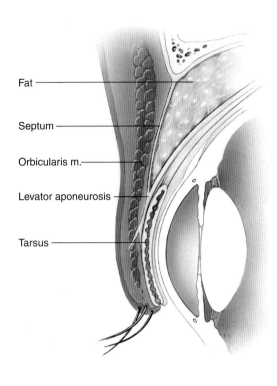

A

B

Figure 7-3 The levator inserts into the dermis, which accounts for the presence of a supratarsal fold in the Caucasian as well as some Asians (**A**). The levator does not insert into the dermis, which accounts for both the creaseless nature of the Asian eyelid as well as the puffiness due to the descent of orbital fat more inferiorly than in the Western eyelid (**B**).

horizontal redundancy of the skin–orbicularis oculi complex at the medial canthus. A broad and heavy epicanthal fold may render the eye smaller and the nose broader and flatter in appearance. Therefore, many surgical techniques have been introduced to alter the epicanthus. The position of the lateral canthus in the Asian has also been recognized to differ from that in the Caucasian in its relative superior location vis-à-vis that of the medial canthus, thus contributing to the observed "slant" of the eye.[17] Surgical alteration of this area is fraught with difficulty, including scarring, an unnatural appearance, and limited aesthetic improvement.

Although the focus of this chapter is almost entirely on the anatomy and surgery of the Asian upper eyelid, a few salient differences in the lower eyelid of the Asian patient should be mentioned for completeness. One cadaveric study found limited to no adhesion of the orbital septum and capsulopalpebral fascia at the lower border of the tarsal plate.[18] In a correlative study using MRI, the orbital fat in the Asian lower eyelid was found to extend further anteriorly with respect to the orbital rim.[19] Second, the orbital fat tended to extend more superiorly to the inferior border of the tarsus in those Asians who did not have a well-defined upper-eyelid crease. The suborbicularis oculi fat (SOOF), however, was found to be similar in both Asians and Caucasians.

Besides eyelid anatomy, the brow constitutes a central component for upper facial rejuvenation in the Asian patient. Brow anatomy in the Asian differs little from that of the Caucasian. Generally, Asians tend to exhibit a similar extent of brow descent as Caucasians and benefit significantly from brow rejuvenation. Conversely, Asians typically do not exhibit the same degree of lower facial aging as Caucasians and may not require any lower facial lifting procedure until they pass 60 years of age or older. Browlift techniques for the Asian patient are the same as for the Caucasian and lie beyond the scope of this chapter.

PREOPERATIVE ASSESSMENT

THE CONSULTATION

Before embarking on a careful physical examination, the surgeon should open the consultation session with a general inquiry as to the patient's motivations, aesthetic desires, fears, and other concerns. The salient points regarding aesthetic and cultural opinions reviewed previously should be kept in mind during the process.

Patients often bring in photographs of professional models to help educate the surgeon as to precisely how they would want to look. Although these photographs can be instructive, they also can be deceptive, especially if the patient is striving to look like the model rather than have only the model's specific eye shape. One author (SML) shows his patients selected model photographs with very different facial features but with the same type of lid-crease shape to help the patient understand the influence that surrounding facial features can have on the aesthetic judgment of the viewer regarding eye shape.

Perhaps the single most important factor in pre-operative planning involves achieving a mutual under-standing of desired lid-crease height. The easiest classification scheme would be to offer the patient a low (3 to 4 mm), medium (5 to 6 mm), or high crease (8 mm or higher). The majority of patients today desire a low crease height with a minority that express interest in a medium crease and very few who desire a high "westernized" crease. To provide the patient with a clear understanding of a desired lid-crease height, several methods can be used. As mentioned, photographs of models can enhance dialogue with the stated caveats recalled. Before-and-after photographs that represent different lid-crease heights can be used for effective communication and to provide concrete evidence of the surgeon's skills. Finally, placement of an open and rounded paper clip, or similar device, pressed into the patient's eyelid to simulate a created lid crease can show the patient in the mirror how a crease would look on his or her face. The patient should always be reminded that use of a paper clip never looks very natural and that the device serves only as an aesthetic guideline for the patient.

EYELID AND FACIAL AESTHETICS

After the patient and surgeon have established a preliminary dialogue about what concerns and desires the patient may have regarding the procedure, the surgeon can evaluate the precise dimensions of the patient's anatomy to determine what eyelid procedure(s) (e.g., partial- versus full-incision, epicanthoplasty, lateral canthoplasty) and related facial procedures (e.g., browlifting, lower-eyelid blepharoplasty, augmentation rhinoplasty) could enhance the result.

The fullness of the patient's eyelid due to adipose tissue should be carefully assessed. The main reason for preoperative analysis of the adipose fullness is to help guide the surgeon's decision concerning how high to place the incision. A patient with significant adipose tissue would require greater removal of fat, which would in turn allow the deflated skin postoperatively to redrape over the incision, as no skin is removed with the limited-incision technique, making the ultimate incision height slightly lower than perhaps originally conceived. Accordingly, the incision may be placed slightly higher (1 to 2 mm) to accommodate the greater skin redrapage that would lower the final postoperative height of the crease. Korean patients tend to exhibit a greater amount of overall adipose compared with other ethnic groups, such as Chinese or Vietnamese.

The greater amount of skin dermatochalasis and brow descent due to aging can make the partial-incision

technique less than ideal. The partial-incision method is particularly well suited for younger patients without evidence of eyelid aging for all the previously enumerated benefits. As mentioned, the full-incision method may be preferable for a more mature patient with evidence of periocular aging to address the dermatochalasis that may be present. However, the surgeon can still offer the patient the partial-incision method in cases of early derma-tochalasis by making the planned incision height again slightly higher to accommodate the excess skin that will redrape over the incision. Ideally, the aging eyelid/brow complex should be addressed in a staged fashion, with browlifting performed first to restore brow height followed by a partial- to full-incision eyelid rejuvenation at a minimum of 6 to 8 weeks after the procedure. The edema and sedation required for a browlift make concurrent double-eyelid blepharoplasty precarious, as the risk of asymmetry is amplified. Convincing Asian patients, especially those who live abroad in Asia or who have recently emigrated to the West, that a staged procedure would be the better solution is often difficult owing to the popularity of double-eyelid surgery alone without browlifting performed in Asia, lack of under-standing of the benefits of a combined procedure, and cost and time considerations. Based on the patient's anatomic findings and surgeon preference and judgment, the proper eyelid and browlift techniques can be determined. Clearly, in the aging Asian eyelid, the etiology of tissue ptosis must be well delineated—pseudoptosis orientalis (due to adipose fullness and a lack of a supratarsal crease), blepharoptosis (due to levator dysfunction that can often arise with age), and brow ptosis—to determine the best procedure(s) for the patient.

Epicanthal shape and extent should also be con-sidered in eyelid and facial analysis. A broad epicanthal web can render the overall eye aperture smaller in appearance and lead to an unbalanced appearance to the eye shape if a double-eyelid procedure is done in isolation, for the increased palpebral aperture that results from a double-eyelid procedure done without epicanthal modulation may render the eye shape overly vertical in dimension and the eye width appear narrower in a relative fashion. Epicanthal advancement can balance the shape and contour of the eyelid in such patients. Because the authors prefer a limited-incision epicanthoplasty, the epicanthal portion of a procedure can be done concur-rently or at a different time from double-eyelid formation. This flexibility permits patients the luxury of choosing to undergo a combined epicanthal advancement and double-eyelid creation or do so during separate sessions. Also, a strong epicanthal fold can make the eye shape appear too narrow when judged by ideal facial proportions: the eye width should be approximately one fifth the total horizontal distance of the face from ear to ear, or more simply, it should match the intercanthal distance. At times, to achieve this desired objective, not only must the epicanthal skin be advanced but the medial canthal ligament may require shortening as well. A broad epicanthal fold can also accentuate a very flat nasal dorsum. Concomitant augmentation rhinoplasty can help restore balance to the eye and nose region with or without epicanthoplasty. As mentioned before, lateral canthoplasty provides limited perceived aesthetic benefit and should only be considered when combined with an epicanthoplasty to attain sufficient opening of the eye aperture in a horizontal dimension.

SURGICAL TECHNIQUE

THE PARTIAL-INCISION METHOD

General Considerations

The first step in surgery is confirmation of the appropriate lid-crease height, especially if some time has elapsed between the initial consultation and procedure. In most circumstances, a crease measured at 8 mm above the ciliary margin will yield a low to medium crease, whereas a 10-mm marking will produce a medium to high crease. Some variability obviously exists, depending on the amount of adipose tissue the patient has—with a greater amount of adipose removal leading to a lower resulting crease— and the amount of extra skin redundancy, which is principally a factor of age, a greater amount of extra skin leading to a lower resulting crease as well. The patient should have the marking performed precisely with Castroviejo calipers and with the eyelid skin stretched taut *until incipient eyelash eversion is noted*. Generally speaking, a measured crease marking will result in a final crease-fold height of about half of the measured distance; thus, a crease marked at 8 mm will give the patient approximately a 4-mm crease height after all edema has resolved (typically 3 months postoperatively). The patient should clearly understand that the exact lid-crease height cannot be determined with absolute precision given the preceding inconsistent anatomic factors, such as the amount of lid skin redundancy and degree of adipose tissue. Of note, the patient should be shown the proposed marking in the seated position using the previously described paper clip, as the skin that folds back over will only do so in the upright posture and not while supine (Fig. 7-4). Also as an aside, the older patient (late 30s and beyond) who exhibits greater skin redundancy should either have a full-incision performed or have the lid crease marking raised to 10 to 12 mm in order to yield a lower final crease height, depending on the degree of brow ptosis and dermatochalasis present.

During the procedure, the patient should have minimal to no sedation because the patient's cooperation with eye opening and closing is a vital component to the success of the operation. The authors prefer no sedation for any phase of the procedure to ensure optimal patient

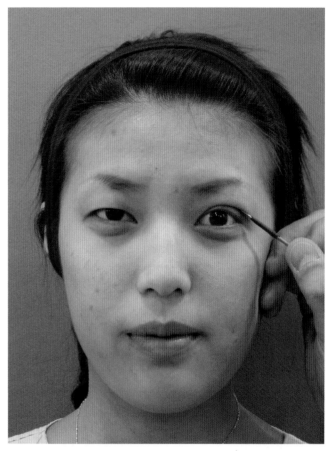

Figure 7-4 The patient shows the characteristic upper eyelid fullness and narrow palpebral aperture on the right side, and the proposed crease formation is shown by using a paper clip pressed into the left upper eyelid as an instructive tool. Given the patient's relatively young age, a partial-incision method has been selected for eyelid crease creation.

compliance. Because the infiltration of anesthesia is quite limited with the partial-incision method, patient discomfort is similarly kept to an acceptable minimum, as compared with the full-incision technique.

Operative Technique

After the patient has corroborated the proposed lid-crease height, the surgeon may begin the marking and execution phase of the procedure. The patient is placed in the supine position, and the surgeon is seated above the patient's head in the midline looking downward for the entire duration of the procedure. The Castroviejo calipers, or a similar measuring device, are used to mark the crease height at the midpupil on each side while the patient's skin is stretched until incipient eyelash eversion (Fig. 7-5). A very fine-tipped, gentian violet surgical marking pen or, alternatively, a fine toothpick dipped in gentian violet should be used for all lid markings. A standard gentian violet marking pen has too broad a nib that leads to imprecision in crease marking and thereby commensurate imprecision when making the incision.

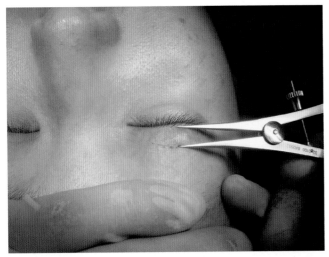

Figure 7-5 The nondominant hand stretches the upper eyelid skin until the eyelashes evert to a perpendicular orientation to the skin. A gentian violet marking pen is then used to indicate a point at this height at the midpupil.

The proposed marking is extended for a total length of 1.5 cm on each eyelid with the medial extent starting approximately at the medial limbus (Figs. 7-5 and 7-6). The Castroviejo calipers should be used to confirm symmetry in three respects: (1) uniform height of the lid crease from the ciliary margin along the entire length, (2) same length of incision (1.5 cm) for both eyelids, and (3) same distance from the medial canthus to the medial limbus, the latter of which again represents the medial extent of the incision line.

When both markings are deemed acceptable (Fig. 7-7), the surgeon may proceed with the infiltration of local anesthesia; 2% lidocaine mixed with 1:50,000 epinephrine is preferred, and a 1-mL syringe outfitted with a 30-gauge needle is used for delivery. The needle is carefully placed in the midline of each marking and

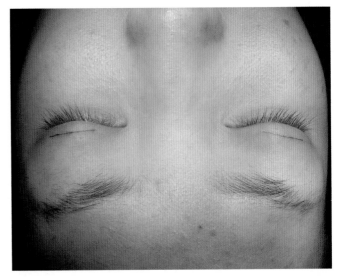

A

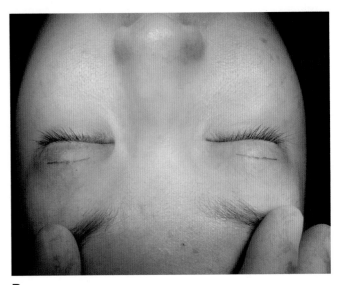

B

Figure 7-7 These photographs show symmetrical markings completed that conform to the specifications outlined in Figure 7-6 with the skin unstretched (**A**) and stretched (**B**).

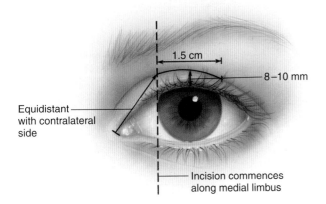

Figure 7-6 This schematic illustration shows the recommended length (1.5 cm) and location (starting at the medial limbus medially and extending laterally from there) of the incision used for the partial-incision method.

1.5 cm

8–10 mm

Equidistant with contralateral side

Incision commences along medial limbus

precisely 0.3 mL of anesthetic is delivered to each eyelid; the needle is not threaded under the skin but held stationary in the midline, and the anesthetic is slowly infiltrated subcutaneously as a wheal (Fig. 7-8). This method minimizes patient discomfort and the risk of hematoma and ecchymosis. The eyelid skin is then gently pinched and rolled between the index and thumb above and below the proposed incision in order to ensure uniform distribution of the anesthetic across the entire length of the incision (Fig. 7-9). After several minutes, the 30-gauge needle can be used to test for adequate anesthesia across the entire length of each proposed incision. If any additional anesthetic is required, the same amount and location of injection should be performed on both eyelids in order to maintain the ability to estimate

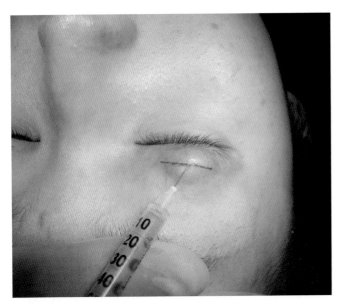

Figure 7-8 Local anesthesia consisting of 2% lidocaine with 1:50,000 epinephrine is infiltrated with a 30-gauge needle and a 1-mL syringe for a total of precisely 0.3 mL by placing the needle in the midline of the incision and raising a wheal.

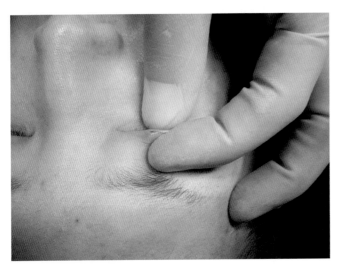

Figure 7-9 After the local anesthesia is infiltrated, the anesthetic is evenly distributed across the entire incision by gently pinching and rolling the incision between the index finger and thumb.

crease symmetry between the two sides: an excessive amount of anesthetic placed on one side will lead to a falsely higher appearance of that lid crease, which will in turn impair the surgeon's ability to judge symmetry.

Povidone-iodine solution is applied topically across both upper eyelids to encompass the forehead and the midface/cheek region, with care taken not to use an excessive amount that would contact the globe and engender conjunctival irritation. The remainder of the face is then covered with sterile drapes following standard operative protocol.

After 10 minutes are allowed to transpire since injection of the anesthetic, the skin incision can be undertaken using a Bard-Parker No.15 blade (Fig. 7-10). Surgery progresses in a symmetrical fashion with incision of each eyelid performed and each step undertaken in tandem, as will be explained. When making each incision, care should be taken to ensure that the marked line is followed precisely in terms of length and height so as to ensure symmetry, which can be facilitated with the upper-eyelid skin placed under tension using the nondominant hand or with the aid of the surgical assistant during the incision.

Both incisions should be carried out through the dermis and muscle. Fine bipolar forceps, needle-point cautery, or customized fine-tip forceps (designed by YKK) to which monopolar cautery is applied can be used to achieve hemostasis before continuing (Fig. 7-11).

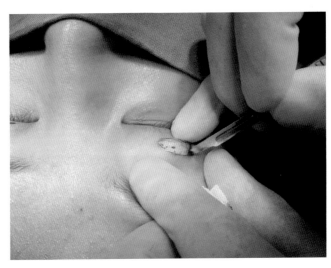

Figure 7-10 The skin and muscle are incised with a No.15 blade.

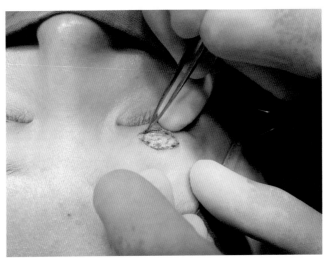

Figure 7-11 As the orbicularis is transected, the orbital septum will become exposed, and additional hemostasis is required before continuing.

The orbicularis oculi is then gently transected on each eyelid with the No.15 blade, and additional cautery is used to attain adequate hemostasis. (The reader is reminded again that both eyelids are operated on in an alternating fashion.)

At this point the orbital septum is encountered; the surgeon should then excise a small wedge of orbital septum laterally to expose the underlying preaponeurotic adipose pocket (Fig. 7-12). Of note, the orbital septum should also be excised as superiorly along the wound edge as possible to avoid injury to the underlying levator and to approach the fat pad more directly. If the adipose tissue does not become immediately apparent, gentle downward pressure on the globe can be applied above and below the wound edges to compel the adipose tissue to herniate through the fenestrated orbital septum. If the adipose tissue is still restricted from full view, then an additional amount of orbital septum may need to be removed. Gentle pressure can again be applied to expose the underlying fat pad. When the fat pad becomes visible through the defect, a pair of forceps can be used to tease the remaining fat out through the fenestration (Fig. 7-13).

A fine pair of straight scissors is then passed with the tines closed through the surgical fenestration from lateral to medial to ensure that there is unrestricted passage of the scissors between the orbital septum above and the adipose tissue below (Fig. 7-14). Then, the remaining orbital septum can be safely transected laterally to medially to permit the remaining adipose tissue to be exposed along the entire incision length (Fig. 7-15).

A cotton-tipped applicator should be used to sweep the adipose tissue away from the underlying levator complex until the glistening white levator aponeurosis is fully in view. At times a thin, filmy layer may remain between the adipose tissue and the true levator, and this attenuated layer must be transected to provide complete and unrestricted access to the levator (Fig. 7-16). If the surgeon is uncertain as to which layer he or she has arrived at, the surgeon should grasp that layer with forceps and ask the patient to open his or her eyes. If the patient cannot open his or her eyes, then the surgeon most likely has grasped the levator and has therefore arrived at the correct depth. Judicious and careful dissection will limit the risk of inadvertent levator injury.

With the adipose tissue and the levator in view, the surgeon should progress to the contralateral side until both structures are similarly exposed. A symmetrical amount (0.1 to 0.2 mL) of 2% *plain* lidocaine should be

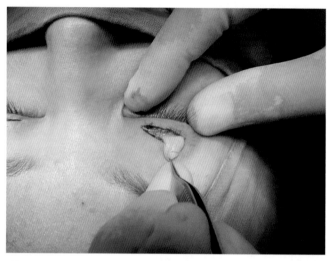

Figure 7-13 When the orbital fat becomes visible, a pair of forceps is used to tease the fat through the orbital-septal fenestration.

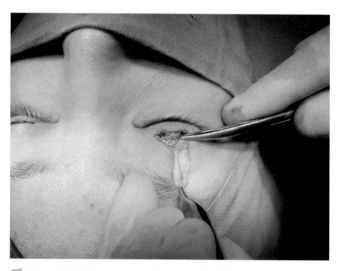

Figure 7-14 The scissors are then passed with tines closed under the remaining orbital septum to ensure that there is a clear plane between the orbital fat and the levator aponeurosis so that inadvertent transection of the levator does not occur. The photograph shows the overlying orbital fat and the glistening white levator below with scissor tips entering immediately below the remaining, untransected orbital septum.

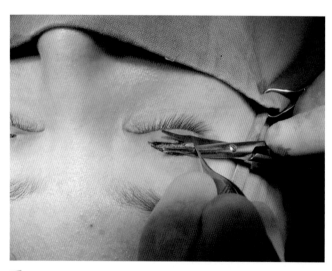

Figure 7-12 Fine scissors should be used to excise a wedge of orbital septum laterally and superiorly along the wound to expose the underlying orbital fat.

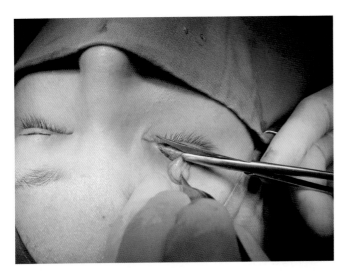

Figure 7-15 The remaining orbital septum can be safely transected laterally to medially to permit the remaining adipose tissue to be exposed along the entire incision length.

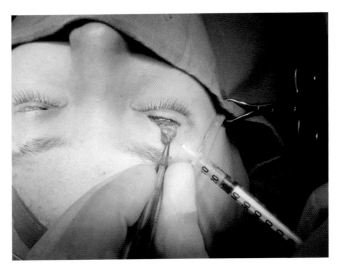

Figure 7-17 After the same technique has been used to expose the contralateral fat pad, both fat pads are anesthetized with 2% plain lidocaine (approximately 0.1 to 0.2 mL).

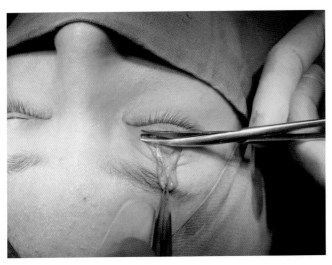

Figure 7-16 Some remaining fibers must be transected in order to attain unrestricted access to the levator aponeurosis.

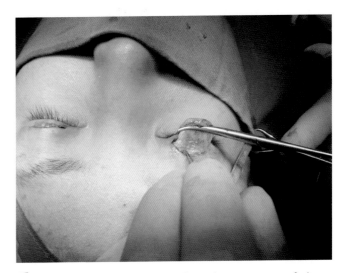

Figure 7-18 The adipose tissue is clamped to permit 1 cm of adipose tissue to remain in situ under the clamp.

infiltrated into each fat pad before resection in order to enhance patient comfort (Fig. 7-17). The surgeon should be careful not to allow any of the lidocaine to trickle onto the underlying levator, which can in turn become anesthetized and not function properly, albeit temporarily. With a temporarily paralyzed levator, determination of symmetry can be quite problematic, and the levator may remain dysfunctional for several weeks postoperatively.

After adequate infiltration of anesthesia directly into the fat pads, the adipose tissue on one side should be clamped with a fine mosquito clamp so that 1 cm of adipose tissue remains under the clamp (Fig. 7-18). The overlying adipose tissue is then removed sharply with scissors (Fig. 7-19), leaving a small cuff of adipose tissue above the clamp to be cauterized (Fig. 7-20). The clamp is removed, and the remaining adipose tissue is carefully

observed for hemostasis. The same technique for adipose resection is then undertaken on the contralateral side. Of note, a symmetrical amount of fat should be retained in situ, whereas it is inconsequential if an asymmetrical amount is removed.

A single levator-to-skin fixation suture is then placed in the central aspect of the incision using a 7-0 nylon (or 8-0 Dexon) in a buried fashion. At first, the needle should pass superiorly to inferiorly (i.e., backhanded) through the inferior wound edge, capturing a full thickness of dermis along with 0.2 to 0.3 mm of the epidermal edge. The surgeon's nondominant index finger should be used to roll out, or evert, the wound edge so that the full thickness of dermis and a small amount of epidermis can be more easily and accurately captured: *Purchase of a small bite of epidermis is a critical component to ensure*

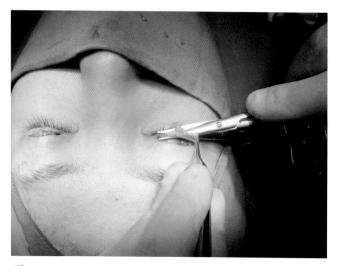

Figure 7-19 The overlying, excess adipose tissue is then sharply removed with scissors.

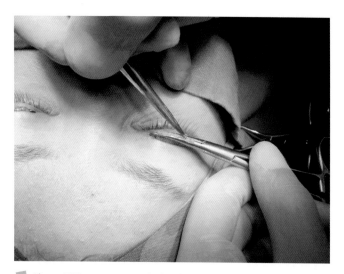

Figure 7-20 Cautery is applied to the clamp before freeing the fat from the clamp.

that a foreign-body reaction occurs and a more permanent lid crease is attained (Fig. 7-21). A second bite is then taken superiorly to inferiorly through the portion of levator that lies superiorly above the initial dermoepidermal bite (Fig. 7-22). The knot is then tied down once (Fig. 7-23*A*); and the patient is asked to open his or her eyes to ensure that the crease height appears adequate and the eyelashes begin to evert (i.e., the eyelashes should be oriented perpendicular, or 90 degrees, to the skin surface) (Fig. 7-23*B*). Conversely, overly or underly everted eyelashes will compromise the surgical outcome. If the foregoing criteria are met, then the suture is tied down with a total of four square knots, and both suture ends are cut with a long tail.

A central fixation suture is then placed in the exact same manner for the other eyelid. If both eyelid creases appear to be symmetrical (Fig. 7-24), then the long

suture tails can be trimmed down to the knot to leave no discernible suture tail. Needle holders that have built-in scissors to allow expeditious and precise trimming of the suture tails. As these sutures remain permanently, it is important that an excessive number of knot throws or long suture tails not be present that would predispose toward suture extrusion over time. If the crease heights do not appear symmetrical, the surgeon should press gently inferiorly on the brow to ensure that the skin above the created creases fold adequately over the crease. If the result still appears asymmetrical, the lower crease can be raised by placing the central suture more superiorly along the levator, or the side with too high a crease, conversely,

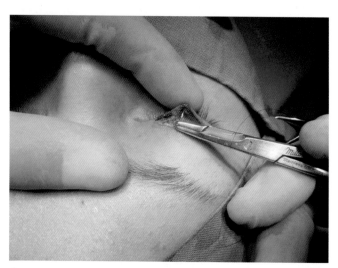

Figure 7-21 A single 7-0 nylon suture is passed through the middle of the incision to capture the full thickness of the dermis by everting the wound edge with the nondominant index finger (**A**). In addition, the suture must also capture 0.2 to 0.3 mm of epidermis as well (**B**). Capturing a small amount of epidermis will help engender a foreign-body reaction and thereby lead to a more tenacious adhesion, which is critical when performing fixation through a limited incision.

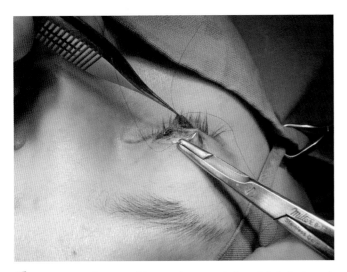

Figure 7-22 The second bite is taken superiorly to inferiorly through the mid-height of the exposed levator directly superior to the skin bite described in Figure 7-21.

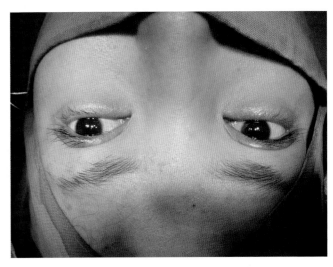

Figure 7-24 The same central suture is placed on the contralateral side, and symmetry is inspected.

lowered by placing the suture more inferiorly along the levator.

After the first levator-to-skin fixation suture has been successfully placed on each side, the remaining fixation sutures can be easily undertaken. The presence of the first fixation suture creates a fanning gullwing-shaped fold in the levator that permits easy placement of the remaining levator sutures through this fold (Fig. 7-25). If the fold is not visible, then an adequate levator-to-skin fixation most likely has not been established, and the first fixation suture should be redone. The manner in which the remaining sutures are placed follows the same method described for the first fixation suture (Figs. 7-26 and 7-27). Each fixation suture should be placed in an

alternating fashion between eyelids, and crease height, confirmed by having the patient open his or her eyes after each fixation suture is placed. A total of approximately five to seven sutures should be placed along the entire length of each incision. It is important not to be tempted to place fewer than this recommended number of sutures, as with fewer sutures, the risk of crease loss over time is amplified.

After all the fixation sutures have been secured, the skin is then closed with three interrupted 7-0 nylon sutures distributed evenly across the wound length and positioned between the fixation sutures (Fig. 7-28).

If asymmetry is noted after skin closure, the levator can be found between the skin sutures and additional

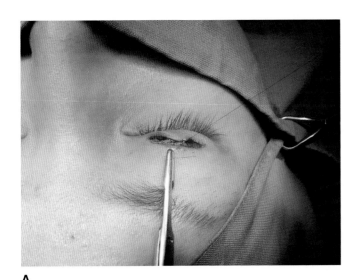

A

B

Figure 7-23 The suture is then tied down with a single knot (**A**). The patient is asked to open his or her eyes to determine proper crease height and the perpendicular orientation of the eyelashes (**B**). If the eyelashes appear overly or underly everted, the suture position of the levator bite should be lowered or raised, respectively.

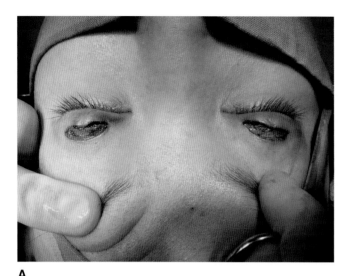

A

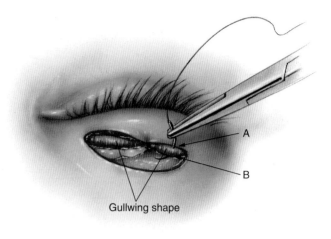

B

Figure 7-25 A properly placed first levator–skin fixation suture will create a gullwing crease configuration in the levator aponeurosis that will guide the remaining fixation sutures (**A**). This schematic illustration shows the gullwing shape that the levator should assume after the first fixation suture is placed (**B**).

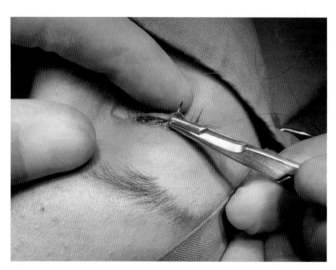

Figure 7-26 The next fixation suture should be placed through the skin for the first bite exactly in the same manner prescribed for the first fixation suture, as described in Figure 7-21.

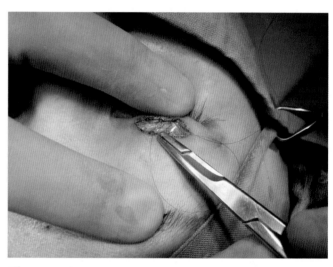

Figure 7-27 The second bite of the next fixation suture should then pass through the gullwing fold in the levator, as diagrammed in Figure 7-25B. A total of five to seven fixation sutures should be placed on each eyelid in an alternating fashion between each side, so the surgeon can verify symmetry with each suture.

fixation sutures can be placed to adjust the lid-crease height: if the surgeon would like to raise a low crease, the surgeon can place new fixation sutures between the *upper* wound edge and the levator until the height of the crease approximates the contralateral side. However, if excessive eyelash eversion arises, then the incision should be opened and the levator-skin fixation sutures replaced.

At the close of the procedure, the patient's face is then cleaned with hydrogen peroxide solution, and the incisions are dressed with Bacitracin ointment. The patient confirms the symmetry of the lid creases in the mirror before ice packs are placed over both eyes to minimize postoperative edema.

THE FULL-INCISION METHOD

General Considerations

The full-incision method that will be described herein follows the principles of levator fixation enumerated in the partial-incision section, including fixation of only the central 15 to 20 mm, as in the partial-incision method.

As with the partial-incision method, marking the appropriate crease height for the patient is an important first step. With the patient sitting upright, the surgeon places a paper clip, or similar device, into the fold to create a natural-appearing crease that appears acceptable to the patient and surgeon alike (Fig. 7-29). The patient

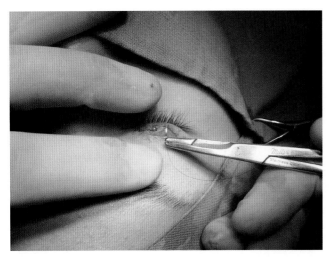

Figure 7-28 After all fixation sutures have been placed, the skin is closed with three interrupted 7-0 nylon sutures. Care should be taken not to transect the fixation sutures with the skin-closure needle, as placement of the skin sutures should be situated between the fixation sutures.

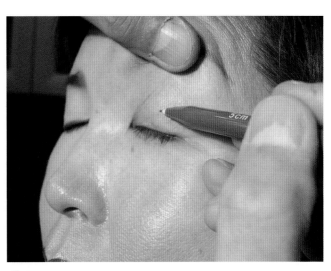

Figure 7-30 The patient is then asked to close his or her eyes with the paper clip left in place, and a surgical marking pen is then used to place a dot at the height of the paper clip in the midpupillary line.

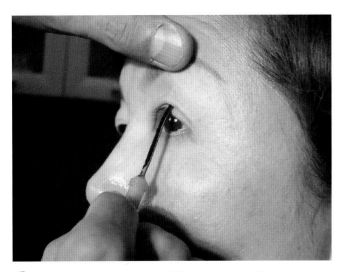

Figure 7-29 The first step in the full-incision method (like in the partial-incision method) for Asian blepharoplasty is placement of an open paper clip, or similar device, into the eyelid to create an eyelid fold.

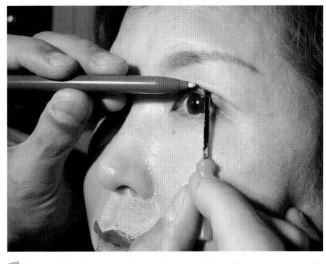

Figure 7-31 The patient is asked to open his or her eyes again and a second dot is placed where the overlapping skin folds over with the paper clip in place at the midpupillary line.

is then asked to close the eyes with the paper clip left in place, and a surgical marking pen is used to place a dot at the height of the paper clip in the midpupillary line (Fig. 7-30). The patient is asked to open the eyes again and a second dot is placed where the overlapping skin folds over with the paper clip in place at the midpupillary line (Fig. 7-31). The patient is asked to close the eyes again, and the surgeon then places a third dot with the marking pen halfway between the two previous dots (Fig. 7-32). The lower dot marks the lower limb of the incision, which is then tapered inferiorly laterally and medially; the incision should end approximately at the lateral canthus laterally and extend to about 5 mm medial to the medial canthus. The superior limb of the incision should follow the third marked dot, the one that lies

halfway between the first two marked dots. Medially, the superior limb should taper to meet the medial point of the inferior limb; laterally, the superior limb should extend to the orbital rim, which is then connected to the lateral extent of the inferior limb with a straight line (Fig. 7-33). The same technique is repeated on the contralateral side and the two sides are compared for symmetry. Castroviejo calipers can be used to verify precise symmetry before continuing.

Operative Technique

After both eyelids are marked appropriately, the patient is administered local anesthesia with a total of 1 mL of 2% lidocaine mixed with 1:50,000 epinephrine on each side from a 1-mL syringe outfitted with a 30-gauge needle. To

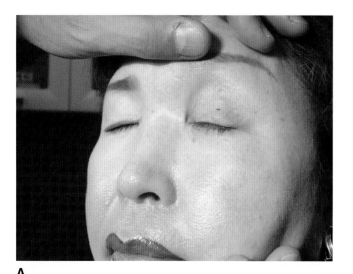

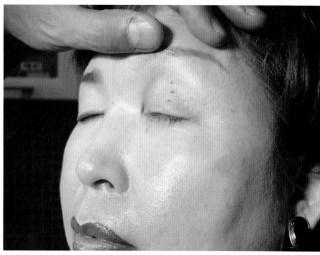

A   **B**

Figure 7-32 The patient is asked to close both eyes again: the two marked dots are shown (**A**). The surgeon then places a third dot with the marking pen halfway between the two previous dots (**B**).

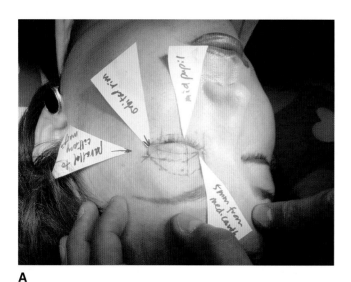

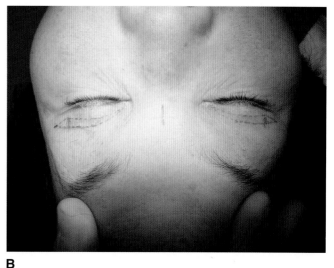

A   **B**

Figure 7-33 The lower dot marks the lower limb of the incision, which is then tapered inferiorly laterally and medially: The incision should end approximately at the lateral canthus laterally and extend to about 5 mm medial to the medial canthus (**A**). The superior limb of the incision should follow the third marked dot, that is, the one that lies halfway between the first two marked dots. Medially, the superior limb should taper to meet the medial point of the inferior limb; laterally, the superior limb should extend to the orbital rim, which is then connected to the lateral extent of the inferior limb with a straight line. The markings are shown to the patient for the full-incision method (**B**).

minimize ecchymosis and patient discomfort, the same technique of raising a subcutaneous wheal (as opposed to tunneling) can be used as described previously in the section on the partial-incision method (Fig. 7-34A and B).

After 10 minutes are allowed to transpire for optimal hemostasis and anesthesia, a No.15 blade is used to incise through the skin and orbicularis muscle (Fig. 7-35). The island of skin and muscle is then dissected free from the underlying orbital septum using tenotomy scissors and then discarded (Fig. 7-36).

Meticulous hemostasis is necessary along the cut edges of the orbicularis muscle in order to minimize

postoperative ecchymosis and to permit ease of further dissection (Fig. 7-37). A small fenestration in the lateral third of the orbital septum is then created by excising a tiny wedge, as described above in the partial-incision method (Fig. 7-38). The fat compartment is then teased out (Fig. 7-39A and B), the orbital septum is incised (Figs. 7-40A and B and 7-41), and the fat is clamped and excised in the same manner prescribed for the partial-incision method. Generally speaking, only the middle third of the levator need be exposed and only the central fat compartment removed, just as described in the partial-incision method. Fixation of the levator proceeds in the

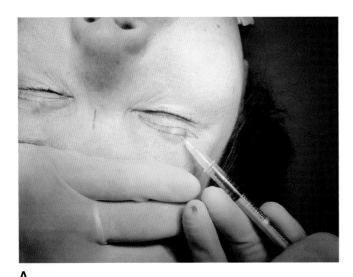

A

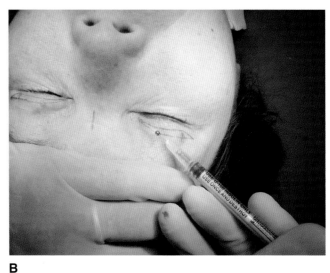

B

Figure 7-34 Subcutaneous wheals are raised with local anesthesia in order to minimize ecchymosis associated with the threading technique (**A** and **B**).

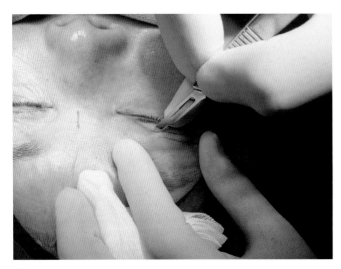

Figure 7-35 After 10 minutes are allowed to transpire for optimal hemostasis and anesthesia, a No.15 blade is used to incise through the skin and orbicularis muscle.

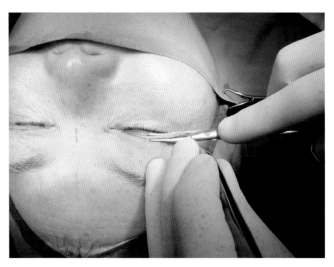

Figure 7-36 The island of skin and muscle is dissected free from the underlying orbital septum using tenotomy scissors and then discarded.

exact manner as described for the partial-incision method—only the central 15 to 20 mm of levator need be fixated for a durable adhesion (Figs. 7-42 to 7-44). After symmetry is confirmed, the skin incisions are closed with a running 7-0 nylon suture that should carefully avoid disturbing any of the fixation sutures (Fig. 7-45). Meticulous surgical execution and attention to symmetry will yield consistently superior aesthetic results (Figs. 7-46 to 7-49).

POSTOPERATIVE CARE

Postoperative care remains essentially the same for the patient undergoing either the partial- or full-incision method. Before the patient is discharged from the operating theater, he or she is reminded that the lid-crease height will appear unnaturally high for several weeks to months (longer with the full-incision method). In addition, symmetry is difficult to assess for the first 2 postoperative weeks owing to resolving edema. The patient is informed as well that he or she may also experience an unusual sensation when opening the eyes for the first few postoperative days, because of suture fixation of the levator. The patient is informed that edema will worsen considerably on the second or third postoperative day and then will begin to dissipate rapidly thereafter. Contact lens use should be restricted for the first 2 postoperative weeks in order to avoid shearing the wound edges open during eyelid manipulation; eyeglasses should be worn instead. All these precautions are preferably declared in the preoperative setting so that the

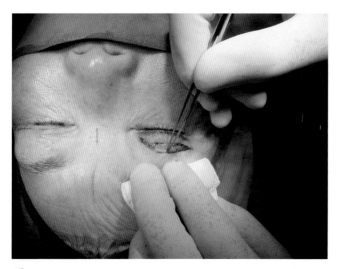

Figure 7-37 Meticulous hemostasis is necessary along the cut edges of the orbicularis muscle in order to minimize postoperative ecchymosis and to permit ease of further dissection.

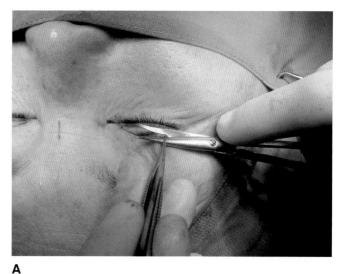

A

B

Figure 7-38 A small fenestration in the lateral third of the orbital septum is then created by excising a tiny wedge of orbital septum (**A**). Additional septum is excised until the fat becomes visible through the defect (**B**).

patient can be comfortable in advance with the postoperative recovery period and plan his or her social/professional calendar accordingly.

The most important aspect for the patient to follow postoperatively is strict adherence to liberal ice application to the surgical site during the first 2 postoperative days; following this policy will expedite resolution of edema. Cold ice packs should be replaced with those that become warm about every 20 to 30 minutes as tolerated, and stressful viewing activity should be kept to a minimum. Ice application thereafter is superfluous, and warm packs should never be used. Perioperative antibiotic usage is not necessary and follows the surgeon's philosophy and preference. Narcotic medication for discomfort is rarely indicated, and significant pain should alarm the surgeon to the evolution of a hematoma.

For the first postoperative week, the patient should gently clean the incision with hydrogen peroxide using a cotton-tipped applicator twice daily followed by application of Bacitracin ointment. Desiccated wounds heal poorly so a generous amount of Bacitracin should be used unless the patient should experience an allergic reaction to the product. Any petroleum-based ointment, such as Aquaphor, can be used as a substitute as needed. It is important that the patient cease all peroxide and Bacitracin application after the first postoperative week, as continued usage only serves to impair wound healing and may lead to wound dehiscence. Skin sutures may be removed from 3 to 7 days postoperatively. On the 10th postoperative day, the patient is encouraged to apply topical vitamin E oil to the incision site twice daily for 2 weeks in order to minimize the risk of scar formation. Thereafter, the patient is free from any postoperative care regimen.

COMPLICATIONS

ASYMMETRY

Perhaps the most common complication following double-eyelid surgery is asymmetry between the created lid creases. Even 1 mm of difference between the eyelids can be glaringly noticeable for the surgeon and patient alike. Therefore, accumulated experience and meticulous surgery will help reduce the incidence of this particular complication. Following the partial-incision method, if asymmetry is noted during the first 2 weeks, no treatment is required, as edema may be accountable for the asymmetry, especially if a small hematoma arose on one side or greater dissection was required on one eyelid. After

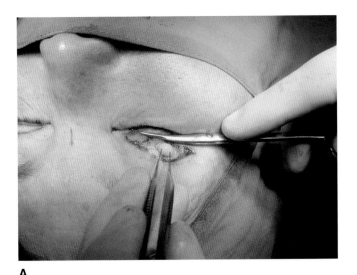
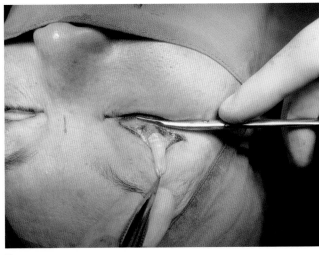

A   **B**

Figure 7-39 The fat compartment is teased out through the defect to expose the levator aponeurosis (**A** and **B**).

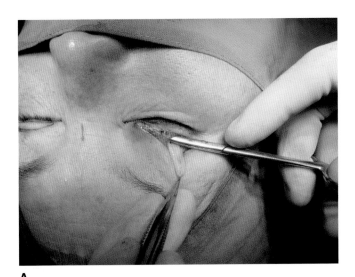
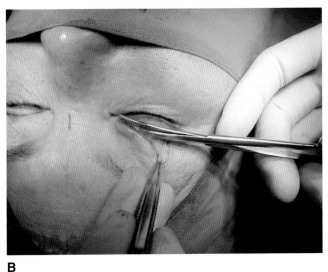

A   **B**

Figure 7-40 The orbital septum is incised with a pair of tenotomy scissors to expose the remaining levator (**A** and **B**).

2 weeks, however, if asymmetry persists, the surgeon should consider elective revision surgery. At this time, revision surgery is quite straightforward, as simple spreading with scissors—after the initial incision is made—will expose the levator quickly. Asymmetry that is noted after that time will require more extensive surgery but remains still relatively less labor intensive than if a full-incision method was undertaken. With the full-incision method, asymmetry may persist for several more weeks and may be entirely accounted for by edema. Therefore, a minimum of 1 month, if not longer, should be taken to attend the resolution of the asymmetry. If asymmetry persists beyond 3 months, the asymmetry most likely is not related to edema but to technical error. *Regardless of surgical technique, the golden rule is to never operate on one single eyelid no matter how tempting, as* *symmetry is impossible to gauge with unilateral, corrective surgery.*

FOLD LOSS

With the partial-incision method, fold loss is higher as compared with the full-incision method because of the more limited distance of fixation, but still less than with the suture-based technique. Fold loss may be due to the technical error of not fixating a small amount of the epidermal edge (as explained before), insufficient number of fixation sutures (five to seven per side), or suture fixation of the false layer above the true levator, among other factors. Careful review of the surgical technique expounded earlier will limit this problem from arising. If fold loss does occur, revision surgery is mandated: Again,

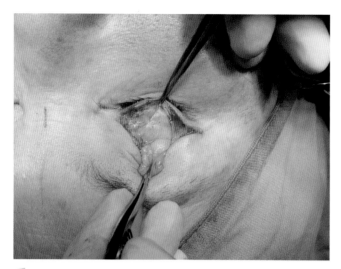

Figure 7-41 The fat and levator are fully exposed after incision of the orbital septum.

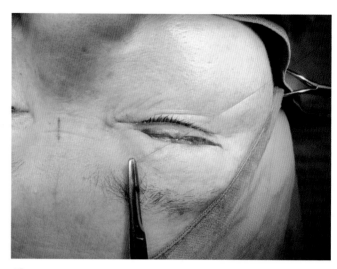

Figure 7-43 The first fixation suture is tied down, and the patient is asked to open the eyes to ensure that the eyelashes appear perpendicularly oriented to the skin.

both eyelids must be operated on in order to ensure symmetry.

SUTURE EXTRUSION

As the authors favor permanent internal fixation sutures, suture extrusion may occur. Burying the knot and minimizing knot throws as outlined in the surgical procedure will help reduce the likelihood of suture extrusion. With either the partial- or full-incision method explained herein, if one or two sutures are lost during the first 3 months, fold loss most likely will not occur.

Nevertheless, if a suture becomes exposed during the initial few months, the surgeon should admonish the patient not to remove the uncovered suture or expect the surgeon to do so in order to minimize the potential for fold loss. After the first 3 months, fold fixation should be more tenacious with the partial-incision method, and removal of any exposed sutures can be safely pursued.

INFECTION

Infection is rare with or without the use of perioperative antibiotics. Typically, if an infection occurs, the situation

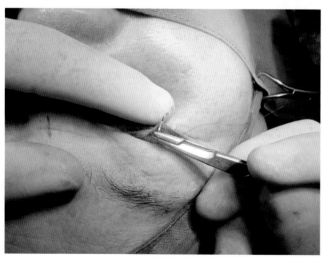

A

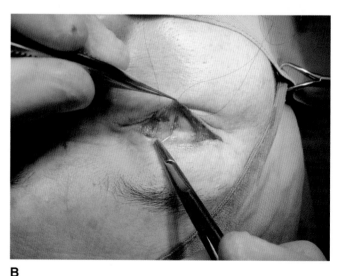

B

Figure 7-42 After the excess fat of the central compartment is excised with a 1-cm cuff left in situ, the first levator to skin fixation suture can be established (**A**). Just like the manner described for the partial-incision method, the full thickness dermis and a small amount of epidermis is taken in the first bite (the skin bite). The second bite is taken through the midportion of the levator (**B**).

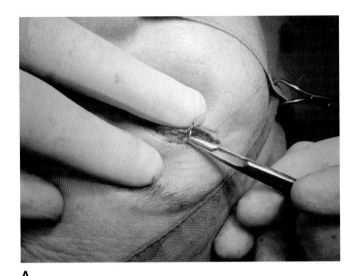

A

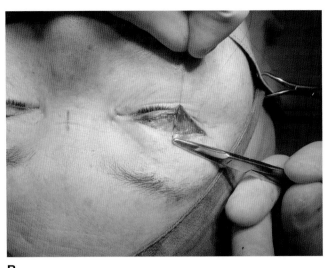

B

Figure 7-44 The second fixation suture is placed in the same manner (**A**). Of note, like in the partial incision method, a gullwing shape should appear in the levator to guide the remaining fixation sutures along this fold in the levator. Like the partial-incision method, fixation sutures can be placed simply along the central 15 to 20 mm of the exposed levator for adequate crease formation (**B**).

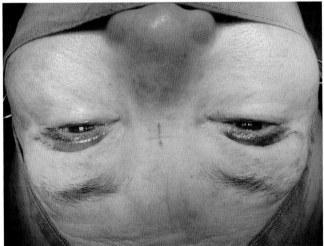

Figure 7-45 After symmetry is confirmed, the skin incisions are closed with a running 7-0 nylon suture that should carefully avoid disturbing any of the fixation sutures.

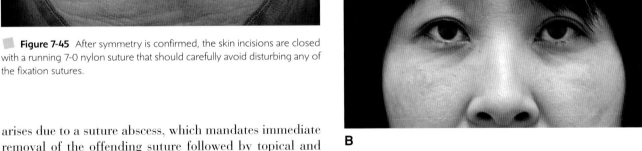

A

B

Figure 7-46 Preoperative (**A**) and postoperative (**B**) views taken of a 41-year-old Japanese woman with the full-incision double-eyelid creation.

arises due to a suture abscess, which mandates immediate removal of the offending suture followed by topical and oral antibiotics until the condition fully resolves. Culture and sensitivity evaluation should be routinely performed, although the causative organism tends to be a constituent of skin flora.

SCARRING

Scarring is quite rare with the partial-incision method, as the incision length is limited and no wound tension is present, and no skin is removed. Hypertrophic scar is most notably problematic along the medial epicanthal region, as may be observed with the full-incision method. Direct, intralesional steroid injection with triamcinolone acetonide (10 mg/mL) can be used to reduce any scar formation. Unless exuberant in nature, the scar should be

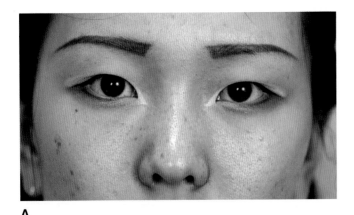

A

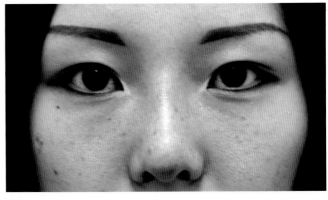

B

Figure 7-47 Preoperative (**A**) and postoperative (**B**) views taken of a 21-year-old Korean woman with the partial-incision double-eyelid creation.

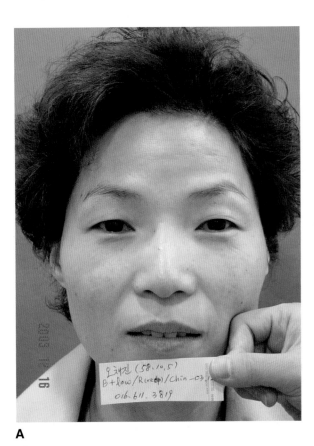

A

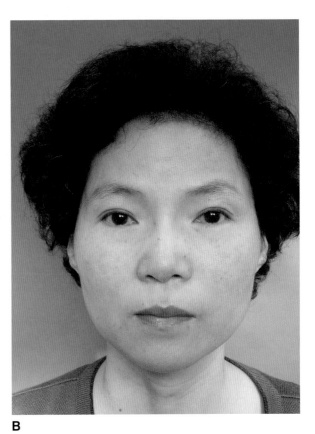

B

Figure 7-48 Preoperative (**A**) and postoperative (**B**) views taken of a 46-year-old woman with the full-incision technique.

left alone for the first few months in order to avoid loosening of the fixation suture during this critical period.

REVISION SURGERY

Fold loss and obvious asymmetry call for revision surgery. As mentioned, during the first 2 postoperative weeks, wound strength is quite low; therefore, revision surgery is relatively facile. Thereafter, dissection through the scarred surgical bed must always be approached carefully and

meticulously: first and foremost, levator injury must be avoided. After the initial incision through the skin, gentle spreading with fine scissors should be undertaken until the levator is exposed. Finding the remaining preaponeurotic fat pad superiorly will help protect the surgeon from inadvertent levator injury, as the levator is always found immediately deep to the adipose tissue. Discovery of any previously placed fixation sutures will also guide the surgeon as to the correct depth. If the surgeon is uncertain, he or she should always verify that

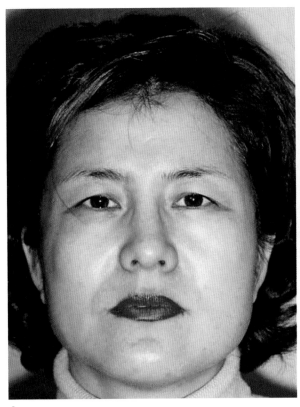
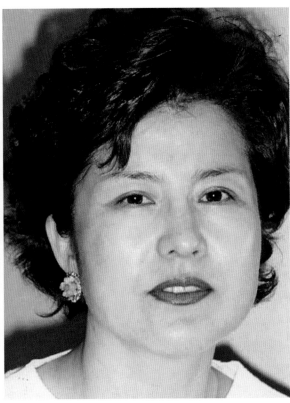

A   **B**

Figure 7-49 Preoperative (**A**) and postoperative (**B**) views taken of a 45-year old woman full-incision technique.

the levator has not been arrived at by grasping the tissue to see whether the patient can open and close the eyes; again, if the patient cannot open the eyes, the surgeon most likely has the levator in his or her grasp.

Future Considerations

Perhaps a look back will help the reader envision what will come. Over the past century, the original suture-based technique has met with the rise of many variations of incisional surgery. Permutations of both major techniques, like the one described herein, are continuing to evolve, and hybrids of suture and incision-based methods have also been explored. Different epicanthoplasty and lateral canthoplasty methods have been introduced as adjunctive measures to the creation of the double eyelid. Surgical techniques that modulate the crease and epicanthus will continue to evolve in the future (as, in fact, the authors are at this time completing work on an original technique for epicanthal advancement). However, no clear trend has arisen, and it is doubtful it will arise, as surgeons will most likely continue to adhere to their own favored method(s). The past decade has witnessed quite a change in aesthetic opinion, moving from the desire for a true "westernization" eyelid appearance to now a low, natural-appearing crease. As the popularity of interracial unions continues to rise and certain cultural boundaries are effaced, a universal aesthetic may propel (or conversely hinder) acceptance of the procedure. Controversy will always surround whether double-eyelid creation represents a denial of one's ethnicity or in fact stems from motivation to emulate a more ideal beauty that is derived from one's own native peers. As notions of fashion, style, and beauty are constantly in flux, the creation of the double eyelid will no doubt be subjected to the same cultural forces.

REFERENCES

1. Lam SM: Mikamo's double-eyelid blepharoplasty and the westernization of Japan. Arch Facial Plast Surg 2002;4:201-202.
2. Mikamo M: Plastic operation of the eyelid. J Chugaii-jishimpo 1896;17:1197.
3. Mikamo M: Mikamo's double-eyelid operation: The advent of Japanese aesthetic surgery: 1896. Plast Reconstr Surg 1997;99:664-669.
4. Fernandez LR: Double eyelid operation in the Oriental in Hawaii. Plast Reconstr Surg 1960;25:257-264.
5. Boo-Chai K: Plastic construction of the superior palpebral fold. Plast Reconstr Surg 1963;31:74-78.
6. Millard DR Jr: The Oriental eyelid and its surgical revision. Am J Opthalmol 1964;57:646-649.

7. McCurdy JA Jr, Lam SM: Cosmetic Surgery of the Asian Face, 2nd ed. New York: Thieme, 2005.

8. McCurdy JA Jr: Upper blepharoplasty in the Asian patient: The "double eyelid" operation. Facial Plast Surg Clin North Am 2002;10:351-368.

9. Lam SM, Kim YK: Partial-incision technique for creation of the double eyelid. Aesthet Surg J 2003;23:170-176.

10. Choi AK: Oriental blepharoplasty: Nonincisional suture technique versus conventional incisional technique. Facial Plast Surg 1994;10:67-83.

11. Homma K, Mutou H, Ezoe K, Fujita T: Intradermal stitch blepharoplasty for Orientals: Does it disappear? Aesthet Plast Surg 2000;24:289-291.

12. McCurdy JA Jr: Cosmetic Surgery of the Asian Face. New York: Thieme, 1990.

13. Jeong S, Lemke BN, Dortzbach RK, et al: The Asian upper eyelid: An anatomical study with comparison to the Caucasian eyelid. Arch Ophthalmol 1999;117:907-912.

14. Hwang K, Kim DJ, Chung RS, et al: An anatomical study of the junction of the orbital septum and the levator aponeurosis in Orientals. Br J Plast Surg 1998;51:594-598.

15. Yuzuriha S, Matsuo K, Kushima H: An anatomical structure which results in puffiness of the upper eyelid and a narrow palpebral fissure in the Mongoloid eye. Br J Plast Surg 2000;53:466-472.

16. Morikawa K, Yamamoto H, Uchinuma E, Yamashina S: Scanning electron microscopic study on double and single eyelids in Orientals. Aesthet Plast Surg 2001;25:20-24.

17. Hanada AL, de Souza EN Jr, Moribe I, Cruz AA: Comparison of palpebral fissure obliquity in three different racial groups. Ophthal Plast Reconstr Surg 2001;17:423-426.

18. Lim WK, Rajendran K, Choo CT: Microscopic anatomy of the lower eyelid in Asians. Ophthal Plast Reconstr Surg 2004;20:207-211.

19. Carter SR, Seiff SR, Grant PE, Vigneron DB: The Asian lower eyelid: A comparative anatomic study using high-resolution magnetic resonance imaging. Ophthal Plast Reconstr Surg 1998;14:227-234.

CHAPTER EIGHT

The Deep Plane Facelift

Calvin M. Johnson Jr., MD • Mark R. Murphy, MD

HISTORY

The signature operation of facial rejuvenation is the rhytidectomy. Of all the procedures designed to remedy the effects of aging, the rhytidectomy has the most profound ability to improve the patient's appearance. The first recorded efforts to surgically rejuvenate the face appeared early in the 20th century.[1-3] The first 50 years of the 20th century saw little advance, burdened by the risks of anesthesia and the lack of medications, such as antibiotics, surgeons were forced to move forward with great trepidation. As technologic advances erupted in the latter half of the 20th century, surgical advances soon followed. In the last 30 years of the century these technologic advances enabled surgeons to provide excellent surgical results to their patients. And the popularity of facial rejuvenation has since exploded. Today, an attractive outward appearance is a sign of strength and health instead of vanity.[4]

The original techniques employed short skin flaps and minimal, if any, manipulation of the underlying soft tissues for fear of damaging the facial nerve. With greater anatomic understanding, the techniques progressed deeper into the ptotic tissues of the aging face. The skin flaps gradually became longer and the manipulations of the underlying soft tissue, the superficial musculoaponeurotic system (SMS), became more aggressive. With these advances new frontiers were crossed and new complications arose. In addition, physicians working in this field have now gained a much greater knowledge and appreciation for other factors that historically had been neglected, especially in regard to lifestyle choices, such as smoking and alcohol intake, and in medications, such as antiplatelet agents.

The field has undergone a fascinating 30-year evolution since the groundbreaking work of Dr. Skoog in the 1970s.[5] Skoog was the first to perform what can be called the deep plane technique; Hamra advanced the concept to include the soft tissues of the midface with his deep plane and composite techniques.[6-9] Today, there is great controversy as to the appropriate technique and plane of dissection for optimal rejuvenation.[4] With the advent of the deep plane facelift technique, rhytidectomy took a quantum leap forward. For decades, the rhytidec-tomy provided the patient with a benefit that often pleased the patient but left the surgeon wanting more. This exciting new technique enabled the surgeon to provide a more lasting, natural result. We propose our techniques described herein not as an answer to these dilemmas but as a proven method to safe, excellent, reproducible results in facial rejuvenation.

PERSONAL PHILOSOPHY

The evolution of our technique was based on several criteria. First, the result with the deep plane technique was superior to that of the SMAS lift plication and imbrication techniques. With a more thorough undermining of the ptotic soft tissues of the face a better postoperative result soon followed, as would be expected. Although the SMAS procedure is excellent for short-term gains in reducing skin laxity and mild improvement of soft tissue ptosis, the majority of the ptotic soft tissue remains fallen. We agree with the previously published viewpoint that "minilifts" or subcutaneous facelift procedures have only dealt with laxity of the skin and do not completely address the ptotic soft tissues of the face.[6,7]

Second, once experience had been gained with this technique the long-term results became evident. In addition, the occurrence of the pulled or "operated look" decreased rapidly with the increased use of this technique. We also believe that with the shorter skin flap and superior blood supply of the deep plane technique, the catastrophic issues of skin loss and poor scar appearance are greatly diminished. With its strict adherence to physiologically sound principles, the effect of the deep plane technique is maintained for a longer period than that of the skin flap techniques. This is due to the composite flap maintaining the viscoelastic properties of the SMAS.[10] Though others have not agreed with these opinions, we maintain our results have improved greatly since the transformation of techniques.[11,12]

Much excitement has been generated over the "weekend" or "mini-facelifts." With the promise of smaller incisions and less downtime, these procedures have received significant attention over the last several years as the popularity of plastic surgery has flourished. These techniques are similar to standard SMAS facelifts and thus are an option for certain patients.

Generally speaking, patients for whom these procedures are devised suffer from lax skin, especially in the lower face. Often, in our practice, these concerns are minor and handled with reassurance. When a patient considers facial cosmetic surgery, we feel the first operation should be the definitive procedure. If the patient has had a "less invasive" procedure in the past, the tissue planes are forever altered, thus making further surgery, when the aging process has come to fruition, much more difficult. This is obviously a matter of personal preference, and some patients will persist in having work done regardless of the surgeon's preferences. This is a matter for each individual practice. For ours, all primary facelifts are done via the deep plane techniques.

A variety of midfacial approaches have been proposed over the last 15 years. The point of origin for most of these procedures is from the work of Tessier.[13] Several variations of this approach have been proposed.[14-26]

We favor the deep plane technique over the subperiosteal midface approach for several reasons. The first is the direct nature in which the deep plane technique addresses the fallen tissue. The focus of midfacial rejuvenation is the suspension of the soft tissues of the midface that have fallen with time. In the deep plane technique, the surgeon may directly manipulate this tissue to the desired location. To state the issue directly, deep plane surgery "works at the level at which mobility and aging laxity are occurring."[27] The tissue to be repositioned in the midface is the cheek fat that rests on the zygomaticus musculature. With elevating the soft tissues off of the zygomatic musculature, the surgeon may now address the nasolabial fold and the descent of the soft tissues in a manner not possible before. A SMAS correction is inherently more effective than a subperiosteal approach in the midcheek because it is closer to the tissue to be repositioned.[28]

In addition, the nerves that innervate the facial musculature enter from below. Thus, it stands to reason that dissection techniques that leave the nervous structures between the plane of dissection and the target tissue leave the nerves at risk from either direct trauma through inadvertent movements of the dissector or, more commonly, through traction neuropraxia. The subperiosteal technique has been reported to have a high rate of facial nerve injuries, implying a steep learning curve.[14]

Edema from periosteal manipulations is significant, and for it to persist for weeks, if not months, is not uncommon.[29-31] To patients who are expecting a "minimally invasive" procedure, this may prove to be a difficult issue. In the subperiosteal approach, the zygomaticus musculature is repositioned to a place it never was before, the intermalar distance is necessarily increased, and frequently manipulation of the lateral canthus is required.[32] Not only is the lateral canthus often altered, but the

resetting of the zygomaticus musculature may also lead to an unwanted alteration of the patient's appearance.[33] One must be concerned about the potential for distortion of the palpebral fissure with many of these procedures.[34-38]

When an open lower lid blepharoplasty approach is incorporated into the subperiosteal midfacial techniques, the lower lid malposition rate has been reported to be as high as 50%.[36]

Our approach to facelifting, as with our overall practice approach, is the attainment of a natural, lasting result via conservative means. We seek to provide the patient with rejuvenation where the observer cannot detect that an operation has occurred. The deep plane technique may not be considered conservative in some quarters, but with the technique performed as described herein, we feel it to be exceedingly safe and well tolerated by the patient.

ANATOMY

The facelift surgeon must be fully versed in the complex anatomy of the face. A complete discussion of the anatomic relationships is beyond the scope of this chapter and the reader is advised to refer to excellent published reports on this challenging territory.[39-41] There are several anatomic keys to the aging face, and specific areas of concern are discussed. As we age, some of the most profound effects are noted in the midface. A key to the deep plane technique is the anatomy of the midcheek and malar region.

The cheek mass descends with age and causes a deepened nasolabial fold inferiorly while creating a depression at the infraorbital rim (Fig. 8-1).[42] The malar fat pad atrophies and descends with age leading to a deepened nasolabial fold, a crescent-shaped hollowness at the lid-cheek interface and nasojugal groove, and lack of cheek prominence, giving a sunken, tired appearance.[43] The effects of gravity are more pronounced on superficial tissues.[29,42]

Another feature of midfacial aging is the buccal fat pad. It provides fullness to the cheek in youth and diminishes, relatively, in size as the patient ages.[44] This fat pad has four major components with the buccal being the largest. On the lateral aspect of the masseter lies this parotid-masseteric fascia, a key structure in the deep plane technique. This fascia layer is found between the overlying SMAS and the underlying branches of the facial nerve (Figs. 8-2 and 8-3). Fortunately, this fascia binds the branches of the facial nerve down, a key factor when placing extreme traction on the SMAS to expose the deep plane. As this fascia continues anteriorly, it shifts superiorly to envelop the buccal fat pad, parotid duct, and buccal branches of the facial nerve.[44-46]

Another important area of the midface is the nasolabial fold.[47-49] The nasolabial fold is a true anatomic

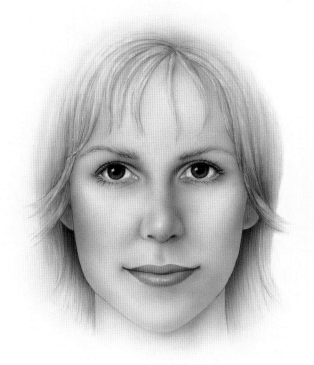

A

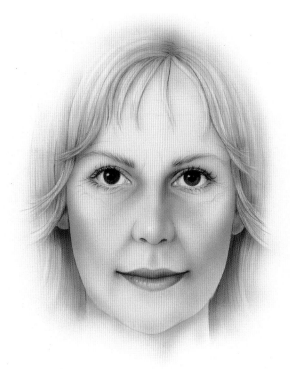

B

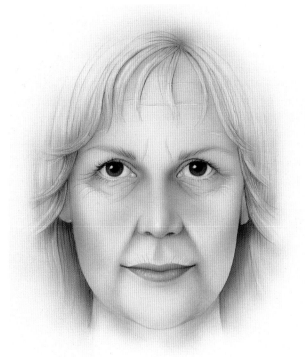

C

Figure 8-1 The graduated stages of the aging face.

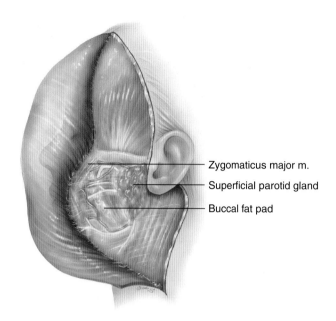

Zygomaticus major m.

Superficial parotid gland

Buccal fat pad

Figure 8-2 A comprehensive view of the important landmarks for the deep plane technique.

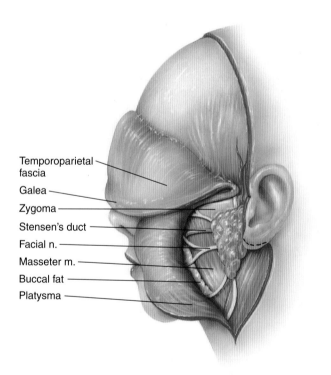

Temporoparietal fascia

Galea

Zygoma

Stensen's duct

Facial n.

Masseter m.

Buccal fat

Platysma

Figure 8-3 The elevated SMAS and its relationship to adjacent structures; note the platysma is continuous with the face as it extends superiorly into the face, a key dissection plane for the deep plane lift. The superior aspect of the anatomic planes is for illustrative purposes alone and is not a component of the deep plane technique

boundary between the fatty cheek above and the upper lip below.[47] As the tissues of the midface become ptotic with age the nasolabial fold deepens and becomes of greater concern to the patient.

The lower aspect of the face is dominated by jowling and submental fat. The jowling that so troubles the aging population results from the descent of the platysma muscle in the neck and face with the associated fat and skin along the mandibular line. The platysma has been described as having a graded aging process.[50,51] The history of submental fat resection is often attributed to the work of Millard and others.[52,53]

The SMAS merits specific discussion. First described by Mitz and Peyronie, the SMAS layer and manipulations thereof have intrigued facial plastic surgeons for 30 years.[54] This layer has been seen as an extension of the platysma into the face (see Figs. 8-2 and 8-3). The SMAS is considered to be a fibromuscular structure that lies in continuity with the platysma and has no bony attachments.[54-60] The layer is thought to consist of connective tissue and muscle. The SMAS has fibrous extensions that connect it to the skin.[61,62] The SMAS is thicker in its lateral aspect over the parotid and tapers as it travels medially.[61] Our experience concurs with this report. There has also been controversy over the relationship of the SMAS to the parotid fascia as to whether they are separate layers or one and the same.[55-59,63,64] Whether they are one and the same or distinct layers means little to the surgeon. The key point is that there is a fascia layer to be raised in this region and its thickness varies from patient to patient. We have found the SMAS to taper as the deep plane dissection is carried medially.

The SMAS is noted to be muscular in its inferior component where the platysma rises into the face and more fibrous as the surgeon goes further cephalad as the platysma tapers. In the more muscular, inferior portion of the SMAS, facial nerve branches are commonly seen traversing the masseter muscle on the floor of the dissection as the deep plane is raised (see Figs. 8-2 and 8-3).

Also of note during our dissection technique are the retaining ligaments of the face. The key ligaments for our procedure are the zygomatic ligament and the masseteric ligaments.[65] The zygomatic ligament may be released as the dissection proceeds to the origin of the zygomaticus major at the anterior aspect of the zygomatic arch. Care should be taken in this area, as it is closely associated with the facial nerve. The masseteric ligaments pose a challenge for the surgeon in that they closely resemble peripheral branches of the facial nerve. When dissecting in the correct plane these ligaments may be safely released.

The vascularity of the deep plane technique is an important concept. Schuster and associates described three concentric vascular arcades.[66,67] The most lateral arcade is drawn from the zygomatico-orbital and transverse facial arteries. The middle arcade consists of the infraorbital and facial artery connected by the middle and posterior jugal branches, and the medial arcade contains the angular artery, superior and inferior labial arteries, and a branch of the ophthalmic artery. When raising a skin flap in the SMAS or skin-only facelift this outermost arcade is traumatized as a random flap is created. As this flap is developed blood must pass through a choke zone as it traverses one arcade to another. The further medial this dissection is carried, the more tenuous the blood supply becomes as the blood must now pass through two choke zones. The deep plane technique avoids this vascular compromise.

There is great concern for the temporal branch and the marginal mandibular branch, due to their respective lack of anastomotic connections, during deep plane rhytidectomy.[68] There are usually four rami of the nerve that cross the zygomatic arch, though this number varies, of course. The most anterior ramus is an average of 2.0 cm posterior to the anterior end of the zygomatic arch. The danger zone is located in a region overlying the zygomatic arch approximately 2.0 cm anterior to the superior attachment of the auricle and 2.0 cm posterior to the bony orbital rim. It is in this area that the nerve is just beneath the subcutaneous fat and directly overlying the bony prominence of the zygoma.[68] When employing the deep plane technique, the surgeon must also be cognizant of the marginal mandibular branch anatomy. As the surgeon aggressively attempts to rid the patient of jowling with an anterior dissection in the lower face he or she must note that the marginal branch is located deep to the platsyma until approximately 2.0 cm lateral to the corner of the mouth. At this point, the nerve takes a more superficial trajectory along the undersurface of the facial mimetic muscles. The facial artery can also be used as a guide. Posterior to the vessels the nerve is generally not in the dissection; however, anterior to the vessels the surgeon must proceed with caution.[69] The most commonly injured nerve in rhytidectomy is the greater auricular. This structure is located approximately 6.5 cm inferior to the bony auditory canal.[70]

PREOPERATIVE ASSESSMENT

Prior to the analysis of the patient's cosmetic desires and possibilities, a thorough history and physical examination must be performed. This is especially true for aesthetic surgery. As an elective procedure there can be no excuse for an overlooked medical issue that can compromise the outcome. General issues that should be investigated include previous surgeries, medications, smoking and alcohol intake, and any coexisting medical conditions. Specific issues to facial rejuvenation surgery such as the use of aspirin and other nonsteroidal anti-inflammatory medications, hypertension, and smoking history should be thoroughly explored and explained to the patient. In addition, there are several medical diseases the facial plastic surgeon must respect. Obviously, any blood dyscrasia must be evaluated with a hematologist. Also, several connective tissue disorders, such as Ehlers-Danlos

syndrome, may compromise the result of an otherwise good operation.

Perhaps of equal importance in the preoperative assessment is the evaluation of the patient's psyche by the surgeon. We make a point to ascertain the patient's motivation for the proposed procedure(s). This is a highly individualized approach that each surgeon must discover for himself or herself. We cannot stress enough the importance of this evaluation. No matter what the technique nor how well it is executed, a psychologically impaired patient will not be pleased.

The surgeon should then evaluate the nature of the skin. Sun damage, smoking history, and Fitzpatrick type are but a few of the skin features that must be assessed during the preoperative consultation process. Fair skin with a moderate amount of sun damage usually heals best, but darker skin types necessitate more caution on the part of the surgeon. The patient should be questioned as to his or her healing history and any preexisting medical conditions or medications that might hinder the healing process.

After the initial examination of the skin we prefer to examine the overall appearance of the face. The patient's ethnicity, body habitus, and age all play a role in this initial assessment. The general proportions of the face should be considered. The face is generally broken down into fifths vertically, based on the width of an eye; and thirds horizontally, as measured from the hairline to the glabella, from the glabella to the subnasale and from the subnasale to the menton. Any facial asymmetries should be noted at this time. All faces have some level of asymmetry. This is normal and should be conveyed to the patient, preoperatively.

The surgeon should then proceed to examine the patient's bony infrastructure. This is the scaffolding on which the soft tissues of the face are suspended. The malar prominence, mandible, and hyoid positions are all examined and palpated. A strong bony structure to the face is obviously the favorable situation.

The soft tissue components of the face are the final facet of the examination. Jowling, buccal fat, the sagging midface and nasolabial fold, infraorbital hollowness, and the aging neck are the focal points of the soft tissue examination. The scope of this chapter is not to elaborate on these components as they are described in other portions of the text.

SURGICAL TECHNIQUE

Nearly all of our deep plane facelifts are performed under general anesthesia. Usually, these procedures are combined with a series of other facial rejuvenation procedures (browlifts, blepharoplasties, etc.). It is certainly acceptable to perform the procedures under local anesthesia with sedation. Our preference for general anesthesia is based on patient comfort and safety, in addition to surgeon preference. We believe that intubation is the safest form of airway management during these long cases when a significant amount of sedation and analgesic agents are administered. It is also an optimal environment for the surgeon, having been relieved of a moving, sometimes talkative, and restless patient. Relieved of the need to constantly monitor the airway and patient comfort, the surgeon may focus on the task at hand.

After administration of the anesthetic the patient is prepped. The first step in our preparation is a minor shaving of hair in the pre- and postauricular areas. The preauricular area is shaved to enable the "bird's beak" incision, which extends horizontally to the temporal hair tuft through the sideburn.[71] The postauricular shaving is performed by noting the superior aspect of the conchal bowl and drawing a straight line in an inferoposterior vector from this point (Fig. 8-4). Regular masking tape is then applied to tuck the remaining hair out of the field.

A thorough injection of local anesthetic (an equal mixture of 0.5% lidocaine with 1:200,000 epinephrine and 0.5% bupivacaine with 1:200,000 epinephrine) is then performed in the subdermal planes of dissection bilaterally. The surgeon should note the character of the skin and dermis during the injection, especially in revision procedures. When performed in conjunction with other procedures, the facelift is always performed last to ensure that a compressive dressing may be placed at the

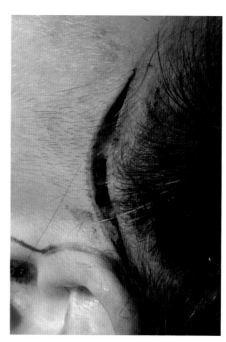

Figure 8-5 The anterosuperior aspect of the incision is made. This incision is beveled, consistent with hair-saving principles.

termination of the case. The face and neck are then prepped and draped in standard surgical fashion and the head is wrapped with a sterile towel and clamped. The endotracheal tube is draped in a sterile stocking.

Our incision placement is dictated by the desire to preserve hair and create the optimal vectors for lifting the tissue in a natural manner. Thus, we choose to bring the anterior and superior aspect of the incision forward, through the sideburn hair with a gentle curve as it progresses anteriorly (Fig. 8-5). Care is taken to maintain an adequate amount of sideburn hair that will grow over and thus mask the scar. In order to maintain a normal hair pattern the preauricular tuft must not be advanced over the level of the supraauricular sulcus.[72] By employing a frontotemporal hairline incision the surgeon may place the vector of lift more superiorly than lateral. It is not a pure vector but we feel it minimizes untoward sequelae.[33,73-75] We agree with others that the classic incision beginning at the superior attachment of the auricle and tracing superior and posterior inherently shifts the hair in unnatural fashion and can be a stigma of facelift surgery.[72,76,77]

The postauricular incision is marked by bisecting the superior aspect of the shaved hair, as noted from the superior conchal bowl vector, to the inferior aspect of the native hairline. The preauricular incision is marked horizontally from the temporal hair tuft, through the sideburn, now shaved, to the bird's beak above the ear. The incision then traverses inferiorly in a native preauricular crease in a pretragal fashion. The preauricular incision then gradually wraps around the lobular attach-

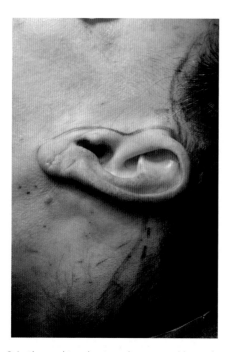

Figure 8-4 The markings begin at the temporal hair tuft and through the sideburn to the bird's beak. The planned incision then traverses the preauricular area, around the lobule, and onto the posterior surface of the auricle. The incision terminates in the postauricular hair-bearing area that has been bisected as shown.

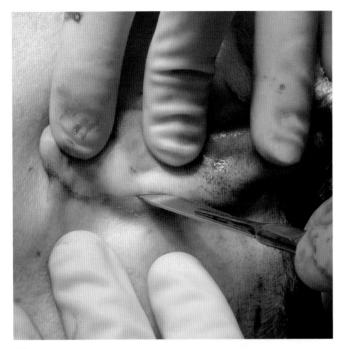

Figure 8-6 The postauricular incision is made slightly onto the posterior aspect of the conchal bowl, out of the sulcus. This position is due to the forward traction placed on the auricle. When released, the incision will rest in the sulcus. The surgeon should not disrupt the perichondrium.

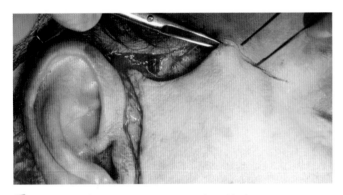

Figure 8-7 The anterior extension may be added in revision cases or in those in whom excess of skin is to be removed. This is generally performed in older patients with an abundance of lines to mask the incision.

ment and slightly onto the posterior aspect of the conchal bowl as it rises to reach the posterior take-off near the superior aspect of the conchal bowl (Fig. 8-6). Occasionally, the anterior aspect of the incision must be extended into the temple region when the surgeon anticipates that a significant amount of skin will be removed. It is vital to place this extension within a natural rhytid emanating from the lateral orbital skin (Fig. 8-7).[78,79] This extension is commonly used in revision procedures and in older patients who have extremely lax skin with multiple fine rhytids.

The lengths of the anterior and posterior components of the incisions are dictated by the anticipated amount of skin mobilization and resection. The function of these

incisions is primarily to manage the dog-ears that occur with the advancement of the flap. The lift is basically a posterior and anterior rotation flap with a central advancement component.[80]

All incisions are made with a No. 10 blade. We prefer the use of these larger blades because with their increased surface area the knife stays sharper for longer periods, an important factor when performing extensive incisions. The incision begins at the anterior/superior aspect and traverses the preauricular portion, around the lobule, and onto the postauricular portion, where it terminates in the hairline. The initial portion of the incision, through the sideburn, should be performed with a beveled blade parallel to the follicles to ensure masking hair growth during the recovery period. The incision is beveled in accordance with accepted hair-saving principles.[81]

Once the incisions have been performed the skin is then elevated. The bird's beak area is grasped with an Adson forceps and using a sharp, fine scissors, the skin elevation is begun. We prefer to use a transillumination technique to ensure proper depth of dissection. The plane of dissection is subdermal, just inferior to the hair follicles. With the transillumination technique the assistant places the overhead lights onto the skin while the operative field has no direct light (Fig. 8-8). This is in direct opposition to the commonly used technique of bright illumination from behind the surgeon's head and onto the field. Once adequate skin has been raised, several different instruments can be used to retract the skin. A thimble with a double prong, a variety of rake retractors, and our preference, the Anderson bear claw, are all acceptable retractors. The skin elevation, as with almost all our dissection maneuvers, requires an excellent assistant to provide countertraction. Other technical

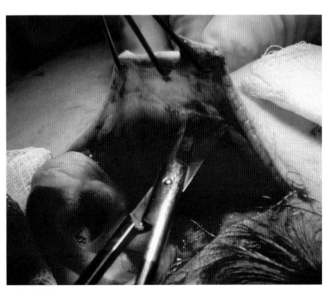

Figure 8-8 The transillumination technique ensures proper depth of dissection.

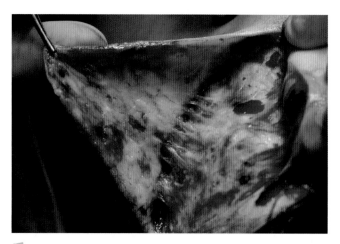

Figure 8-9 The postauricular skin is raised, displaying the thin flap and adherent fascia overlying the sternocleidomastoid muscle.

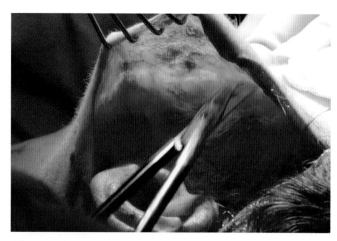

Figure 8-10 The extent of skin dissection using the transillumination technique.

aspects worthy of mention include the dissection over the sternocleidomastoid musculature. The fascia in this area can be very adherent leading to injury of the great auricular nerve if care is not taken (Fig. 8-9).[82] After discerning the plane, we change scissors from sharp-tipped to dull. Many surgeons will perform a blunt dissection of the subdermal plane, which is definitely acceptable. But in this day and age of minimal downtimes and the need for expedient recoveries, we have found our technique to be less traumatic to the tissues and thus our postoperative edema is considerably less than if we employed the blunt dissection techniques.

The subdermal elevation is continued for approximately 5 to 6 cm from the incision points (Figs. 8-10 and 8-11). This dissection may be carried slightly more anterior in the region of the malar eminence, where the dissection turns deeper as the deep plane is raised.

In the inferior aspect of the dissection, the subdermal plane is raised until the surgeon reaches the angle of the mandible. At this point, a lighted retractor is used to dissect the posterolateral portion of the platysma (Fig. 8-12). The overhead lights used for transillumination are now removed from the field. The subdermal dissection should be relatively bloodless as long as adequate local has been injected and sufficient time has transpired.

Once the edge of the platysma has been identified, the plane can be rapidly developed with broad spreading movements of the dissecting scissors. The preplatysma dissection may require the use of extra long scissors to dissect to the midline. We try to lift all of the subdermal fat off the muscle, leaving a clean plane of muscle at the floor of the dissection.

We infrequently perform liposuction of the neck, though it is a viable option in select cases. We prefer direct excision of fat. We concur with other authors that liposuction can lead to several postoperative issues that are exceedingly difficult to remedy. As with many other issues in plastic surgery, it is best to underdo this portion of the

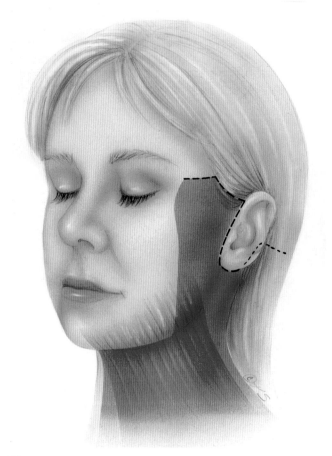

Figure 8-11 The shaded area depicts the extent of the subcutaneous dissection.

procedure than to try to attain the "perfect" result, which can lead to drastic, difficult postoperative issues.[83,84]

After completely elevating the skin and subcutaneous tissue from the platysma, the surgeon pays attention to the deep plane. We prefer to enter this plane 2 to 3 cm anterior and slightly superior to the angle of the mandible

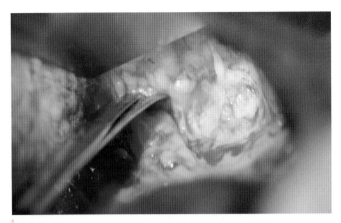

Figure 8-12 The lateral aspect of the platysma is dissected. The red muscle is seen on the floor of this dissection.

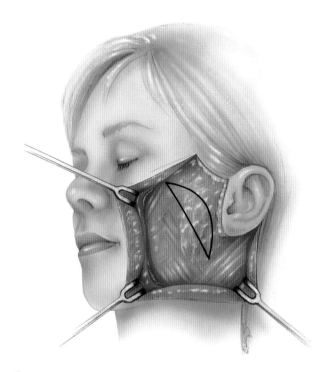

Figure 8-14 The deep plane incised. The outlined portion illustrates the amount of tissue excised when the flap is suspended.

inferiorly (Figs. 8-13 and 8-14). A line may be marked for the incision into the deep plane from just above the angle of the mandible to the junction of the zygomatic arch and body. This incision, as with all others in the deep plane technique, is performed with the No. 10 blade. The incision into the deep plane is generally placed near the anterior aspect of the parotid gland. By placing the incision this far forward with a curve at the superior aspect, the frontal branch of the facial nerve is avoided in the dissection because it is posterior and superior to the incision into the deep plane (Fig. 8-15).

The lighted retractor, preferably with nonlacerating teeth, is used to gain a purchase of the SMAS and the surgeon's wrist is turned to place the SMAS under tension. The assistant provides countertraction similar to that provided when raising the skin flap. This can be awkward

for the surgeon and assistant until the move is learned. Patience is encouraged in attaining the proper balance of retraction between surgeon and assistant.

With the SMAS held taut by the lighted retractor and the countertraction provided by the assistant the plane is incised with the No. 10 blade (Fig. 8-16). Almost immediately after opening this plane, the surgeon will note the SMAS lifted up with the retractor at the roof of the dissection while the masseteric fascia falls to the floor, broadly displaying the deep plane (Figs. 8-17 and 8-18). Occasionally, facial nerve branches can be seen traversing this fascia (Fig. 8-19). The surgeon can take great comfort in that as long as the masseteric fascia is seen, the facial nerve branches are intact. Once opened, the plane can be developed with either a scissors in a spreading fashion or with the No. 10 blade in a pushing motion. We prefer to use the No. 10 blade to push down the connective tissue attachments from the undersurface of the flap (Fig. 8-20). The muscle fibers of the platysma are usually seen on the undersurface of the flap and are used as guide for the dissection. The blade should be positioned so as to peel fibers from the undersurface as opposed to using the knife from the floor of the dissection and pushing the fibers up to the undersurface of the platysma. The surgeon must be mindful of the position of the mandible as the dissection continues anteriorly and inferiorly so as not to risk injury to the marginal mandibular nerve.

After mobilization of the inferior aspect of the flap, attention is then directed to the superior portion of the

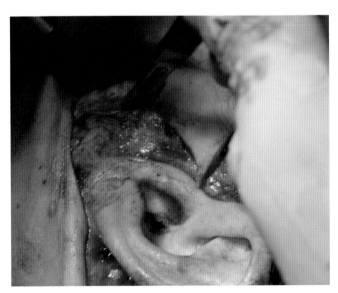

Figure 8-13 The inferior portion of the deep plane is entered over the masseter muscle approximately 2 to 3 cm anterior and slightly superior to the angle of the mandible.

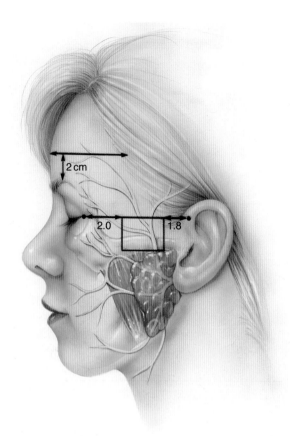

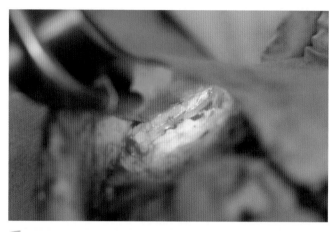

Figure 8-17 The deep plane has been exposed and tension, with the lighted retractor, must be utilized to further dissect the plane. The retractor is placed immediately superficial to the incision and elevated away from the face. The assistant provides vital countertraction (note the fingers of the assistant) and the plane is dissected.

Figure 8-15 The trajectory of the frontal branch of the facial nerve is depicted. Note that the placement of the incision into the deep plane is anterior to these rami and thus protects the nerve from injury.

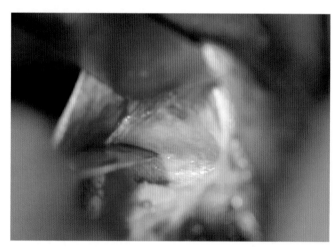

Figure 8-18 With adequate traction, and countertraction, the plane immediately shows itself.

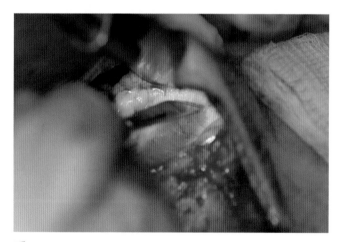

Figure 8-16 The superior aspect of the incision is made and the flap is raised. Note the near pure anterior vector of the incision over the zygoma, as the incision is directly over the bone.

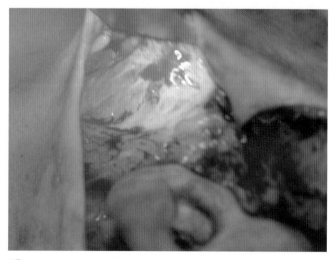

Figure 8-19 The masseteric fascia ensures the underlying facial nerve branches are intact.

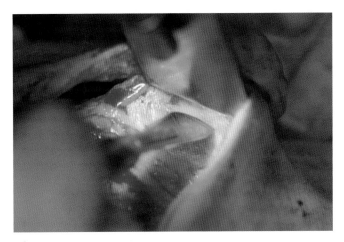

Figure 8-20 The blade is angled superficially and the connective tissue is pushed down from the undersurface of the flap.

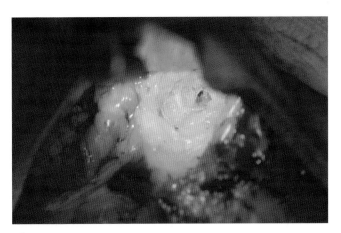

Figure 8-22 The origin of the zygomaticus major is seen as the red muscle in the distal aspect of the dissection

dissection. With a finger, the surgeon palpates the zygomatic arch to ascertain the location of the notch on the inferior aspect of this bone. With the No. 10 blade, he or she makes an incision approximately 1 to 2 cm in front of this landmark.

The zygomatic major muscle is the key structure to be identified (Figs. 8-21 to 8-23). Often, a small, perforating branch of the transverse facial artery will be encountered before the zygomaticus is completely identified. This is carefully addressed with bipolar cautery. Discerning the zygomaticus from the lateral, inferior aspect of the orbicularis is often difficult, and the surgeon should consider the depth of the dissection to ensure proper identification, the orbicularis being the more superficial of the two muscles.

Once free, the zygomaticus provides an excellent landmark as the surgeon continues freeing the soft tissues of the midface anteriorly while safeguarding the facial

nerve branches deep to the muscle.[46] It is often necessary to incise the tissue anterior to this muscle to completely mobilize it. Superior dissection is generally avoided secondary to the persistent edema that results from surgical manipulation in this region. This edema persists

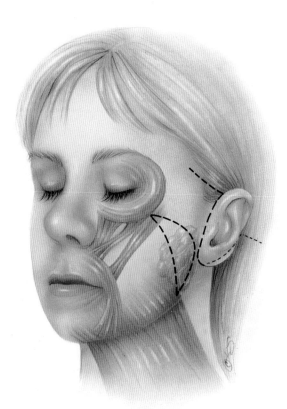

Figure 8-23 The key anatomic relationships of the deep plane dissection are depicted. The superior aspect of the dissection is at the superior segment of the zygomaticus major. The zygomaticus serves as a safe guide for the dissection as it progresses anteriorly. The inferior aspect of the deep plane is anterior to the mandible, at the posterior end of the platysma.

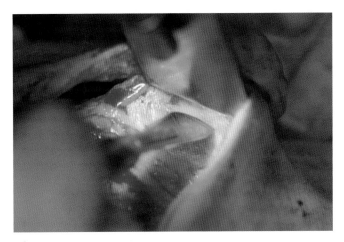

Figure 8-21 Once incised the upper portion of the deep plane is dissected to the origin of the zygomaticus major medially.

longer than any other in the deep plane facelift and can be most troublesome to patients. Thus, we have diverged from the composite technique as described by Hamra.[7,32,85,86] We prefer to perform our periorbital dissection in the blepharoplasty component of our facial rejuvenation. This is in contrast to others favoring the deep plane technique, where the periorbital rejuvenation is incorporated into the facelift component of the rejuvenation. Our preference to avoid dissection in the periorbital area is shared by others.[87] Our rationale is similar, to avoid excessive postoperative edema and recovery periods and the difficult issues that often arise with periorbital manipulation. Grounded in the excellent anatomic work of Pessa, we do not dissect superior to the caudal margin of the orbicularis oculi so as not to disrupt the malar septum.[40,41]

When this dissection is complete the surgeon will have the flap raised in two sections with an intervening ridge of adherent tissue between two well-developed planes (Fig. 8-24). The ligamentous attachments in this area are densely adherent. With the two well-developed portions of the plane as a guide, the surgeon may confidently use the No. 10 blade in a pushing fashion similar to that done with the inferior and superior aspects of the flap (Fig. 8-25). It is not recommended to dissect only the superior or inferior portion of the flap and then free this area. After dissecting the inferior plane the surgeon may be tempted to continue the dissection superiorly. The surgeon should avoid this temptation because it is easy to be led deep to the zygomaticus musculature and into the facial nerve branches. It is by connecting the tunnels that the surgeon may move forward with the dissection in a safe manner.

As the plane elevation continues the lighted retractor must be advanced with the advancing dissection to maintain appropriate tension at the point of dissection.

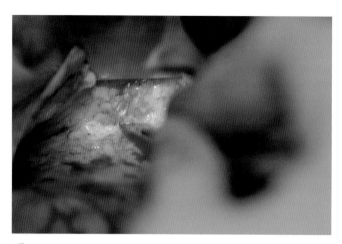

Figure 8-25 The medial aspect of the deep plane is raised using sharp dissection. Please note that the suspensory ligaments shown here must be released for a maximum lift.

The surgeon must retain focus on elevating the flap at the appropriate depth. It is common to migrate superficially as the flap is dissected anteriorly. This risks perforating the flap and limiting the tension that may be placed upon it when suspending the fallen tissues. There is no definitive anterior limit to the dissection. We generally try to free the flap to within 1 to 2 cm of the nasolabial fold.

Once raised, the surgeon may address the buccal fat pad if necessary. We generally do not perform resection of the buccal fat pad, but it is in the center of the field at the end of this dissection if the surgeon chooses to alter it. Care should be exercised here as this is deeper than the plane of dissection and the facial nerve branches are at greater risk.

The submental region poses unique challenges. Some patients may require no intervention in this region, others need submental liposuction, and yet others benefit from a submental incision with direct fat excision and platysmaplasty or platysmaplasty without fat excision.[78] When performing liposuction without platysmaplasty we create two small, 1-cm incisions within a native crease. When combining platysmaplasty either with direct submental fat excision or liposuction the approach is via a 2- to 3-cm incision in a natural submental crease. The planned incision is injected with local anesthetic and the incision is made. A small subcutaneous dissection is performed until the medial aspects of the paired platysma muscles are defined (Fig. 8-26). The medial edges of these muscles, or bands, are completely freed and the dissection is carried laterally to meet with the previously undermined skin in the neck. This dissection is performed with a headlight. There are a variety of rakes and retractors that can be utilized for this step of the procedure. We prefer a small fine rake followed by a malleable retractor. Again, the use of countertraction by the assistant greatly facilitates this dissection.

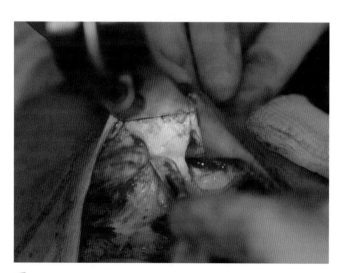

Figure 8-24 The intervening bridge of tissue separating the superior and inferior portions of the deep plane is dissected using the push-down technique.

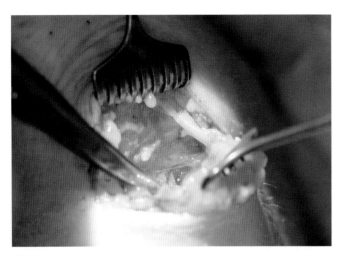

Figure 8-26 The medial aspects of the paired platysma muscles are dissected via a submental incision in a natural skin crease.

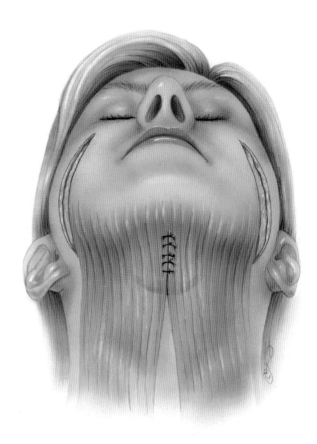

Figure 8-27 The medial edges of the trimmed platysma muscles are bound with permanent suture.

After the medial aspects of the muscles are freed, the flaccid medial components, bands, are grasped with an Allis clamp. A Kelly clamp is then placed parallel to the excess musculature being retracted by the Allis. This excess tissue is then sharply excised and the clamp is released. Care should be exercised so as not to pull on the tissues excessively with the Allis to make sure that an excess of platysma is not removed. There is little need for hemostasis as the clamp is released. After the excess platysma is removed, the free ends are then bound with buried 3-0 Prolene (Fig. 8-27). This closure should be tensionless so that when the tissue is suspended in the superolateral vector the bound platysma muscles do not shred. The surgeon must be cautious not to remove too much platysma, as the actual mechanism of tightening the neck is from the superolateral movement of the deep plane and skin, not the midline binding of the muscle. The bound muscles act as a sling to lift the submental region.

After completing the platysmal portion of the procedure, fat may then be directly excised from the undersurface of the skin and subcutaneous flap with standard facelift scissors or by meticulous liposuction under direct visualization. We use both direct and submental liposuction to remove excess fat in this area depending on the severity of the amount of fat. We prefer, as do others, direct lipectomy for removal of significant amounts of fat. With the direct exposure the surgeon may comfortably remove adequate fat while maintaining the masking properties of this fat layer.[88]

The surgeon should display extreme caution in this aspect of the case. This is not a fat removal procedure. Although there is a strong temptation to aggressively utilize this technique many patients may develop profound anterior banding because the cushioning padding of fat has been removed. At the far end of this spectrum is the "cobra" deformity which manifests as a deep submental concavity as a result of oversuctioned fat.[83,88] Once this deformity is created it is exceedingly difficult to remedy.

The surgeon can sculpt the preexisting fat but should avoid operating on patients with an excessive amount of fat in the submental area. It is recommended to have the patient lose the excess weight prior to any surgical manipulation. Before closure, the surgeon should reassess the area to make sure a smooth contour surface exists with no irregularities. A suction drain is then placed in the preplatysmal plane and suspension of the flaps is begun.

The drain serves two purposes. The first is to limit postoperative hematoma formation. Although no drain prevents, or resolves, a true hematoma, a drain can minimize the extent of the complication. The other purpose of the drain is to evacuate normal fluid that accumulates under the flap and prolongs the healing process. While these collections are generally physiologically benign, in this era a premium is placed on a speedy recovery and return to normal activity. With the drain, this recovery is hastened.

At this point, the lateral aspect of the deep plane flap is grasped and pulled in a superolateral vector and sutured in the preauricular area (Fig. 8-28). The surgeon should attempt to move the flap as superior as possible and avoid a lateral pull as that leads to the "operated

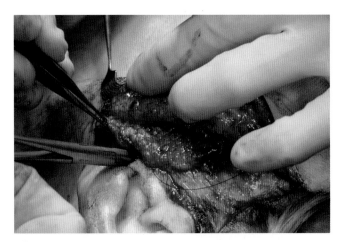

Figure 8-28 The deep plane flap is grasped near the angle of the mandible and using a near vertical vector is suspended superiorly with a buried 3-0 Prolene suture.

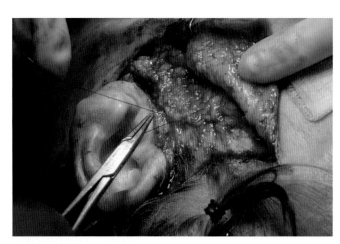

Figure 8-29 The last of several suspension sutures is placed.

look" dreaded by surgeon and patient alike. When suspending the deep plane, the surgeon should minimize tension. If not, the SMAS will elongate over time and the improvement will be gradually lost.[89]

As desirable as a purely vertical vector is in facelifting, when oblique traction is applied to the lateral face the distortions that are produced with a purely vertical lift are minimized, such as crowding of tissue at the lateral orbital rim.[27] The superior vector is usually limited with a dog-ear of the deep plane and skin flaps anteriorly. The flap is then sutured in place with buried 3-0 Prolene sutures. We choose Prolene less for its permanent effect than for its excellent biocompatibility and inert nature. We have rarely had any of our deep Prolene sutures spit.

Infrequently, we need to incise the posterior aspect of the deep plane flap to redrape it behind the ear to the mastoid tip. The suture suspensions track from the mastoid tip to the superoanterior aspect of the flap near the zygomatic arch (Fig. 8-29). In the region of the zygomatic arch we often use a smaller caliber suture, 4-0 or 5-0 Prolene, depending on the nature of the flap and overlying skin. If the tissue lying between the sutures is rough and will be palpable through the overlying skin, we will run a 4-0 or 5-0 caliber suture through these areas to smooth them. When suspending the inferior aspects of the flap, near the lateral edge of the platysma, the surgeon should take care not to place excessive tension on one side of the flap. This is to avoid difficulties in suspending the contralateral, lower region of the flap. Here the surgeon is basically pulling against himself or herself.

When the flap suspension is complete, the surgeon will more often note puckering at the interface of the skin flap and deep plane. With a sharp scissors, he or she should free these regions with caution. It is possible to perforate the deep plane flap when performing this tailoring if the surgeon migrates deeply. This can be fixed

with a 4-0 Prolene, but it is obviously best to avoid this problem with a careful dissection technique.

The skin flap is then tailored and sutured into place. The first step in this process is to grasp the flap and redrape it along a superolateral vector and secure it to the region immediately above the ear. With the tissue firmly held with an Adson forceps, a No. 11 blade is then used to incise the skin at the point of approximation between the flap and area superior to the auricular root. As with draping of the deep plane flap, the primary vector should be superior and limited by the amount of dog-ear formation anteriorly. The anterior aspect of our incision is a more favorable vector for tissue suspension.[75]

Once incised, a key suture is placed to reapproximate the opposing edges (Fig. 8-30). At this point the surgeon will have a dog-ear anteriorly between the suture and the most anterior component of the incision, near the anterior portion of the sideburn. This dog-ear is marked and

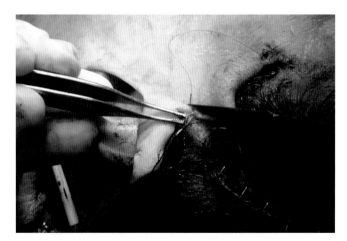

Figure 8-30 The first skin suspension suture is placed. The skin flap is suspended in a superolateral vector. The flap is incised with a No. 11 blade as it is held in the desired location with an Adson forceps.

excised and the opposing skin edges are stapled (Figs. 8-31 and 8-32). We prefer stapling rather than suturing in this area because the staples are masked by the hair and we believe the staples cause less constriction of the blood vessels, thus maximizing blood supply to the regenerating hair follicles.

The next key suture is the postauricular tacking stitch. The skin flap is grasped in the postauricular region and draped in an almost direct superior vector. As opposed to the preauricular tacking suture a No. 11 blade is not needed to incise the flap. In actuality, the surgeon is grasping tissue that previously lay at the level near the lobule and advancing it to the turnoff point of the postauricular incision as it turns posterior into the hairline. This will leave a dog-ear in the hair-bearing area. This is marked, excised, and stapled in an identical fashion to the preauricular dog-ear (Fig. 8-33).

At this juncture the fashioning of the preauricular incision is performed. The surgeon should grasp the skin

with an Adson forceps in front of the ear, and using the inferior conchal bowl as a guide the surgeon cuts the skin with a scissors to the area immediately inferior to the tragus. The preauricular skin is then tailored, with this mark as a guide (Fig. 8-34). When excising the excess skin the surgeon should leave a 2- to 3-mm gap between the opposing skin edges (Fig. 8-35) to compensate for the inherent residual laxity that causes a sheared appearance to the scar as it heals. Obviously care must also be taken to avoid leaving too large a gap and thus creating a situation of extreme tension at the closure site, especially at the lobule where a satyr's ear may result. The skin closure is performed with 5-0 Prolene in a running, locking fashion that is begun at the lobular attachment with a vertical mattress suture (Fig. 8-36). Another vertical mattress suture is placed adjacent to this one and a running, locking suture is performed on the posterior aspect of the closure (Figs. 8-37 and 8-38). If a submental approach was performed, this incision is closed with interrupted vertical mattress sutures.

After closure is complete, the wounds are coated with antibiotic ointment and a nonadherent Telfa dressing is placed over the incisions. The wounds are then dressed in a light compressive dressing of fluffed cotton and Kerlix. Figures 8-39 and 8-40 demonstrate preoperative and postoperative photographs of individuals who have undergone deep plane facelift procedures.

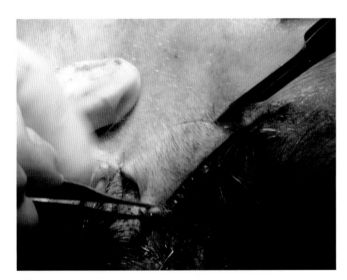

Figure 8-31 The anterior dog-ear is excised.

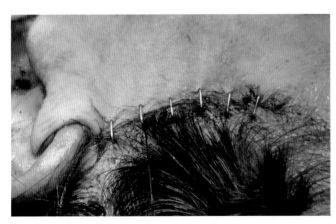

Figure 8-32 The anterior aspect of the incision is closed with staples.

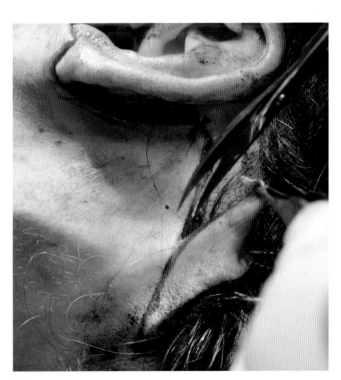

Figure 8-33 The posterior dog-ear is excised. This area is closed in a similar fashion to the anterior dog-ear.

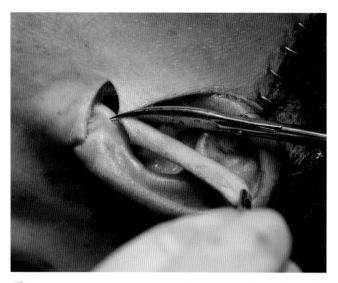

Figure 8-34 The preauricular excess skin is removed. Note the guiding cut at the inferior aspect of the tragus.

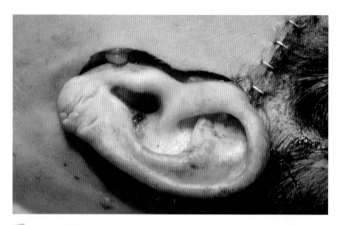

Figure 8-35 A 2- to 3-mm gap is ideal to compensate for postoperative skin laxity.

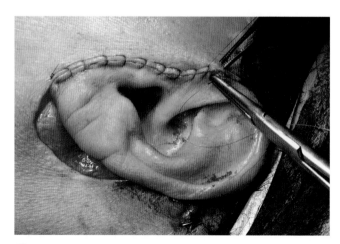

Figure 8-36 The preauricular closure is begun with a vertical mattress suture and completed in a running, locking fashion.

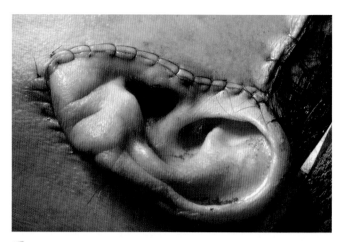

Figure 8-37 The complete closure. The postauricular incision is closed in an identical manner to the preauricular portion, starting with a vertical mattress and completed in a running, locking fashion.

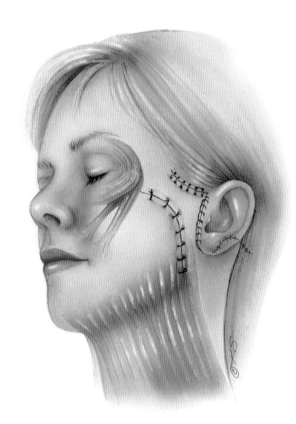

Figure 8-38 The complete closure is shown with the deeper suspension sutures.

POSTOPERATIVE CARE

The patient undergoing facial rejuvenation is very concerned about the night of his or her surgery. By keeping the patient within our facility, with our personnel, the patient is reassured of attendant care in a manner not possible in a hospital. And even though it is certainly acceptable to send the patient home, or to a hotel, on the night of the procedure with trained personnel, if a

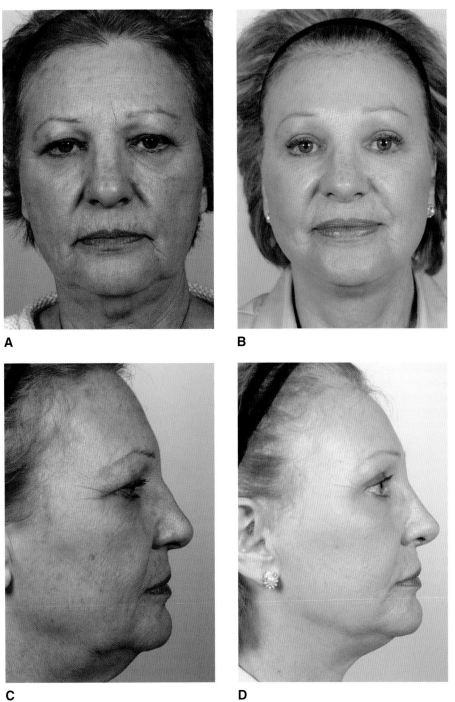

A

B

C

D

Figure 8-39 Preoperative frontal (**A**) and lateral (**C**) views of a 67-year-old woman. Postoperative frontal (**B**) and lateral (**D**) views of a 67-year-old woman after a tricophytic browlift, upper lid blepharoplasty, transconjunctival lower lid blepharoplasty with skin pinch, and deep plane facelift.

problem arises it is optimal to have the facilities to deal with such an issue immediately.

The following morning all drains are removed and a lighter compression dressing is placed. This lighter dressing is removed by the patient, at home, on the following day. The patient is instructed to maintain meticulous care of the incisions with 50% hydrogen peroxide and antibiotic ointment. On postoperative day 3 or 4 the preauricular and submental sutures are removed and the incisions are immediately taped with flesh tone tape after the application of an adhesive. The postau-

ricular sutures and staples are removed 1 week after the surgery, followed by the application of tape and adhesive. The tape remains on the incisions 24 hours a day for 1 week. After this period, depending on the patient's healing, we continue taping only at night for up to a month. We advise patients that they can return to nonstrenuous work within 1 week, though most patients choose to take 2 weeks off. The patient is also instructed that he or she may comfortably go out in public within 10 to 14 days. Strenuous activity may slowly commence 3 to 4 weeks from the procedure.

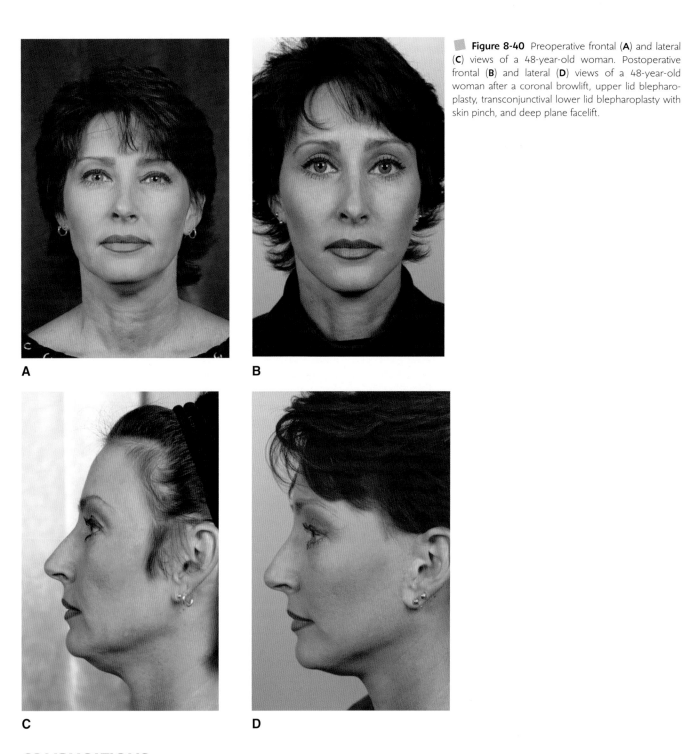

A

B

C

D

COMPLICATIONS

The most common risk with this technique, as with all facelifts, is hematoma formation. Hematomas predominantly occur within the first 6 to 12 hours after the procedure; thus our preference for keeping our patients within our facility. The only factor proved to increase the incidence of hematoma is preoperative hypertension.[90] The incidence of hematomas in facelift surgery has been reported between 0.3% and 15% with a variety of operative techniques.[90-96] For deep plane techniques, the incidence has been reported at 2.2% for major hematomas and 6.65% for minor hematomas. It should be noted that none of the hematomas in this report were in the deep plane, thus confirming the premise that this is a relatively avascular plane.[96] Left untreated, a facial hematoma can have catastrophic consequences.[97] The damage incurred with hematomas is greatly lessened when the issue is promptly noted and treated.

Other, less common issues may also occur. Skin loss is exceedingly rare with the enhanced vascularity seen with our technique. Infection is also very rare secondary to the excellent vascular supply to the face as a whole. Hypertrophic scarring in our practice is most commonly seen in the postauricular region and is managed with monthly Kenalog-10 injections and massage. These scars usually resolve given the appropriate time.

The most feared complication of the deep plane technique is facial nerve paralysis. In the senior author's practice of a decade with the technique described herein no permanent nerve injuries have occurred (unpublished data). Kamer has recently reported no facial nerve injuries in over 2600 cases with a similar deep plane technique.[98] Reports in the literature range from 0.4% to 2.6% for various techniques.[46,93,99-102] Although it seems counterintuitive, we feel that dissecting in a deeper plane is safer than other procedures. The surgical planes are very well delineated using our technique. It is not uncommon to notice a mild paresis within the first 6 hours after surgery. Calm should be maintained as this is most likely secondary to the use of local anesthesia. If the paresis exists beyond this time, patience must be practiced by both the physician and the patient, as the issue will likely resolve, albeit slowly.

The most common nerve injury is iatrogenic trauma to the greater auricular nerve.[103] Of the motor branches of the facial nerve, the frontal and marginal branches are at the greatest risk for a functional deficit. This is due to the lack of a significant anastomotic network.[46] For the deep plane and subsequent composite techniques, the reported rates of facial nerve injuries were 0.99% and zero percent, respectively, with no permanent weakness.[67]

approaching the midface through the lower lid must be weighed against the morbidity incurred.[106]

Our approach to facelifting, as with our overall practice approach, is the attainment of a natural result via conservative means. We seek to provide the patient with a lasting, natural result where the observer cannot detect that an operation has occurred. The deep plane technique may not be considered conservative in some quarters but with the technique performed as described herein we feel it to be exceedingly safe and well tolerated by the patient.

Various modalities have been recommended to address, and complement, trouble areas of facial rejuvenation such as the nasolabial folds. Fat grafting, soft tissue fillers, and alloplastic implants are all adjunctive methods that may be utilized by the surgeon to attain the optimal result. It is beyond the scope of this chapter to discuss, in detail, each of these methods. Each has its own strengths and weaknesses. Fat grafting is highly variable and there are donor site issues that must be considered. Soft tissue fillers do not have donor site considerations but there is the question of longevity, infection, and injection technique, which can be painful even with regional blocks. The more permanent tissue fillers can potentially cause palpable abnormalities. Alloplastic implants are a consideration, but unless the original issue was a hypoplastic malar eminence on retrognathia the surgeon must question what he or she is treating.

We have followed with great interest the progress of the invasive, minimally invasive, and endoscopic approaches to midfacial rejuvenation.[34,107-109] We feel, as do others, that an ideal midfacial rejuvenation procedure has yet to be determined (see Figs. 8-39 and 8-40).

Future Considerations

Long-standing improvement in the midface continues to be an elusive goal for the facial cosmetic surgeon. It has been found that after 12 years the improvement in the jawline is superior to that found in midface, as noted by improvement in the nasolabial fold. It should be noted in this report that the sample size was small, 20 patients, and that all patients were pleased with their results. Within this field of surgery patient satisfaction must be recognized and honored.[104,105]

We would suggest that this is not a technical fault, but merely that the patient does continue to age and that different components of the face age differently. An improvement that lasts for years should not be dismissed in this realm of surgery, especially with patients' understanding that they will continue to age and that we have an arsenal of techniques to deal with aging after the original procedure. We feel our techniques minimize the common sequelae of the standard facelift.[33,74]

To minimize the "lateral sweep," we prefer a prehairline incision in the temple region to make the vector more vertical.[29,74]

We have discussed the subperiosteal and composite techniques previously in this chapter. The benefits of

REFERENCES

1. Joseph J: Hangewangenplastik (Melomioplastik). Dtsch Med Wochenschr 1921;47:287.
2. Joseph J: Verbesserung meiner Hangewangenplastik (Melomioplastik). Dtsch Med Wochenschr 1928;54:567.
3. Passot R II: La correction chirurgicale des rides duvisage. Bull Acad Natl Med 1919;82:1120.
4. Larson DL: An historical glimpse of the evolution of rhytidectomy. Clin Plast Surg 1995;22:207.
5. Skoog T: Plastic surgery: The aging face. In Skoog TG: Plastic Surgery: New Methods and Refinements. Philadelphia: WB Saunders, 1974, p 300
6. Hamra ST: The deep plane rhytidectomy. Plast Reconstr Surg 1990;86:53.
7. Hamra ST: Composite rhytidectomy. Plast Reconstr Surg 1992;90(1):1.
8. Kamer FM: One hundred consecutive deep plane face lifts. Arch Otol Head Neck Surg 1996;122:17.
9. Godin MS, Johnson CM: Deep plane/composite rhytidectomy. Facial Plast Surg 1996;12:231.
10. Saulis AS, Lautenschlager EP, Mustoe TA: Biomechanical and viscoelastic properties of skin, SMAS, and composite flaps as they pertain to rhytidectomy. Plast Reconstr Surg 2002;110(2):590.

11. Becker FF, Bassichis BA: Deep-plane face-lift vs. superficial musculoaponeurotic system plication face-lift. Arch Facial Plast Surg 2004;6:8.

12. Ivy EJ, Lorenc ZP, Aston SJ: Is there a difference? A prospective study comparing lateral and standard SMAS face lifts with extended SMAS and composite rhytidectomies. Plast Reconstr Surg 1996;98(7):1135.

13. Tessier P: Lifting facial sous-perioste. Ann Chir Plast Esthet 1989;34:193.

14. Psillakis JM, Rumley TO, Carmargos A: Subperiosteal approach as an improved concept for correction of the aging face. Plast Reconstr Surg 1988;82:383.

15. Ramirez OM: The subperiosteal approach for the correction of the deep nasolabial fold and the central third of the face. Clin Plast Surg 1995;22(2):341.

16. Ramirez OM, Maillard GF, Musolas A: The extended A subperiosteal facelift: A definitive soft tissue remodeling for facial rejuvenation. Plast Reconstr Surg 1991;88:227.

17. Dempsey PD, Oneal RM, Izenberg PH: Subperiosteal brow and midface lift. Aesthet Plast Surg 1995;19:59.

18. Byrd HS, Andochick SE: The deep temporal lift: A multiplanar, lateral brow, temporal, and upper face lift. Plast Reconstr Surg 1996;97:928.

19. Ramirez OM: Endoscopic full facelift. Aesthet Plast Surg 1994;18:363.

20. Anderson RD, Lo MW: Endoscopic malar/midface suspension procedure. Plast Reconstr Surg 1998;102:2196.

21. Hester TR, Codner MA, McCord CD: The centrofacial approach for correction of facial aging using the transblepharoplasty subperiosteal cheek lift. Aesthet Surg Q 1996;16:51.

22. Hester TR, Codner MA , McCord CD, et al: Transorbital lower-lid and midface rejuvenation. Oper Tech Plast Reconstr Surg 1995;5:163.

23. Yaremchuk MJ: Subperiosteal and full-thickness skin rhytidectomy. Plast Reconstr Surg 2001;107(4):1045.

24. Ramirez OM: Fourth-generation subperiosteal approach to the midface: The tridimensional functional cheek lift. Aesthet Surg J 1998;18:133.

25. Hobar PC, Flood J: Subperiosteal rejuvenation of the midface and periorbital area: A simplified approach. Plast Reconstr Surg 1999;104:842.

26. Heinrichs HL, Kaidi AA: Subperiosteal face lift: A 200 case, 4-year review. Plast Reconstr Surg 1998;102:843.

27. Mendelson BC: Surgery of the superficial musculoaponeurotic system: Principles of release, vectors, and fixations. Plast Reconstr Surg 2001;107(6):1545.

28. Mendelson BC: Extended sub-SMAS dissection and cheek elevation. Clin Plast Surg 1995;22(2):325.

29. De Cordier BC, de la Torre JI, Al-Hakeem MS, et al: Rejuvenation of the midface by elevating the malar fat pad: Review of technique, cases, and complications. Plast Reconstr Surg 2002;110(6):526.

30. Mendelson BC: Volumetric perceptions in midfacial aging with altered priorities for rejuvenation and three-dimensional rejuvenation of the midface: Volumetric resculpture by malar imbrication (discussion). Plast Reconstr Surg 2000;105:286.

31. Sasaki GH, Cohen AT: Meloplication of the malar fat pads by percutaneous cable-suture technique for midface rejuvenation: Outcome study (392 cases, 6 years' experience). Plast Reconstr Surg 2002;110(2):635.

32. Hamra ST: The zygorbicular dissection in composite rhytidectomy: An ideal midface plane. Plast Reconstr Surg 1998;102(5):1646.

33. Hamra ST: Correcting the unfavorable outcomes following face lift. Clin Plast Surg 2001;28(4):621.

34. Hester TR, Codner MA, McCord CD, et al: Evolution of technique of the direct transblepharoplasty approach for the correction of lower lid and midfacial aging: Maximizing results and minimizing complications in a five-year experience. Plast Reconstr Surg 2000;105:393.

35. Scheflan M, Maillard GF, Cornette de St. Cyr B, Ramirez OM: Subperiosteal facelifting: Complications and the dissatisfied patient. Aesthet Plast Surg 1996;20:33.

36. Hurwitz DJ, Ruskin EM: Reducing eyelid retraction following subperiosteal facelift. Aesthet Surg J 1997;17:149.

37. Hester TR, McCord CD, Nahai F, et al: Expanded applications for transconjunctival lower lid blepharoplasty. Plast Reconstr Surg 2001;108(1):271.

38. Hester TR Jr: Evolution of lower lid support following lower lid/midface rejuvenation: The pretarsal orbicularis lateral canthopexy. Clin Plast Surg 2001;28:639.

39. Mendelson BC, Muzaffar AR, Adams WP Jr: Surgical anatomy of the midcheek and malar mounds. Plast Reconstr Surg 2002;110:885.

40. Pessa JE, Garza JR: The malar septum: The anatomic basis of malar mounds and malar edema. Aesthet Surg J 1997;17:1.

41. Pessa JE, Zadoo VP, Adrian EK, et al: Anatomy of a "black eye": A newly described fascial system of the lower eyelid. Clin Anat 1998;11:157.

42. Yousif NJ: Changes of the midface with age. Clin Plast Surg 1995;22(2):213.

43. Muenker R: Problems and variations in cervicofacial rhytidectomy. Facial Plast Surg 1992;8(1):33.

44. Stuzin JM, Wagstrom L, Kawamoto HK, et al: The anatomy and clinical applications of the buccal fat pad. Plast Reconstr Surg 1990;85(1):29.

45. Grodinsky M, Holyoke EA: The fasciae and fascial spaces of the head, neck, and adjacent regions. Am J Anat 1938;63:367.

46. Baker DC, Conley J: Avoiding facial nerve injuries in rhytidectomy. Plast Reconstr Surg 1979;64:781.

47. Barton FE, Ildiko G: Anatomy of the nasolabial fold. Plast Reconstr Surg 1997;100(5):1276.

48. Yousif NJ, Gosain A, Matloub HS: The nasolabial fold: An anatomic and histologic reappraisal. Plast Reconstr Surg 1994;93(1):60.

49. Rubin LR, Mishriki Y, Lee G: Anatomy of the nasolabial fold: The keystone of the smiling mechanism. Plast Reconstr Surg 1989;83:1.

50. Kamer FM, Letkoff LA: Submental surgery. Arch Otolaryngol Head Neck Surg 1991;117(1):40.

51. Dedo DD: Preoperative classification of the neck for cervicofacial rhytidectomy. Laryngoscope 1980;40:1894.

52. Millard DR Jr: Mandibular lipectomy. Plast Reconstr Surg 1968;41:513.

53. Millard DR Jr, Garst WP, Beck RL, et al: Submental and submandibular lipectomy in conjunction with a face lift in the male or female. Plast Reconstr Surg 1972;49:385.

54. Mitz V, Peyronie M: The superficial musculo-aponeurotic system (SMAS) in the parotid and cheek area. Plast Reconstr Surg 1976;58:80.

55. Yousif NJ, Mendelson BC: Anatomy of the midface. Clin Plast Surg 1995;22(2):227.

56. Thaller SR, Kim S, Patterson H, et al: The submuscular aponeurotic system (SMAS): A histologic and comparative anatomy evaluation. Plast Reconstr Surg 1990;86:690.

57. Jost G, Wassef M, Levet Y: Subfascial lifting. Aesthet Plast Surg 1987;11:163.

58. Jost G, Levet Y: Parotid fascia and face lifting: A critical evaluation of the SMAS concept. Plast Reconstr Surg 1984;74:42.

59. Gosain AK, Yousif NJ, Madiedo G, et al: Surgical anatomy of the SMAS: A reinvestigation. Plast Reconstr Surg 1993;192:1254.

60. Cardoso de Castro C: Superficial musculoaponeurotic system-platysma: A continuous study. Ann Plast Surg 1991;26:203.

61. Gardetto A, Dabernig J, Rainer C, et al: Does a superficial musculoaponeurotic system exist in the face and neck? An anatomical study by the tissue plastination technique. Plast Reconstr Surg 2003;111(2):664.

62. Owsley JQ Jr: SMAS-platysma face lift. Plast Reconstr Surg 1983;71:573

63. Levet Y: Surgical anatomy of the SMAS: A reinvestigation (discussion). Plast Reconstr Surg 1993;92(7):1264.

64. Jost G, Lamouche G: SMAS in rhytidectomy. Aesthet Plast Surg 6:69,1982.

65. Furnas DW: The retaining ligaments of the cheek. Plast Reconstr Surg 1989;83:11.

66. Schuster RH, Gamble WB, Hamra ST, Manson PN: A comparison of flap vascular anatomy in three rhytidectomy techniques. Plast Reconstr Surg 1995;95(4):863.

67. Whetzel TP, Mathes SJ: The arterial supply of the face lift flap. Plast Reconstr Surg 1997;100(2):480.

68. Larrabee WF Jr, Makielski KH, Cupp C: Facelift anatomy. Facial Plast Surg Clin North Am 1993;1(2):135.

69. Larrabee WF Jr, Makielski KH: Surgical Anatomy of the Face. New York: Raven Press, 1992, p 77.

70. McKinney P, Gottlieb J: The relationship of the greater auricular nerve to the SMAS. Ann Plast Surg 1985;14:310.

71. Webster R: Personal communication, 1980.

72. Brennan HG, Toft KM, Dunham BP, et al: Prevention and correction of temporal hair loss in rhytidectomy. Plast Reconstr Surg 1999;104(7):2219.

73. Hamra ST: A study of the long-term effect of malar fat repositioning in face lift surgery: Short-term success but long-term failure. Plast Reconstr Surg 2002;110(3):940.

74. Hamra ST: Frequent face lift sequelae. Hollow eyes and the lateral sweep: Cause and repair. Plast Reconstr Surg 1998;102:1658.

75. Furnas DW: Correction of the nasolabial fold: Extended SMAS dissection with periosteal fixation (discussion). Plast Reconstr Surg 1992;89(5):834.

76. de Castro CC: Preauricular and sideburn operating procedures for natural look in facelifts. Aesthet Plast Surg 1991;15:149.

77. Ellenbogen R: Avoiding visual tipoffs to face lift surgery. Clin Plast Surg 1992;19:447.

78. Johnson CM: Personal communication, 2004.

79. Johnson CM, Godin MS: The anterior extension face-lift. Arch Otolaryngol Head Neck Surg 1995;121:613.

80. Kamer FM: Sequential rhytidectomy and the two stage concept. Otolaryngol Clin North Am 1980; 12(2):305.

81. Kridel RW, Liu ES: Techniques for creating inconspicuous face-lift scars: Avoiding visible incisions and loss of temporal hair. Arch Facial Plast Surg 2003;5(4):325.

82. Larrabee WF: Facelift anatomy. Facial Plast Surg Clin North Am 1993;1:415.

83. Kamer FM, Minoli JJ: Postoperative platysmal band deformity: A pitfall of submental liposuction. Arch Otolaryngol Head Neck Surg 1993;119:193.

84. Dedo DD: Management of the platysma muscle after open and closed liposuction of the neck in facelift surgery. Facial Plast Surg 1986;45:47.

85. Hamra ST: The role of the septal reset in creating a youthful eye-lid cheek complex in facial rejuvenation. Plast Reconstr Surg 2004;113:2124.

86. Hamra ST: Repositioning of the orbicularis oculi in composite rhytidectomy. Plast Reconstr Surg 1992;90:14.

87. Owsley JQ Jr, Zwiefler M: Midface lift of the malar fat pad: Technical advances. Plast Reconstr Surg 2002;110(2):674.

88. Kamer FM: Isolated platysmaplasty: A useful procedure but with important limitations. Arch Facial Plast Surg 2003;5:184.

89. Har-Shai Y, Bodner SR, Egozy-Golan D, et al: Mechanical properties and microstructure of the superficial musculoaponeurotic system. Plast Reconstr Surg 1996;98:59.

90. Straith R, Raghava R, Hipps C: The study of hematomas in 500 consecutive face lifts. Plast Reconstr Surg 1977;59:694.

91. Larrabee WF Jr, Ridenour BD: Rhytidectomy: Technique and complications. Am J Otolaryngol 1992;13:1.

92. Rees TD, Aston SJ: Complications of rhytidectomy. Clin Plast Surg 1978;5:109.

93. Baker DC: Complications of cervicofacial rhytidectomy. Clin Plast Surg 1983;10:543.

94. Perkins SW, Williams JD, Macdonald K, Robinson EB: Prevention of seromas and hematomas after face-lift surgery with the use of postoperative vacuum drains. Arch Otolaryngol Head Neck Surg 1997;123:743.

95. Adamson P, Moran M: Complications of cervicofacial rhytidectomy. Facial Plast Surg Clin North Am 1993;1:257.

96. Kamer FM, Song AU: Hematoma formation in deep plane rhytidectomy. Arch Facial Plast Surg 2000;2:240.

97. Rees TD, Barone CM, Valauri FA, et al: Hematomas requiring surgical evacuation following face lift surgery. Plast Reconstr Surg 1994;93:1185.

98. Kamer FM: Evolution of my facelift technique. American Academy of Facial Plastic and Reconstructive Surgery Annual Fall Meeting, New York, NY, 2004.

99. Baker TJ, Gordon HL: Complications of rhytidectomy. Plast Reconstr Surg 1967;40:31.

100. Cohen SR, Webster RC: Primary rhytidectomy— Complications of the procedure and anesthetic. Laryngoscope 1983;93:654.

101. Leist F, Masson J, Erich JB: A review of 324 rhytidectomies, emphasizing complications and patient dissatisfaction. Plast Reconstr Surg 1977;59:535.

102. Lemmon ML, Hamra ST: Skoog rhytidectomy: A five-year experience with 577 patients. Plast Reconstr Surg 1980;65:283.

103. Pitanguy I, Cervello MP, Degand M: Nerve injuries during rhytidectomy: Consideration after 3,203 cases. Aesthet Plast Surg 1980;4:257.

104. Hamra ST: Rejuvenation of the midface by elevating the malar fat pad: Review of technique, cases and complications (discussion). Plast Reconstr Surg 2002;110(6):1537.

105. Hamra ST: A study of the long-term effect of malar fat repositioning in face lift surgery: Short term success but long-term failure. Plast Reconstr Surg 2002;110(3):940.

106. Stuzin JM, Baker TJ, Baker TM: Midface lift of the malar fat pad: Technical advances (discussion). Plast Reconstr Surg 2002;110(2):686.

107. Ramirez OM: Three-dimensional endoscopic midface enhancement: A personal quest for the ideal cheek rejuvenation. Plast Reconstr Surg 2002;109:329.

108. Owsley JQ, Fiala TGS: Update: Lifting the malar fat pad for correction of prominent nasolabial folds. Plast Reconstr Surg 1997;100:715.

109. Little JW: Three-dimensional rejuvenation of the midface: Volumetric resculpture by malar imbrication. Plast Reconstr Surg 2000;105:267.

CHAPTER NINE

Lateral SMASectomy Facelift

Daniel C. Baker, MD

HISTORY

My first experience with rhytidectomy was during my residency in the late 1970s. At that time, the emphasis was on extensive defatting of the neck with complete platysma muscle transection, plicating medial borders and pulling laterally. However, several years of patient complaints, complications, and overoperated necks led me to modify this technique. With the advent of liposuction in the 1980s, I found that I could obtain excellent neck contouring in many patients utilizing liposuction combined with strong lateral platysmal suturing.

When superficial musculoaponeurotic system (SMAS) dissection first became popularized in 1976, it became fashionable to include a dissection of the lateral SMAS directly overlying the parotid gland. I initially utilized this form of SMAS dissection beginning in the late 1970s and continuing into mid-1980s but overall was disappointed with the effects of a simple elevation and tightening of the lateral superficial fascia. Specifically, I saw little difference in overall facial contour whether I had performed a lateral SMAS dissection or had omitted it.

As I gained greater experience with SMAS dissection, it became obvious that for the superficial fascia to produce any effective contour change in facelifting, it was necessary to elevate the SMAS anterior to the parotid gland. The problem of more extensive SMAS dissection is that facial nerve branches are placed in greater jeopardy. I also noted that the superficial fascia tends to thin out as it is dissected more anteriorly, making the SMAS easy to tear. A SMAS dissection that is not raised as a continuous fascial sheet but rather is raised with several tears in it is a poor substrate for holding the tension of contouring the face. For these reasons, I felt that an extensive SMAS dissection was not warranted in most patients and offered little long-term benefit when compared with SMAS plication.

In 1992, I realized that an alternative to formal elevation of the superficial fascia was a "lateral SMASectomy," removing a strip of SMAS in the region directly overlying the anterior edge of the parotid gland, and extending to the lateral canthus. Excision of the superficial fascia in this region secures mobile anterior SMAS to the fixed portion of the superficial fascia overlying the parotid. The direction in which the SMASectomy is performed is oriented so that the vectors of elevation following SMAS closure lie perpendicular to the nasolabial fold, thereby producing improvement not only of the nasolabial fold but also of the jowl and jawline. In 2001, this technique was further developed and refined into the minimal incision rhytidectomy (short scar facelift).

PERSONAL PHILOSOPHY

For many years I have listened to panels and presentations and have read articles about the "super-SMAS," "deep-plane," "subperiosteal," and various other extended rhytidectomy procedures. In their search for the penultimate facelift, these pioneering surgeons demonstrate superb anatomic studies, beautiful illustrations, and impeccable photographs. Their presentations are well organized, stimulating, and seductive.

I have always considered myself to be a bold and aggressive surgeon, and the temptation to utilize these new, deeper dissections is extremely appealing. However, I am reluctant to employ them, and I keep asking myself why? The explanation is partly that I am not convinced that the results are superior to those obtained by the standard SMAS-platysma techniques. More important, I do not yet believe that the implied "benefits" outweigh the increased morbidity and risks, especially to the facial nerve.

The presentations on deep dissection and subperiosteal rhytidectomies recall the period between 1976 and 1980 when virtually all panels and courses were advocating complete platysma muscle transactions and a multitude of platysma flaps. As a plastic surgeon just completing residency, I was highly impressed; I became a believer and a convert: The only way to get the "best result" in rhytidectomy was with these techniques. However, many years of patient complaints, complications, and overoperated necks occurred before most of these techniques were abandoned. I can only speculate on whether the deep-plane rhytidectomy techniques will have a similar evolution.

In the 21st century the consumer's preference has been for minimally invasive and noninvasive techniques: fillers, Botox, endoscopy, and limited incision aesthetic surgery. The rationale for any minimal incision surgery is evident: less invasiveness, less bleeding, presumably less pain, faster healing, and less scarring. The primary advantages of minimal incision rhytidectomy, however, are that it preserves the posterior hairline and avoids retroauricular scars, which are particularly important for a woman with a pulled-up or swept-back hairstyle. It is a ponytail-friendly facelift.

The primary goal of any surgeon performing rhytidectomy should be to utilize a technique giving consistently good results with minimal risk, complications, morbidity, and a speedy postoperative recovery.

My intention is not to discredit these deep dissection techniques nor to deplete the splendor of creative surgery. Their contribution is already evident: an increased and clearer knowledge of facial anatomy, muscle function, and human expression. I am certain that some aspect of these techniques will be incorporated by many plastic surgeons. The questions that remain to be answered are (1) What are the indications for these newer techniques? (2) How great are the risks and complications? and most important, (3) Do the benefits significantly outweigh the risks to justify using these techniques routinely?

There are several advantages of lateral SMASectomy in comparison with traditional SMAS elevation. First, because the procedure does not require traditional SMAS flap elevation, there is less concern about tearing of the superficial fascia. Second, the potential for facial nerve injury is lower because most of the deep dissection is over the parotid gland. If the SMASectomy is performed anterior to the parotid, the deep fascia will similarly provide protection for the facial nerve branches as long as the resection of the superficial fascia is done precisely and the deep fascia is not violated. Third, because SMAS flaps have not been elevated, they tend to hold suture fixation more strongly, and the potential for postoperative dehiscence and relapse of contour is decreased.

There are certainly other rhytidectomy techniques that produce excellent results. Each surgeon must adopt a technique that serves his or her patients best. Ideally, the technique should be safe, consistent, easily reproducible, and applicable to a variety of anatomic problems. The surgeon also must have the versatility to adapt and modify his or her technique to the needs and desires of each patient. At present, the lateral SMASectomy provides this for most of my patients. In the future, as endoscopy and fixation techniques advance, I will seek to modify and further improve my present rhytidectomy operation.

It must be emphasized that I do not perform SMASectomy in every rhytidectomy. Patients with thin faces and minimal subcutaneous fat undergo simple plication or imbrication.

SURGICAL TECHNIQUE

ANESTHESIA

Virtually all my facelifts are performed with the patient under monitored intravenous propofol sedation. Patients are given oral clonidine, 0.1 to 0.2 mg, 30 minutes before surgery to control their blood pressure. The face and neck are infiltrated with local anesthesia, 0.5% lidocaine with 1:200,000 epinephrine, through use of a 22-gauge spinal needle. I inject the face before I scrub to provide the requisite 10 minutes for vasoconstriction.

INCISIONS

When the temporal hairline shift is assessed as minimal, the preferred incision is well within the temporal hair. With this incision, it is often necessary to excise a triangle of skin below the temporal sideburn at the level of the superior root of the helix.

However, when larger skin shift is anticipated (frequently the lift is more vertical with minimal incision rhytidectomy) or the distance between the lateral canthus and temporal hairline is greater than 5 cm, I prefer an incision a few millimeters within the temporal hairline (Figs. 9-1 to 9-3). Although this is a compromise, the

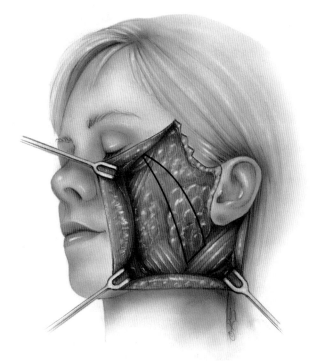

Figure 9-1 Lateral SMASectomy dissection. The temporal hairline incision allows for a more vertical elevation of the facial flap that is usually required in a short scar rhytidectomy. Subcutaneous dissection is performed extending across the zygoma to release the zygomatic ligaments but stops several centimeters short of the nasolabial fold. The SMAS resection is performed on a tangent from the lateral malar eminence to the angle of the mandible in the region along the anterior edge of the parotid gland. The width depends on the laxity of the tissues and the desired elevation. Vectors are perpendicular to the nasolabial fold. A platysma flap is elevated and secured to the mastoid periosteum.

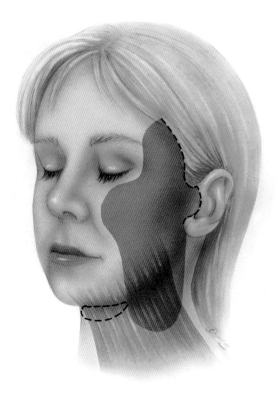

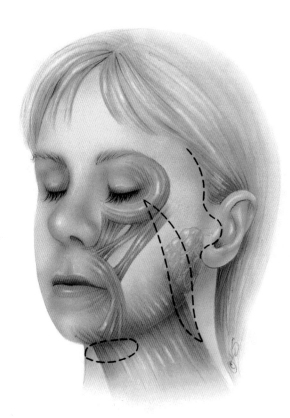

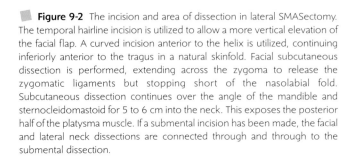 **Figure 9-2** The incision and area of dissection in lateral SMASectomy. The temporal hairline incision is utilized to allow a more vertical elevation of the facial flap. A curved incision anterior to the helix is utilized, continuing inferiorly anterior to the tragus in a natural skinfold. Facial subcutaneous dissection is performed, extending across the zygoma to release the zygomatic ligaments but stopping short of the nasolabial fold. Subcutaneous dissection continues over the angle of the mandible and sternocleidomastoid for 5 to 6 cm into the neck. This exposes the posterior half of the platysma muscle. If a submental incision has been made, the facial and lateral neck dissections are connected through and through to the submental dissection.

Figure 9-3 Outline of the SMAS excision. The SMAS resection is performed on a tangent from the lateral malar eminence to the angle of the mandible in the region along the anterior edge of the parotid gland. Continuous with the lateral SMASectomy is the resection of a strip of posterior platysma muscle several centimeters long over the tail of the parotid and anterior border of the sternocleidomastoid.

alternative of a receding temporal hairline is never acceptable to a female patient. When the incisions are executed properly, these scars heal well and are easy to revise or camouflage. The only exception might be in a patient with deeply pigmented skin in whom the scar will contrast and appear as a white line. The temporal hairline incision should be made parallel to the hair follicle and no higher than the frontotemporal hairline.

The temporal hairline incision allows for the more vertical elevation of the facial flap that is usually required in a short scar rhytidectomy. Other indications for this incision are a receding hairline from previous facelifts and a fine, fragile hairline.

The choice of preauricular incision is up to the surgeon. When executed properly, all these incisions heal well and are imperceptible. I usually prefer a curved incision anterior to the helix and continue inferiorly anterior to the tragus in a natural skinfold. This preserves the thin, pale, hairless tragal skin and its demarcation from the usual coarser, thicker, darker cheek skin with its lanugo hairs. I perform intratragal incisions in patients in whom the cheek and tragal skin are similar and the tragal cartilage is not sharp or prominent. Closure must be without tension and the flap overlying the tragus defatted to dermis.

In minimal incision rhytidectomy, efforts are made to end the incision at the base of the ear lobe. This is usually possible in young patients, but sometimes a short retroauricular incision is necessary to correct a dog-ear after the facial flap rotation.

SKIN FLAP ELEVATION

All skin flap undermining is carried out under direct vision (with scissors dissection) to minimize trauma to the subdermal plexus and preserve a significant layer of subcutaneous fat on the undersurface of the flap (see Fig.

9-2). I prefer subcutaneous dissection in the temporal region because the skin seems to redrape better. (I believe that hair loss results primarily from tension rather than superficial undermining.) Subcutaneous dissection in the temporal region must be performed carefully to avoid penetrating the superficial temporal fascia that protects the frontal branch of the facial nerve. All dermal attachments between the orbicularis oculi muscle and the skin are separated up to the lateral canthus.

Dissection extends across the zygoma to release the zygomatic ligaments but stops several centimeters short of the nasolabial fold. I have never felt that further dissection provides significant benefit; on the contrary, the only result is increased bleeding. In the cheek, dissection releases the masseteric-cutaneous ligaments and, if necessary, the mandibular ligaments.

Subcutaneous dissection continues over the angle of the mandible and sternocleidomastoid for 5 to 6 cm into the neck. This exposes the posterior half of the platysma muscle. If a submental incision has been made, the facial and lateral neck dissection is connected through and through to the submental dissection.

DEFATTING THE NECK AND JOWLS

Whenever possible, I prefer closed suction-assisted lipoplasty in the neck and jowls. I use a 2.4-mm Mercedes tip cannula, keeping it under constant, steady motion in the subcutaneous space. I attempt to leave a layer of subcutaneous fat on the undersurface of the cervical skin. If I suction the jowls, this is always done conservatively. I never suction or remove subplatysmal fat because (1) the facial nerves run just beneath the platysma and (2) any patient with significant subplatysmal fat probably has a fat, round face, so removing subplatysmal fat could create an overoperated look.

I usually perform lipoplasty before elevating the skin flaps. In doing so, I am careful not to oversuction the portion of the SMAS-platysma that will be elevated over the mandible with the lateral SMASectomy.

OPEN SUBMENTAL INCISION WITH MEDIAL PLATYSMA APPROXIMATION

After many years, I had almost stopped opening the neck, except in unusual cases, because I found that I could accomplish excellent results with closed lipoplasty and strong lateral platysma pull. With short scar rhytidectomy there is limited access to the platysma and the lateral vector has changed. Therefore, in patients with active platysma bands on animation, the medial approximation provides another vector to enhance the cervicomental recontouring (Fig. 9-4).

The submental incision is made either in the submental crease or just anterior to it. The subcutaneous dissection is performed with the neck hyperextended, and

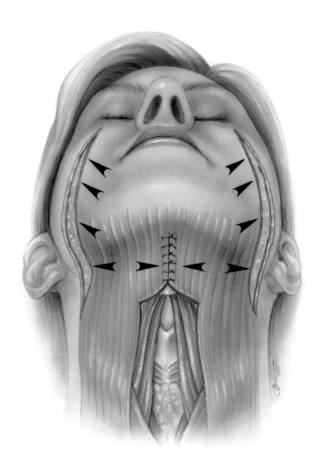

Figure 9-4 Medial platysma approximation. Subcutaneous dissection through a submental incision is performed with the neck hyperextended. The dissection usually extends to the level of the thyroid cartilage and angle of the mandible. Suction-assisted lipoplasty is then performed. The medial borders of the platysma muscle are elevated for several centimeters. To break the continuity of the bands, a wedge of muscle is removed at the level of the hyoid. The medial borders of the muscle are then sutured together.

undermining is usually to the level of the thyroid cartilage and angle of the mandible. Suction-assisted lipoplasty is then performed with a large, single-hole cannula under direct vision. Direct fat excision is carried out if necessary, but to avoid depressions, subplatysma fat is rarely removed.

The medial borders of the platysma muscle are identified and elevated for several centimeters. To break the continuity of the bands, a wedge of muscle is removed at the level of the hyoid. The medial borders of the muscle are then sutured together with interrupted buried 4-0 PDS (Ethicon, Inc., Somerville, NJ).

The submental incision is left open to allow for final hemostasis and recontouring after communication with the facial dissection and completion of the lateral SMASectomy.

LATERAL SMASECTOMY INCLUDING PLATYSMA RESECTION

The outline of SMASectomy is marked on a tangent from the lateral malar eminence to the angle of the mandible, essentially in the region along the anterior edge of the parotid gland (see Figs. 9-1 and 9-3). In most patients, this involves a line of resection extending from the lateral aspect of the malar eminence toward the tail of the parotid gland. Usually, a 2- to 3-cm segment of superficial fascia is excised, depending on the degree of SMAS-platysma laxity.

In SMAS resection, I like to pick up the superficial fascia in the region of the tail of the parotid, extending the resection from inferior to superior in a controlled fashion. When SMAS resection is being performed, it is important to keep the dissection superficial to the deep fascia and avoid dissection into the parotid parenchyma. Note that the size of the parotid gland varies from patient to patient; consequently, the amount of protection for the underlying facial nerve branches will also vary. Despite this, as long as one carries the dissection superficial to the deep facial fascia, ensuring that only the superficial fascia is resected, facial nerve injury as well as parotid gland injury will be prevented. In essence, this is a resection of the superficial fascia in the same plane of dissection in which one would normally raise the SMAS flap.

Continuous with the lateral SMASectomy is the resection of a strip of posterior platysma muscle several centimeters long over the tail of the parotid and anterior border of the sternocleidomastoid. The facial nerves are protected here.

VECTORS

The various vectors accomplish correction of the anterior neck, the cervicomental angle, the jowls, and the nasolabial fold. The first key suture grasps the platysma at the angle of the mandible and advances it in a posterosuperior direction; it is secured with 2-0 Maxon (United States Surgical Corp., Norwalk, CT) to the fixed lateral SMAS overlying the parotid (Figs. 9-3 and 9-4). This lifts the cervical platysma and cervical skin.

After SMAS resection, interrupted 3-0 PDS buried sutures are used to close the SMASectomy, fixed lateral SMAS being evenly sutured to more mobile anterior superficial fascia (Fig. 9-5). Vectors are perpendicular to the nasolabial fold. The last suture lifts the malar fat pad, securing it to the malar fascia. It is important to obtain a secure fixation to prevent postoperative dehiscence and relapse of facial contour.

If firm monofilament sutures are used, such as PDS or Maxon, the sutures should be buried and sharp ends on the knot trimmed. Final contouring of any SMAS or fat irregularities along the suture line is completed with scissors. Fat can also be trimmed at the sternomandibular trough, final contouring being accomplished with lipoplasty.

For the neck, a flap of the lateral platysma is developed in the region inferior to the mandibular border. After this lateral platysma flap is raised, the platysma is

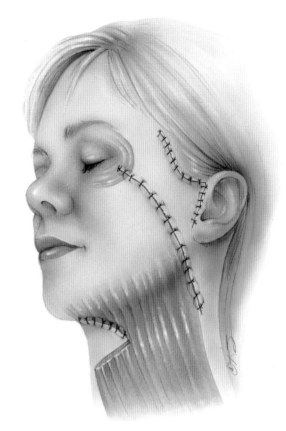

Figure 9-5 SMAS, platysma, and skin closure in lateral SMASectomy.

secured to the mastoid periosteum with figure-of-eight 2-0 Maxon sutures to help define the jawline and improve contouring in the submandibular region. This is the basic rhytidectomy operation that I have performed since July 1992.

SKIN CLOSURE, TEMPORAL AND EARLOBE DOG-EARS

After SMAS and platysma approximation, some tethering of the skin might appear at the anterior extent of the subcutaneous dissection because of the pull of the underlying SMAS. This can also occur in the lower eyelid with elevation of the malar fat pad. Further subcutaneous undermining is necessary to free these tethers, allowing the skin to redrape.

The first key skin suture rotates the facial flap vertically and posteriorly to lift the midface, jowls, and submandibular skin. Suture fixation is at the level of the insertion of the superior helix. I like to use a buried 3-0 PDS through the temporal fascia with a generous bite of dermis on the skin flap. Closure is under minimal to moderate tension. Staples are used to close any incisions in the hair. A wedge is usually removed at the level of the sideburn to preserve the hairline. If an anterior hairline incision has been made, I like to close it with buried 5-0 Monocryl sutures (Ethicon, Inc., Somerville, NJ) and 5-0

Nylon sutures. Extra time and attention must be spent on this closure to eliminate any dog-ears and obtain the finest scar. Excess skin is then trimmed from the facial flap so that there is no tension on the preauricular closure. Wound edges should be "kissing" without sutures.

In short scar rhytidectomy trimming at the earlobe must be without tension, and the skin flap is tucked under the lobe with 4-0 PDS sutures, taking a bite of earlobe dermis, cheek flap dermis, and conchal perichondrium to minimize any tension. A small dog-ear might be present behind the earlobe; this is easily trimmed and tailored into a short incision in the retroauricular sulcus. A closed suction drain is usually brought out through a separate stab in the retroauriculus sulcus. Figures 9-6 and 9-7 are representative pre- and postoperative photos of patients who have undergone lateral SMASectomy.

POSTOPERATIVE CARE

For the first 48 hours of the postoperative period, blood pressure monitoring is continuous to avoid systolic spikes and potential bleeding. Treatment of rising blood pressure is essential to minimize hematoma formation.

Figure 9-6 Preoperative (**A** and **C**) and postoperative views (**B** and **D**) after lateral SMASectomy and chin implant.

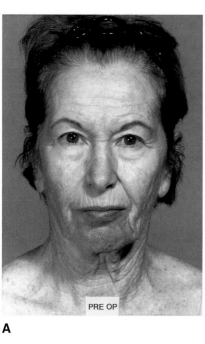

A

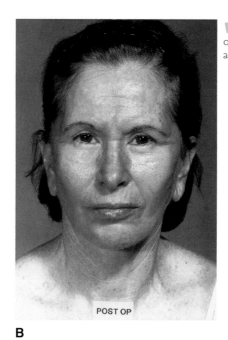

B

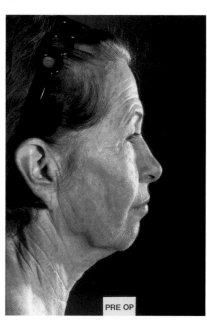

C

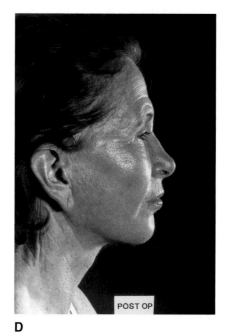

D

I usually utilize suction drains and a soft head dressing to cover the flaps and incisions. Although drains never prevent expanding hematomas, I prefer to remove serosanguineous fluid in this manner. Sutures are removed on the 7th and 10th postoperative days.

When large hematomas are recognized early, they are usually successfully managed at the bedside with sedation, blood pressure control, and irrigation.

The overall incidence of hematoma for women is about 1.5%; for men it is 4%.

COMPLICATIONS

Table 9-1 summarizes the complications of this technique, which are consistent with other standard

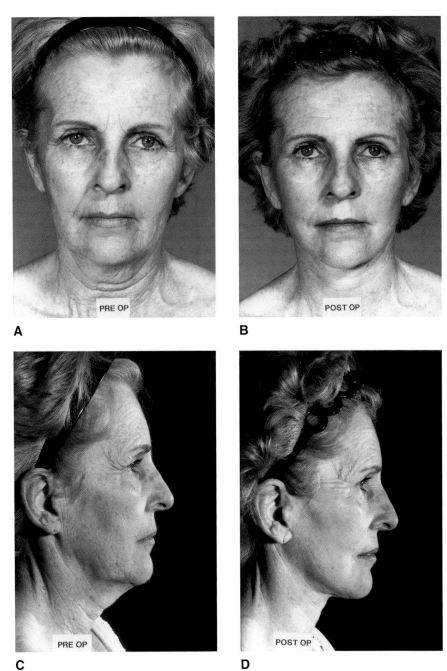

Figure 9-7 Preoperative (**A** and **C**) and postoperative views (**B** and **D**) after lateral SMASectomy.

A   B

C   D

Table 9-1   Complications Associated with 3,500 Lateral SMASectomy Facelifts

Complication	Incidence (%)
Hematoma	1.5
Facial nerve weakness	0.1 *
Earlobe scar revision	2.0
Skin slough	2.0
Retroauricular and temporal scar revisions	2.0
Infection	1.0
"Minilift" after 1 year	2.0

*All resolved in 6 months.

facelift operations. Despite special attention to blood pressure control in the postoperative period, the hematoma rate is still 1.5%. The most common problems are minor revisions of earlobe and temporal hairline scars. Secondary lifts are occasionally performed, but I require all patients to allow healing for 1 year before considering any revisions. My goal is to keep the occurrence of all revisions to less than 5%. When revisions exceed this limit, I know I must re-evaluate my technique.

SUGGESTED READING

Baker DC, Aston SJ, Guy CL, Rees TD: The male rhytidectomy. Plast Reconstr Surg 1977;60:514.

Baker DC, Conley J: Avoiding facial nerve injuries in rhytidectomy. Anatomical variations and pitfalls. Plast Reconstr Surg 1979;64:781.

Baker DC: Anatomy and injuries of the facial nerve in cervicofacial rhytidectomy. In Kaye BL, Gradinger GP (eds): Symposium on Problems and Complications in Aesthetic Plastic Surgery of the Face. St. Louis: CV Mosby, 1984.

Baker DC, Rees TD: Complications of cosmetic facial surgery. In Lewis JR (ed): Aesthetic Plastic Surgery. Boston: Little, Brown, 1989.

Baker DC: Deep dissection rhytidectomy: A plea for caution. Plast Reconstr Surg 1994;93(7):1498–1499.

Baker DC: Lateral SMASectomy. Plast Reconstr Surg 1997; 100(2):509–513.

Baker DC: Rhytidectomy with lateral SMASectomy. Facial Plast Surg 2000;16(3):209–213.

Baker DC: Minimal incision rhytidectomy (short scar facelift) with lateral SMASectomy: Evolution and application. Aesthet Surg J 2001;21(1):68–79.

Baker DC, Chiu ES: Bedside treatment of early acute rhytidectomy hematomas. Plast Reconstr Surg 2005;115(7):2119–2222.

Baker DC, Stefani WA, Chiu ES: Reducing the incidence of hematomas requiring surgical evacuation following male rhytidectomy: A thirty year review of 985 cases. Plast Reconstr Surg 2005;116(7):1973–1985.

CHAPTER TEN

Short-Flap SMAS Rhytidectomy

Babak Azizzadeh, MD, FACS • Tessa A. Hadlock, MD • Mack L. Cheney, MD, FACS

HISTORY

The facelift operation has evolved over the past century. During the early 20th century, aesthetic procedures were not well accepted socially. The early facelift surgeons performed skin excisions that did not have long-lasting results. As the field of aesthetic surgery matured, physicians and patients demanded more reliable and longer lasting results. In 1919, Bettman and Bourget simultaneously presented their experience with subcutaneous rhytidectomy.[1,2] Despite limited anatomic understanding, facelift surgeons were performing extensive skin undermining, which increased the complication rates and produced minimal aesthetic improvement.

In 1960, Aufricht was the first to describe plication of the tissue deep to the superficial fat plane.[3] Webster and other facelift surgeons used similar techniques of suturing the "deeper layers" to improve their results.[4,5] During the same period Skoog had started performing facelifts utilizing the skin and platysma as a musculocutaneous advancement flap.[6] In 1976, Mitz and Peyronie advanced the rhytidectomy procedure into the modern era by describing the anatomy of the superficial musculoaponeurotic system (SMAS).[7] They showed that a deeper fascial tissue layer exists between the subcutaneous fat and the parotidomasseteric fascia. Their anatomic studies established that the SMAS invests the muscles of facial expression and is contiguous with the frontalis and platysma muscles. Following Mitz and Peyronie's description, the incorporation of the SMAS layer in cervicofacial rhytidectomy gained popularity.[8-14] In the 1980s and 1990s, the deep plane facelift[15-20] and subperiosteal facelift[21-30] were increasingly utilized. However, variations of the SMAS facelift continued to be the most commonly performed technique.

Today, most types of SMAS facelifts and subcutaneous rhytidectomies incorporate extensive skin undermining in hopes of achieving better results. Advocates of extensive dissections believe that the release of the osteofasciocutaneous ligaments is necessary to obtain better results.[31-37] Facelifting with limited skin undermining was first advocated by Richard Webster.[5,38-41] Webster published several papers demonstrating that the results of facelifts with conservative skin undermining and SMAS plication were no different than more aggressive surgery.

He also demonstrated intraoperatively that this method not only decreased wound tension in facelifts but also increased the strength of facial suspension. Webster believed that the longevity of facelifts would be improved if a significant portion of the dermal-SMAS attachments were maintained. McCollough, who further advocated the approach of maintaining the skin adipose-SMAS attachments, coined the term "suspension rhytidectomy."[42] In 1993, Burgess confirmed some of Webster's findings in a cadaveric study comparing different types of SMAS facelifts. In this study, he demonstrated that wound tensions significantly increased with more extensive skin undermining when compared to short skin flaps.[43]

PERSONAL PHILOSOPHY

Having performed numerous facelift techniques including the standard (long flap) SMAS, deep plane, and tuck-up "mini-facelifts," we have come to the conclusion that a modified version of the Webster SMAS facelift with limited skin undermining is a valuable option for many of our patients. The key components of our "short-flap SMAS rhytidectomy" include limited skin undermining in the facial region, SMAS imbrication, platysmaplasty, and judicious cervical suction-assisted lipectomy. By limiting the facial skin flap dissection, we maintain the anterior dermal-SMAS attachments, which allow aggressive suspension of the face without significant tension on the skin. The SMAS serves as the carrier of the facelift flap. Unlike the deep plane facelift, the SMAS is not undermined past the parotid gland, thereby limiting the risk for facial nerve injury and postoperative edema.

The short-flap rhytidectomy provides some advantages over other facelift techniques. We have found a significant reduction in the duration of procedure, rate of complication, and postoperative recovery time. By limiting the subcutaneous dissection, the risk of hematoma formation and facial nerve injury is reduced. Short skin flaps diminish the chance of flap necrosis in patients who have compromised vascularity, such as smokers, diabetics, and elderly patients.[44,45] We have also seen less long-term skin atrophy and telangectasias. The undissected areas could safely also undergo simultaneous fat grafting or resurfacing.

A significant advantage of the short-flap rhytidectomy is patient satisfaction and aesthetic outcome. Some have criticized the concept of performing operations that do not restore the face to its original anatomic and aesthetic ideals, despite high patient and surgeon satisfaction.[46] Our philosophy for elective aesthetic surgery is to obtain outstanding results, reduce the risk of perioperative complications, and allow our patients to return to their normal activity in a reasonable time. Most of our patients return to their normal routine within 8 to 10 days. In addition to the shortened recovery period, most patients are extremely pleased with the long-term surgical outcome. We have not found any difference between the longevity of our short-flap rhytidectomy technique versus more extensive facelift procedures.

SMAS facelifts impact the jowls and lower face but do not always transmit well to the nasolabial fold. Most SMAS facelifts, including the short-flap rhytidectomy, obtain only modest midface enhancement. The short-flap rhytidectomy, therefore, does not address several important issues such as the double cheek convexity, infra-orbital rim hollowness, tear-trough deformity, facial volume loss, and deep nasolabial folds. Dermal fillers (calcium hydroxylapatite, hyaluronic acids), subcutaneous volumizers (poly-L-lactic acid), and fat grafting can be used to address moderate midface ptosis and volume loss. Submalar implants are utilized for significant volume deficits in patients who do not desire temporary fillers.[47] Endoscopic subperiosteal midface lifts are reserved for motivated patients with advanced midface ptosis and prominent nasolabial folds. The reader must, however, be cautious about the use of endoscopic midface lifts because of the higher risk for facial nerve injury, steep learning curve, prolonged postoperative edema, as well as temporary changes in the patient's lateral canthal contour. Nevertheless, several authors have had excellent outcome with minimal complications when utilizing this approach.[22-30]

The majority of our patients only desire injectables or fat grafting to address the midface. Webster was one of the first proponents of utilizing bovine collagen to enhance the appearance of the nasolabial folds.[48] Although injectables do not provide permanent improvement in the area, patients are quite pleased with the outcome and are usually willing to have intermittent in-office procedures. A new generation of long-lasting fillers and volumizers will continue to give our patients more options in this arena.

Long-flap facelifts (SMAS or subcutaneous techniques) incorporate extensive skin undermining in order to release the fascioosteocutaneous ligaments.[31-37] In attempting to accomplish the ligamentous release, extensive flap elevation in the subcutaneous plane can destroy the dermal-SMAS attachments, hence invalidating the SMAS support for the lift. Anatomic studies by Muzaffar and Mendelson have also demonstrated that the release of retaining ligaments in the prezygomatic space through extensive subcutaneous dissection can potentially cause nerve injury to the motor branch of the orbicularis oculi.[36,37] It is also well known that the facial nerve has a more superficial course near the oral commissure and midportion of the zygomatic arch, placing it at risk during the dissection of long skin flaps.[49] The deep plane facelift does not incorporate extensive skin undermining like the short-flap rhytidectomy. Deep plane facelifts, however, utilize a sub-SMAS composite musculocutaneous advancement flap. The results of the deep plane facelift in the lower face (jowls and neck) are consistent because the SMAS is utilized as a carrier of the facelift, just like the short-flap rhytidectomy. Midface enhancement of the deep plane facelift is more controversial. Owsley and others have shown that in order to truly obtain nasolabial effacement, the SMAS must be totally released anteriorly beyond the melolabial fold over the zygomaticus muscle.[50-53] A lengthy anteromedial dissection is hence necessary and can cause extensive postoperative edema as well as place the branches of the facial nerve at significant risk. Furthermore, similar to the short-flap rhytidectomy, the deep plane facelift does not truly address the volume deficits associated with the aging process. In our experience as well as that of others, the difference in the aesthetic outcome between the deep plane and SMAS rhytidectomy is not significant except in older patients with extensive rhytidosis.[54-55] The results of the subperiosteal facelift are better for patients who have midface ptosis.

In the past decade, patient demands for decreased downtime has fueled the resurgence of "limited" or "mini-facelift" surgery. The short-flap rhytidectomy is not a mini-facelift as it entails a critical amount of cervicofacial dissection and SMAS imbrication. In our experience, mini-facelifts are indicated only for a limited number of patients who have minimal signs of facial aging or those who require minor facelift revisions.[55-58] The postoperative recovery of mini-facelifts is shorter than most standard rhytidectomy procedures, but the results are not as dramatic. Our patient population has a much higher rate of satisfaction with the short-flap rhytidectomy.

ANATOMY

The salient features of the facial anatomy have been discussed in detail in other chapters. The most important aspect of the anatomy relating to our current technique has been elegantly described by Webster and McCollough.[38-42] They believed that the guiding principle for safe and long-lasting rhytidectomy is for the skin and the SMAS to function as a unit; therefore, if you separate the unit, the SMAS will not truly have any functional support of the skin. In fact, it is this same principle of maintaining the skin-SMAS unit that guides the excellent results achieved by sub-SMAS dissection employed in deep plane facelifts.[15-20] In the short-flap rhytidectomy, the SMAS is not undermined extensively beyond the parotid. Subcutaneous, long-flap SMAS and extended SMAS facelifts widely separate the skin from the SMAS, thereby disrupting the skin-SMAS attachments. This separation does not allow the SMAS to serve as a foundation for the facelift. If the attachments of the skin and SMAS are maintained, imbrication of the SMAS will suspend the entire complex. These attachments are main-tained only in short-flap rhytidectomy and deep plane facelifts.

The pathophysiology of midface aging involves both inferomedial descent as well as well as atrophy of the soft tissue (Fig. 10-1). The nasolabial fold is an area where

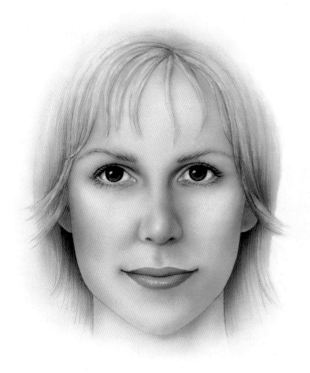

A

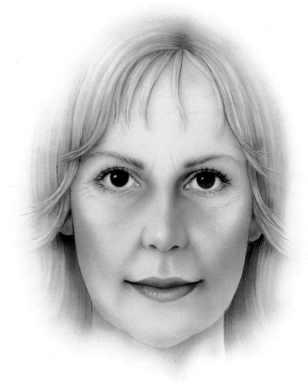

B

Figure 10-1 The progression of the aging face. The aging process is illustrated in this individual in her 20s (**A**), 40s (**B**), and 60s (**C**). The face continuously and gradually changes, resulting in prominent nasolabial folds, jowl formation, marionette furrows, neck laxity, volume loss, and rhytids in the perioral and periorbital region.

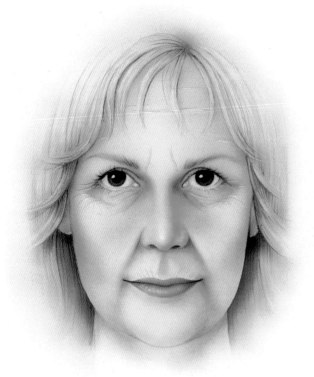

C

the cutaneous insertions of the lip elevators fuse onto to the ligamentous structure formed by the SMAS and deeper facial fascia. Studies have shown that the nasolabial fold becomes more prominent as the malar fat pad and suborbicularis oculi fat (SOOF) begin to descend.[59] Also, a progressive atrophy of the midface muscles and subcutaneous fat results in cavitary depressions and midfacial flatness contributing to the overall aging process.

The safety of the facial nerve is perhaps the most important aspect of facelift surgery. The facial nerve exits the stylomastoid foramen and enters the body of the parotid gland (Fig. 10-2). Within the parotid gland it bifurcates into an upper and lower division. It further divides into five main branches, including the temporal (frontal), zygomatic, buccal, marginal mandibular, and cervical. Permanent iatrogenic facial paralysis is rare owing to the extensive arborization of the facial nerve branches. The frontal branch is a terminal branch with limited arborization. Injury to the frontal branch has the highest risk of causing permanent paralysis. The overall risk of permanent facial nerve paralysis in standard rhytidectomy is between 0.53% and 2.6%.[45,60-61] There have been very few reports in the literature regarding the risk for facial nerve injury associated with more invasive facelifting procedures. The short-flap rhytidectomy significantly limits the risk for facial nerve injury by limiting facial subcutaneous and SMAS dissection. This is the primary reason that the short-flap rhytidectomy is an extremely safe procedure.

Finally, the skeletal anatomy of the face and neck is extremely important in obtaining satisfactory results in

cervicofacial rhytidectomy. The key skeletal regions include the malar-submalar region, dental occlusion, chin projection, prejowl sulcus, and the position of the hyoid. Patients with prominent malar prominence and submalar fullness will obtain better results from short-flap rhytidectomy. If these areas are extremely underdeveloped or atrophied, the patient must be consulted for skeletal and soft tissue volume enhancements. Individuals with poor chin projection and prominent prejowl sulcus will also require further evaluation for simultaneous chin augmentation to enhance the results of the rhytidectomy. Finally, patients with low and anteriorly positioned hyoid bone will not obtain satisfactory results in the neck.[62] Unlike the other skeletal regions, the hyoid cannot be manipulated during the rhytidectomy procedure.

PREOPERATIVE ASSESSMENT

The short-flap rhytidectomy is typically indicated for patients with moderate facial aging as manifested by jowl formation, neck banding, and early midface aging changes. Patients are typically between 45 and 65 years old. A complete history and physical examination are performed. The most important aspect of the consultation is to understand the patient's aesthetic and functional goals. Mirror and photographic facial analysis are utilized. Comprehensive facial analysis is prerequisite for a successful surgical outcome. Please refer to Chapter 1 for an overview of the aging face consultation and facial analysis.

Following the facial analysis, a treatment plan is formulated for the patient. The first feature of the treatment protocol will focus on preventive measures to slow the aging process. Antiaging regimen, skin care consultation, sun protection, and tobacco cessation are discussed with every patient at this time. In the second phase of the consultation, nonsurgical procedures that could improve the facial appearance are considered. Skin resurfacing, soft tissue fillers, and botulinum toxin type A are discussed at length. The third feature of the consultation focuses on areas of the face that will benefit from facial plastic surgical intervention. All regions of the face will be evaluated in order to achieve a balanced and aesthetically pleasing outcome. Box 10-1 highlights the surgical and nonsurgical options discussed with every patient. We invite the patients back for a second consultation to further discuss the risks, alternatives, incisions, aesthetics, and perioperative course of the short-flap rhytidectomy and adjunctive procedures. Photographs are reviewed in detail with patients at that time.

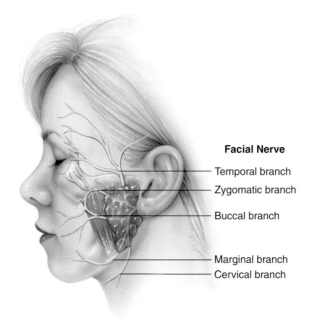

Facial Nerve

Temporal branch

Zygomatic branch

Buccal branch

Marginal branch

Cervical branch

Figure 10-2 The facial nerve. The facial nerve bifurcates in the parotid into an upper and lower division. It then divides into five main branches: temporal (frontal), zygomatic, buccal, marginal mandibular, and cervical.

SURGICAL TECHNIQUE

The short-flap rhytidectomy is typically performed at a certified ambulatory surgical center under general anesthesia. Local anesthesia with sedation may be offered as an alternative. The patients are encouraged to avoid a number of medications starting 2 weeks prior to the surgical date (Box 10-2). All herbal products are discontinued at the same time. The patients are started on arnica and Bromolin starting 3 days prior to the surgery. Although there are very few studies available, we have found that this regimen helps the patients prepare psychologically for their surgery as well as reduce the perioperative bleeding, edema, and ecchymoses.

In the preoperative area, ice packs are applied to the facial region. The markings for short-flap rhytidectomy,

blepharoplasty, and endoscopic browlift as well as important landmarks are placed with the patient in the sitting position. Patients are given a mirror to view the proposed incisions. We take extreme care to mark the patient preoperatively, because the facial landmarks are distorted once the patient is supine and local anesthesia has been infiltrated.

The patients are placed under general anesthesia or propofol sedation. A midline endotracheal tube is tied to the lower teeth with a 2-0 silk suture in patients who are under general anesthesia. Cefazolin and decadron are administered. Foley catheter and lower extremity pulsatile compression stockings are placed in all patients. Ice gloves are applied to the areas of the face and eyes that are not in the immediate operative field. Lidocaine 1% with 1:100,000 epinephrine is infiltrated into all the pertinent regions prior to the preparation. This will allow ample time for the vasoconstrictive actions of the epinephrine. A 3-mL syringe and 27-gauge needle are used for face and brow infiltration. A 1-mL syringe with 30-gauge needle is utilized for the blepharoplasty injection. Autoclave tape is applied to the hair 2 to 4 cm posterior to the hairline (Fig. 10-3). The entire face and anterior hairline are cleaned with 3% hexachlorophene. Sterile blue towel is stapled to the autoclave tape and the endotracheal tube is wrapped in a sterile manner. This is an effective and rapid method of preparing the patient.

Box 10-3 outlines the specific order of procedures in patients who are undergoing multiple facial rejuvenation procedures. Prior to each portion of the procedure, a second round of local anesthetic using 0.5% lidocaine with 1:200,000 epinephrine is administered. The facelift procedure generally begins with suction-assisted lipectomy of the neck region. A 5-mm incision in the submental crease is utilized to access the region. If platysmaplasty or chin implants are to be performed, a 1- to 2-cm incision is utilized. A 3-mm flat liposuction cannula is used for the

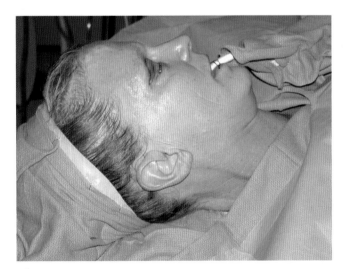

Figure 10-3 The preparation. Autoclave tape is applied to the hair 2 to 4 cm posterior to hairline. Sterile towel is then stapled to the autoclave tape, and the endotracheal tube is wrapped in a sterile manner.

Box 10-3   Sequential Procedure Order

1. Transconjunctival lower blepharoplasty
2. Endoscopic browlift
3. Endoscopic midface lift
4. Upper blepharoplasty
5. Lower pinch blepharoplasty
6. Submental liposuction
7. Platysmaplasty
8. Chin implant
9. Rhytidectomy

aspiration. The subcutaneous region is cannulized first without suction, after which suction assistance is used. Extreme caution is utilized to avoid excessive removal of fat, which will increase the risk of cobra neck deformity. The opening of the liposuction cannula should always face away from the dermis. A fan-shaped region is aspirated (Fig. 10-4). The body of the mandible is avoided in order to minimize the risk of marginal mandibular facial nerve injury.

Using an Aufricht retractor, we commonly identify the medial borders of the platysma in order to perform the platysmaplasty (Fig. 10-5). Vertical spreading with the facelift scissors allows easy identification of the platysma. Once the medial borders are identified, further subcutaneous dissection is performed laterally in both directions. A small portion of the platysma muscle's medial border is excised. This allows better adhesion after the two bellies are sewn together and approximated. Three to six buried interrupted 3-0 Mersilene sutures (Ethicon, Inc., New Brunswick, NJ) are utilized to plicate the two muscles. The first suture is placed at the most anterior portion of the platysma where the two sides are closest to one another. Instrument ties are utilized to tie the sutures in this small incision. Three to six sutures are placed to approximate the muscles. The thyroid cartilage generally marks the inferior limit. Back cuts in the platysma are rarely utilized. Platysmal approximation allows the lateral SMAS/platysma imbrication to lift the neck as a sling and create a more defined cervicomental angle. If necessary, chin augmentation is performed at this point of the operation.

The lateral facelift portion is then initiated. The facelift starts as a 2- to 3-cm incision in the anterior temporal hair tuft (Figs. 10-6 and 10-7). The incision curves back to meet the root of the helix and follows the preauricular contour down to the tragus. The incision continues in the retrotragal region and follows the natural crease of the lobule posteriorly onto the postauricular conchal bowl. In men, a pretragal incision is utilized to avoid placing the beard inside the ear. The postauricular incision is not made directly onto the postauricular crease but about 3 mm onto the conchal bowl up to the point where the helix meets the occipital hair tuft. The incision takes a soft turn back into the occipital hair tuft for about

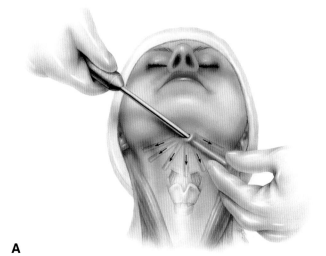

A

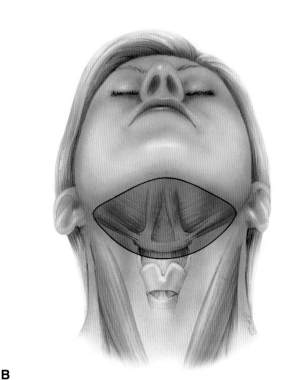

B

Figure 10-4 Submental suction-assisted lipectomy. Fan-shaped aspiration in the submental area is shown in **A**. The outlined area in **B** can be safely aspirated.

3 cm. The occipital incision is at a 45-degree angle and does not follow the hairline because of increased visibility. The postauricular incision is generally very well camouflaged because of the high placement and is rarely a source of concern to our patients. We occasionally perform a short-scar facelift in selected patients using a limited postauricular incision.

The flap elevation starts at the temporal hair tuft and facial region in the subcutaneous plane. A Brown-Adson forceps and No. 15 blade are utilized to begin the dissection (Fig. 10-8). Double hooks or three-prong cat-paws are utilized with Metzenbaum scissors for the

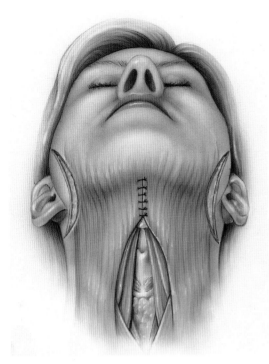

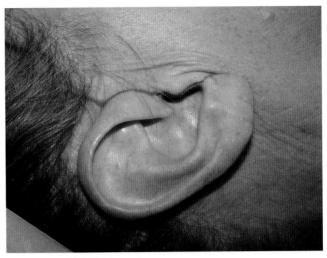

A

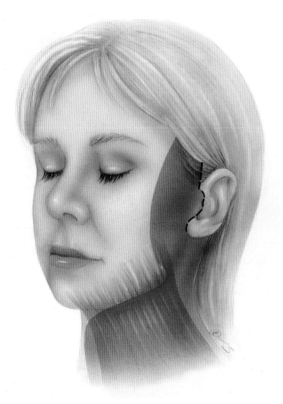

Figure 10-5 Platysmaplasty. Platysmaplasty allows the lateral SMAS/platysma imbrication to lift the neck as a sling and create a more defined cervicomental angle. Three to six buried interrupted 3-0 Mersilene sutures are utilized to plicate the muscles together. The first suture is placed at the most anterior portion of the platysma.

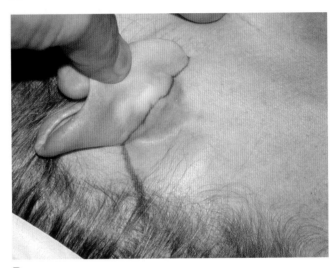

B

Figure 10-7 Intraoperative markings for incisions: preauricular (**A**) and postauricular (**B**) incision.

Figure 10-6 The incision and area of dissection in short-flap rhytidectomy. The temporal and occipital incisions are limited. A retro-tragal route is utilized. The facial region is dissected for 4-5 cm. The neck is widely dissected to the submental region.

majority of the undermining. Retraction by the assistant is of utmost importance to allow a safe and predictable depth of dissection. At the level of the tragus, we initially dissect a thick flap just above the perichondrium for 8 to 10 mm. The facial skin is much thicker than the native tragal skin; this maneuver in addition to aggressive thinning of the tailored skin at the end of the procedure significantly limits postoperative tragal fullness.

The skin elevation is performed for only 4 to 5 cm in the facial region. This limited skin dissection is the most important variation of the short-flap rhytidectomy as compared to other SMAS facelift procedures. Lower facial dissection at the angle of the mandible is not performed until posterior (occipital) neck elevation is completed, thereby decreasing the risk of marginal mandibular injury. The temporal area also needs to be dissected with extreme care in the subcutaneous plane as the frontal branch can have a superficial course over the zygomatic arch (Fig. 10-9). After the facial dissection is completed,

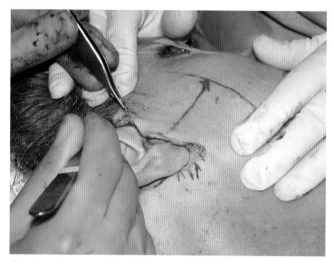

A

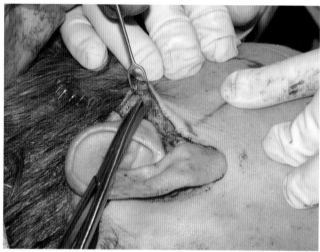

B

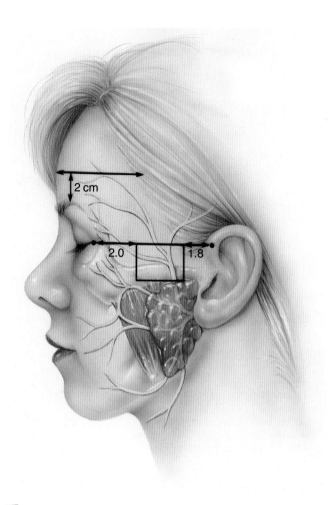

Figure 10-9 Danger zone for the frontal branch of the facial nerve. Typically four rami of the frontal branch of the facial nerve pass over the zygomatic arch. The most anterior ramus runs about 2 cm posterior to the anterior zygomatic arch. The branch is almost always anterior to the superficial temporal vessels.

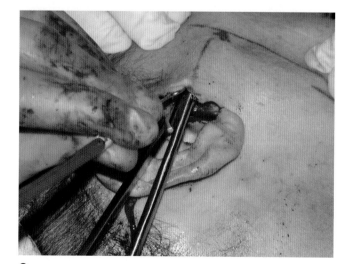

C

Figure 10-8 Facial subcutaneous dissection. The flap elevation starts at the temporal hair tuft (**A**). Brown-Adson forceps and No. 15 blade are utilized to start the dissection. A double hook is utilized with Metzenbaum scissors for the majority of the undermining (**B** and **C**). The assistant retracts the facial skin centrally at all times.

the posterior occipital area is elevated initially with a No. 15 blade (Fig. 10-10). This dissection is more fibrous and difficult than the anterior dissection. The subcutaneous plane is more difficult to ascertain. Facelift scissors are utilized to complete the cervical dissection. We perform an extensive cervical dissection. The lateral cervical dissection is united with the central dissection, which was created for the platysmaplasty and suction-assisted lipectomy. The inferior limit of the dissection is 4 to 5 cm below the angle of the mandible and at the level of thyroid notch. The surgeon must be cognizant of the external jugular as well as the great auricular nerve, as they can be easily injured. Complete cervical dissection is necessary in patients with significant laxity to obtain exceptional aesthetic results.

The lower facial subcutaneous elevation at the level of the angle of the mandible is performed once the cervical and superior facial dissections are completed (Fig. 10-11). Hooks are placed on the facial and cervical regions as the ear and facial skin are retracted in opposite direction.

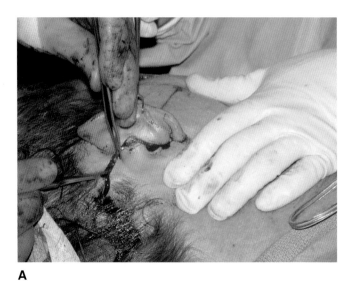

A

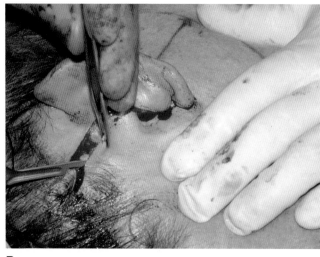

B

Figure 10-10 Postauricular skin flap elevation. This posterior dissection is more fibrous and difficult than the anterior dissection. The inferior limit of this dissection is 4 to 5 cm below the angle of the mandible. An extensive cervical elevation is performed in order to join the submental dissection.

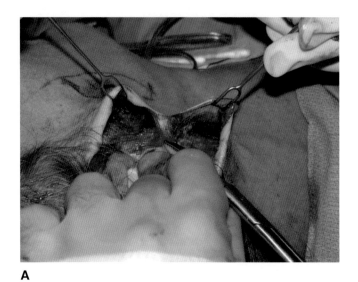

A

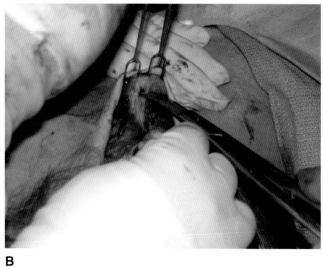

B

Figure 10-11 The upper facial dissection and cervical dissection are joined. Once the cervical and superior facial dissections are completed, the lower facial subcutaneous elevation at the level of the angle of the mandible is performed. Hooks are placed on the facial and cervical regions as the ear and facial skin are retracted in opposite directions. The dissection is usually carried out for 4 to 5 cm.

C

Babak Azizzadeh • Tessa A. Hadlock • Mack L. Cheney

This maneuver helps to further protect the marginal mandibular nerve because the subcutaneous plane is easily dissected. The anterior limit of this dissection is 4 to 5 cm. Facial liposuction is strictly avoided because of unpredictable results.

At this time, a segment of SMAS is excised using a Brown-Adson forceps and facelift scissors (Figs. 10-12 and 10-13). The excision starts 1 to 2 cm anterior to the

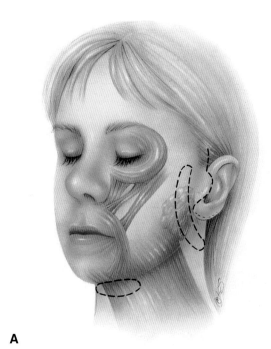

A

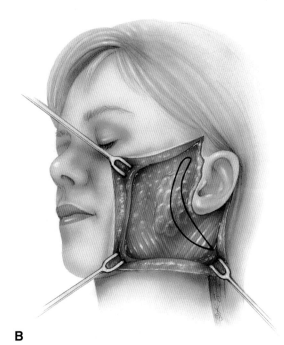

B

Figure 10-12 Outline of the SMAS excision. A segment of SMAS (**A**) is excised 1 to 2 cm anterior to the preauricular incision at the level of the root of the helix and extends inferiorly down to the infra-auricular platysma (**B**).

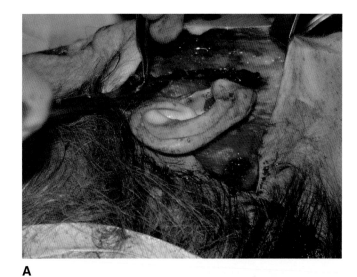

A

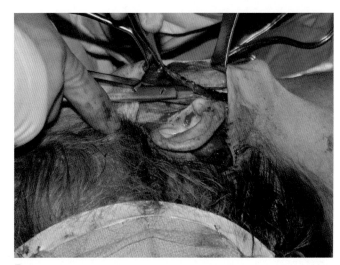

B

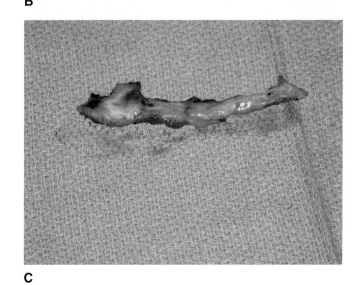

C

Figure 10-13 Intraoperative excision of SMAS. A segment of SMAS is excised using Brown-Adson forceps and facelift scissors (**A** and **B**). The excision starts 1 to 2 cm anterior to the preauricular incision at the level of the root of the helix and extends inferiorly down to the infra-auricular platysma. A segment of SMAS after excision is shown in **C**.

preauricular incision at the level of the root of the helix and extends inferiorly down to the infraauricular platysma. The anterior segment of the SMAS is then elevated to the anterior border of the parotid using Metzenbaum scissors (Fig. 10-14). The SMAS and platysma are imbricated with buried 3-0 Mersilene sutures, thereby suspending the anterior facial tissues. Multiple buried horizontal mattress sutures are placed. The vector of the SMAS imbrication is in a posterosuperior direction.

Excess skin is then tailored. Our goal is to minimize tension in the facial region and maximize tension in the occipital hair tuft. Skin tailoring can be challenging; thus, we have created a simple method for consistent results. Several anchor points are created (Fig. 10-15). The skin between these anchor points can subsequently be easily trimmed. A Brown-Adson forceps is utilized to place tension on the skin and calculate the exact distance for skin excision. The anchor points are all closed in two layers. The root of the helix serves as the first anchor point (AP-1). Once this location has been set, excess temporal

hair tuft superior to AP-1 is excised. To avoid a "dog-ear" deformity, closure is performed toward AP-1. Because our temporal incision is not extensive, we rarely find any significant change in hair position.

The second anchor point is at the level of the antitragus (AP-2). The intervening skin between the first and second anchor point can now be safely tailored. Extreme caution is used not to remove too much skin in this area because excess tension can widen the scar and pull the tragus anteriorly. The tragus is an extremely important landmark, and a natural pretragal cleat should be created in order to reduce the detection of the facelift incision. Using facelift scissors and curved iris scissors, the surgeon thins the newly positioned facial skin over the tragus. A Vicryl suture is then placed in the skin flap to recreate a natural tragal notch and secure to the underlying tissue. The suture has to penetrate the dermis in order to accomplish its goal. This deep suture additionally prevents the anterior pull of the tragus during the secondary healing phase.

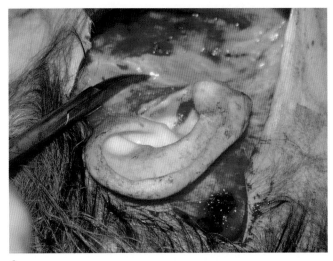

A

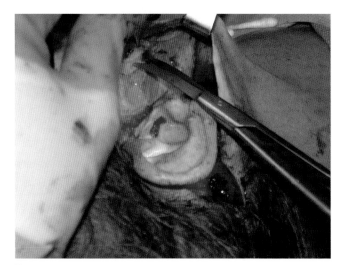

B

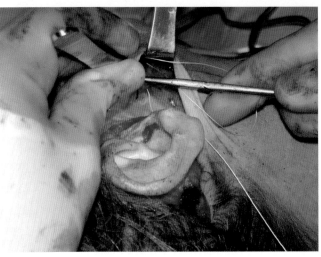

C

 Figure 10-14 SMAS imbrication. The anterior segment of the SMAS is elevated up to the anterior border of the parotid gland (**A** and **B**). The SMAS is imbricated with buried 3-0 Mersilene sutures (**C**). Multiple buried horizontal mattress sutures are placed. A posterosuperior vector is used for the SMAS imbrication.

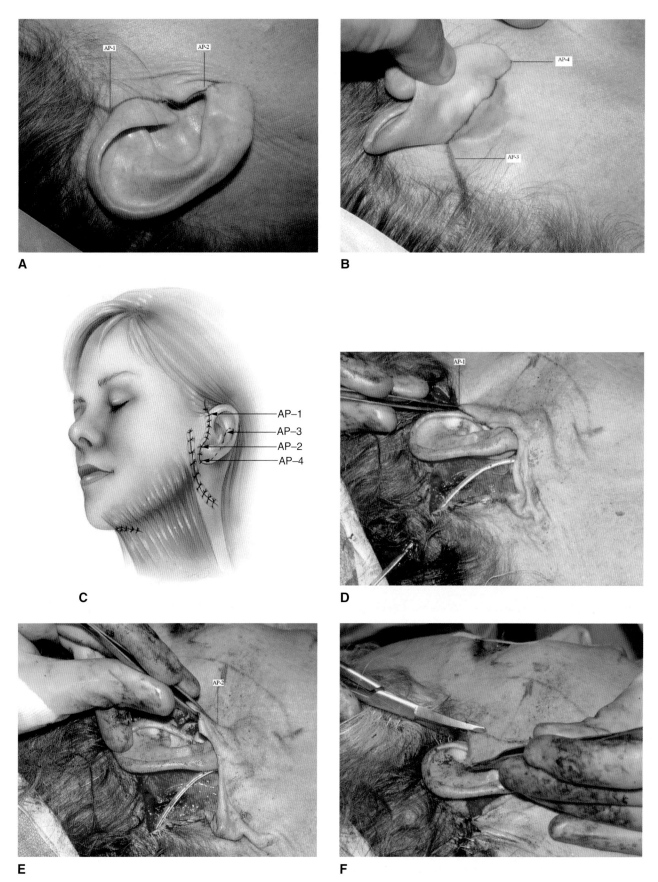

Figure 10-15 Skin tailoring. Several anchor points are utilized for tailoring the skin (**A–C**). The root of the helix (AP-1) serves as the first anchor point (**D**). Once this location has been set, excess temporal hair tuft superior to AP-1 is excised and staples are used for closure. The second anchor point (AP-2) is at the level of the antitragus (**E**). The intervening skin between the first and second anchor point is removed (**F**).

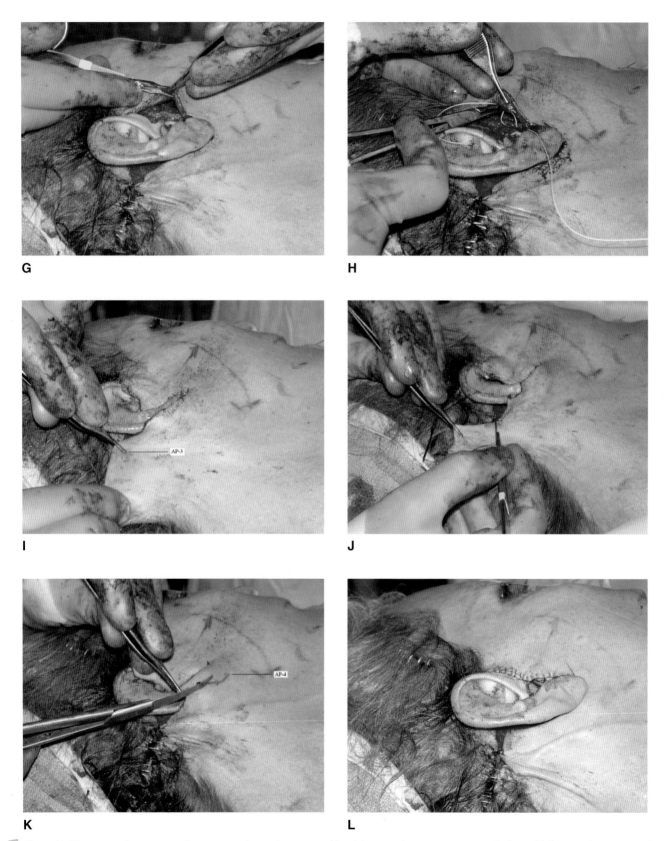

G   H

I   J

K   L

Figure 10-15 *Continued.* Using curved iris scissors, the newly positioned facial skin over the tragus is aggressively thinned (**G**). A Vicryl suture is used to create a pretragal cleat; it penetrates the dermis of the facial skin and is secured to the pretragal tissue (**H**). The third anchor point (AP-3) is the apex of the postauricular incision (**I**). Excess occipital skin is excised with the help of a hook (**J**). The occipital hairline is aligned with deep dissolvable sutures. The intervening tissue between AP-2 and AP-3 is draped over the ear lobule (**K**). The inferior border of the lobule is then used to make a split into this intervening skin. The apex of this incision becomes the anchor point of lobule attachment (AP-4). The excess skin between AP-2 and AP-4 is excised. In the postauricular area, the skin between AP-3 and AP-4 is also trimmed conservatively. The preauricular incision is closed with a 6-0 nylon in a running locking manner (**L**).

Once the anterior facial skin has been tailored, we turn our attention to the posterior skin. The third anchor point (AP-3) is the apex of postauricular incision. After the anchor point is set, excess occipital skin is excised with the help of a single hook. The occipital hairline is aligned with deep dissolvable sutures. Staples are then utilized to close the hair-bearing occipital hair tuft. The intervening tissue between AP-2 and AP-3 is draped over the ear lobule. The inferior border of the lobule is then used to make a split into this intervening skin. This incision must be performed in a precise manner, as the apex will become the anchor point of lobule attachment (AP-4). Pixie ear deformity is avoided by limiting the tension at this anchor point. Excess skin between AP-2 and AP-4 is excised. In the postauricular area, the skin between AP-4 and AP-3 is also trimmed conservatively, completing the skin tailoring in the cervicofacial region.

The preauricular incision is then closed with running locking 6-0 nylon or Prolene suture between AP-1 and AP-4. In the postauricular region, 4-0 fast-absorbing gut suture is used for closure. Staples are used for the temporal and occipital hair tufts. Small drains are placed prior to closure. If the patient is agreeable, Tisseel fibrin sealant (Baxter, Mississauga, ON Canada) can be used prior to closure and eliminates the need for drains. The submental incision is closed with a 6-0 nylon. A pressure dressing is applied and the patient is extubated and transferred to the recovery room. Ice gloves are used throughout the procedure to promote vasoconstriction and limit perioperative ecchymoses.

POSTOPERATIVE CARE

The patients typically stay in an aftercare facility for 12 to 48 hours where registered nurses attend to their special needs. Some patients choose to recover at home. We recommend continuous use of cool compresses in the first 72 hours. Patients are encouraged to have their head elevated. Antibiotics, analgesics, sleep, and antinausea medications are prescribed to the patients.

On the first postoperative day, the dressing and drains are removed. Hydrogen peroxide and antibiotic ointments are utilized to keep the incisions clean and moist for the first 5 days. An Ace wrap is then used when the patient is at home and at night for the first week. Patients are encouraged to take light showers starting on the second postoperative day. The preauricular sutures are removed on the third or fourth postoperative day, and Steri-Strips (3M, St. Paul, MN) are applied. Staples are removed on the sixth or seventh postoperative day. The patients are

seen again at the 4-week mark. During this visit, dermal fillers, volumizers, and botulinum toxin type A are utilized to address the midface as well as the perioral and periorbital rhytids (Figs. 10-16 to 10-18).

COMPLICATIONS

Box 10-4 summarizes potential complications associated with the short-flap rhytidectomy. We have not performed a prospective randomized study to ascertain the exact complication rate with the short-flap rhytidectomy. However, our experience has shown that the short-flap rhytidectomy lowers the risk for facial hematoma, flap necrosis, and facial nerve palsy when compared to other rhytidectomy techniques. The rates of cervical hematoma, postauricular skin necrosis, alopecia, and numbness is similar to those for other facelift methods. We have not noted an increase in the rate of revision surgery with this technique.

Future Considerations

Patients' desires for less invasive procedure have become a common trend during the last decade of aesthetic plastic surgery. Mini-facelifts, "thread lifts," and other limited procedures dominate the television and print media. The future of facial rejuvenation will likely converge on combining a variety of surgical and nonsurgical modalities. Longer lasting fillers, volumizers, and new noninvasive technology will likely reduce the number of patients who will opt for surgical intervention. Time-tested procedures such as facelifts, blepharoplasty, and browlifts will however continue to be very important tools for facial rejuvenation. Volume restoration will have an even a more prominent role in the treatment of the aging face and eyes.

Box 10-4   Complications Associated with Short-Flap Rhytidectomy

1. Cervicofacial hematoma
2. Alopecia
3. Scar
4. Skin slough
5. Infection
6. Numbness
7. Need for revision surgery
8. Facial nerve injury

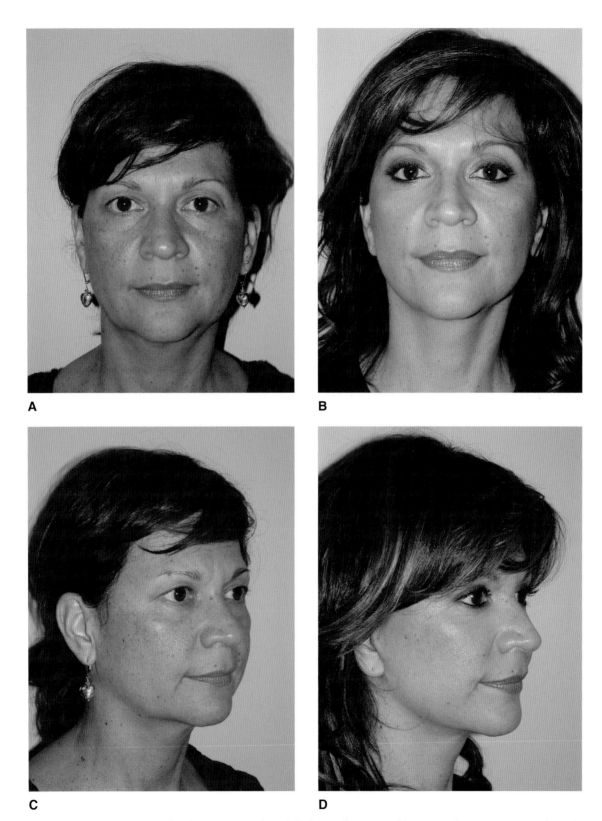

A

B

C

D

Figure 10-16 Preoperative (**A** and **C**) and early postoperative (**B** and **D**) photos of a 37-year-old woman with premature aging who underwent short-flap SMAS rhytidectomy and upper blepharoplasty.

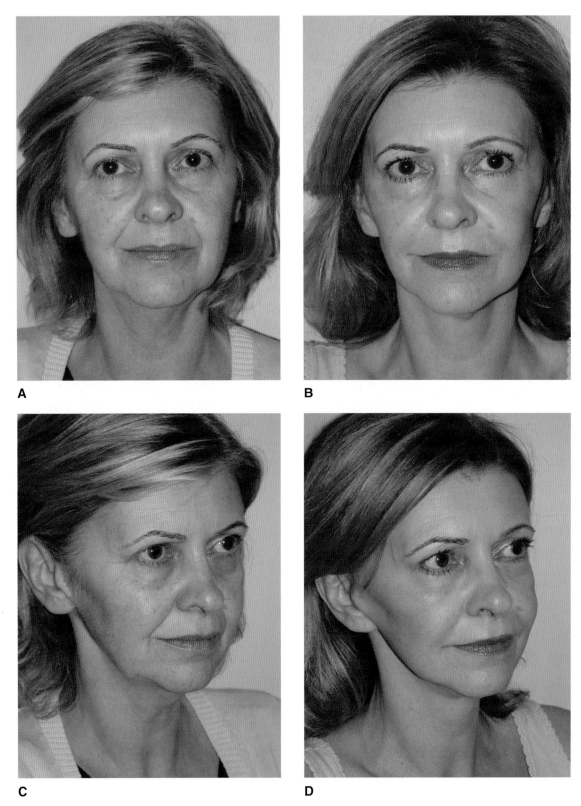

A

B

C

D

Figure 10-17 Preoperative (**A, C,** and **E**) and 7-month postoperative (**B, D,** and **F**) photos of a 52-year-old woman who underwent short-flap SMAS rhytidectomy and pinch lower blepharoplasty. The patient also had calcium hydroxylapatite (Radiesse) injections to the nasolabial folds and botulinum toxin type A (Botox) treatment for her periorbital rhytids in the immediate postoperative period.

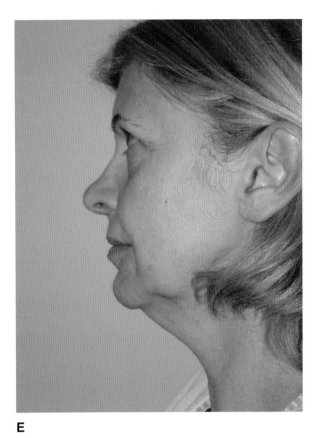

E

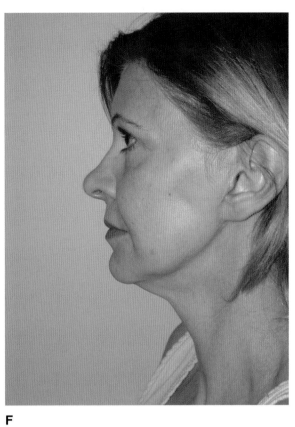

F

Figure 10-17 *Continued.*

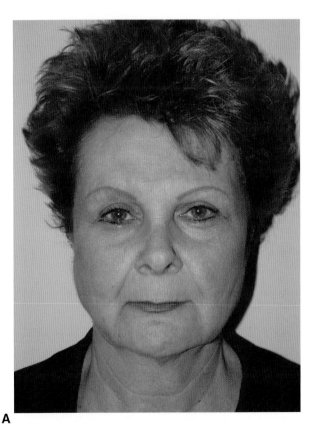

A

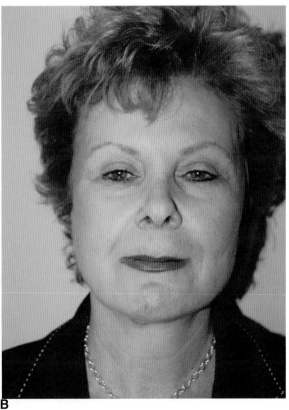

B

Figure 10-18 Preoperative (**A, C,** and **E**) and 8-month postoperative (**B, D,** and **F**) photos of a 67-year-old woman who underwent short-flap SMAS rhytidectomy, endoscopic browlift, blepharoplasty, and 30% trichloroacetic acid peel. The patient also had calcium hydroxylapatite (Radiesse) injections to the nasolabial folds and marionette furrows in the immediate postoperative period.

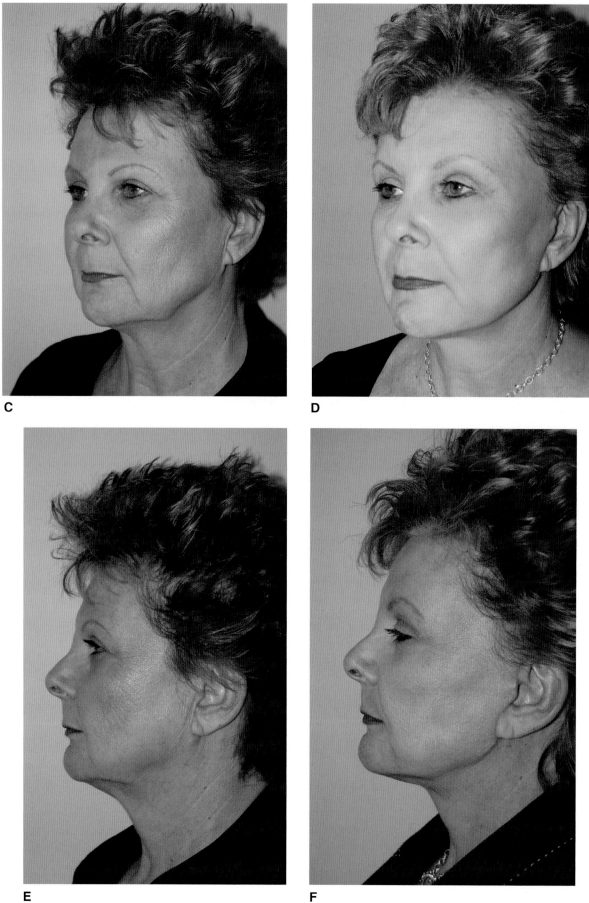

C

D

E

F

REFERENCES

1. Bettman A: Plastic and cosmetic surgery of the face. NW Med 1920;19:205.

2. Bourget J: La disparition chiurgicale des rides et plis du visage. Bull Acad Med (Paris) 1919;82:183.

3. Aufricht G: Surgery for Excessive Skin of the Face. Transactions of the Second International Congress of Plastic Surgery. Edinburgh: Livingstone, 1960, p 495.

4. Guerrero-Santos J, Espaillat L, Morales F: Muscular lift in cervical rhytidoplasty. Plast Reconstr Surg 1974;54:127.

5. Webster RC, Smith RC, Papsidero MJ, et al: Comparison of SMAS plication with SMAS imbrication in face lifting. Laryngoscope 1982;92:901.

6. Skoog T: Plastic Surgery: New Methods and Refinements. Philadelphia: WB Saunders, 1974.

7. Mitz V, Peyronie M: The superficial musculoaponeurotic system (SMAS) in the parotid and cheek area. Plast Reconstr Surg 1976;58:80.

8. Owsley JO Jr: SMAS-platysma face lift. Plast Reconstr Surg 1983;71(4):573.

9. Fodor PB: Platysma-SMAS rhytidectomy—A personal modification. Aesthet Plast Surg 1982;6(3):173.

10. Jost G, Lamouche G: SMAS in rhytidectomy. Aesthet Plast Surg 1982;6(2):69.

11. Kamer FM, Halsey W: The two-layer rhytidectomy. Arch Otolaryngol 1981;107(7):450.

12. Adamson JE, Todsu AE: Progress in rhytidectomy by platysma-SMAS rotation and elevation. Plast Reconstr Surg 1981;68(1):23.

13. Rees TD, Aston SJ: A clinical evaluation of the results of submusculo-aponeurotic dissection and fixation in face lifts. Plast Reconstr Surg 1977;60(6):851.

14. Baker DC: Lateral SMASectomy. Plast Reconstr Surg 1997;100(2):509.

15. Hamra ST: The deep plane rhytidectomy. Plast Reconstr Surg 1990;86(1):53-61, discussion 62.

16. Hamra ST: Composite rhytidectomy. Plast Reconstr Surg 1992;90(1):1.

17. Kamer FM: One hundred consecutive deep plane face lifts. Arch Otolaryngol Head Neck Surg 1996;122:17.

18. Godin MS, Johnson CM: Deep plane/composite rhytidectomy. Facial Plast Surg 1996;12(3):231.

19. Alsarraf R, Johnson CM: The Aging Face: A Systematic Approach. Philadelphia: WB Saunders, 2002.

20. Baker SR: Triplane rhytidectomy. Combining the best of all worlds. Arch Otolaryngol Head Neck Surg 1997;123:1167.

21. Tessier P: Lifting facial sous-perioste. Ann Chir Plast Esthet 1989;34:193.

22. Psillakis JM, Rumley TO, Carmargos A: Subperiosteal approach as an improved concept for correction of the aging face. Plast Reconstr Surg 1988;82:383.

23. Ramirez OM: The subperiosteal approach for the correction of the deep nasolabial fold and the central third of the face. Clin Plast Surg 1995;22(2):341.

24. Ramirez OM, Maillard GF, Musolas A: The extended subperiosteal facelift: A definitive soft tissue remodeling for facial rejuvenation. Plast Reconstr Surg 1991;88:227.

25. Ramirez OM: Endoscopic full facelift. Aesthet Plast Surg 1994;18:363.

26. Ramirez OM: Three-dimensional endoscopic midface enhancement: A personal quest for the ideal cheek rejuvenation. Plast Reconstr Surg 2002;109(1):329-40, discussion 341.

27. Quatela VC, Choe KS: Endobrow-midface lift. Facial Plast Surg 2004;20(3):199.

28. Williams EF 3rd, Vargas H, Dahiya R, et al: Midfacial rejuvenation via a minimal-incision brow-lift approach: critical evaluation of a 5-year experience. Arch Facial Plast Surg 2003;5(6):470.

29. Quatela VC, Jacono AA: The extended centrolateral endoscopic midface lift. Facial Plast Surg 2003;19(2):199.

30. Isse NG: Endoscopic facial rejuvenation: endoforehead, the functional lift. Aesthet Plast Surg 1994;18:21.

31. Furnas DW: The retaining ligaments of the cheek. Plast Reconstr Surg 1989;83(1):11.

32. Stuzin JM, Baker TJ, Gordon HL: The relationship of the superficial and deep facial fascias: Relevance to rhytidectomy and aging. Plast Reconstr Surg 1992;89(3):441.

33. Hoefflin SM: The extended supraplatysmal plane (ESP) face lift. Plast Reconstr Surg 1998;101(2):494.

34. Mendelson BC: SMAS fixation to the facial skeleton: Rationale and results. Plast Reconstr Surg 1997;100(7):1834-1842.

35. Ozdemir R, Kilinc H, Unlu RE, et al: Anatohistologic study of the retaining ligaments of the face and use in face lift: Retaining ligament correction and SMAS placation. Plast Reconstr Surg 2002;110(4):1134.

36. Mendelson BC, Muzaffar AR, Adams WP: Surgical anatomy of the midcheek and malar mounds. Plast Reconstr Surg 2002;110:885.

37. Muzaffar AR, Mendelson BC, Adams WP: Surgical anatomy of the ligamentous attachments of the lower lid and lateral canthus. Plast Reconstr Surg 2002;110:873.

38. Webster RC, Davidson TM, White MF, et al: Conservative face lift surgery. Arch Otolaryngol 1976;102(11):657.

39. Webster RC, Smith RC, Smith KF: Face lift, Part I: Extent of undermining of skin flaps. Head Neck Surg 1983;5:525.

40. Webster RC: Facelifts: Conservative vs. radical. In Ward P, Berman W (eds): Plastic and Reconstructive Surgery of the Head and Neck. St. Louis: CV Mosby, 1984, pp 363-382.

41. Webster RC, Hamdan U, Fuleihan N, et al: The considered and considerate facelift. Am J Cosmet Surg 1985;2:1.

42. McCollough EG, Perkins SW, Langsdon PR: SASMAS suspension rhytidectomy. Arch Otolaryngol Head Neck Surg 1989;115:228.

43. Burgess LP, Casler JD, Kryzer TC: Wound tension in rhytidectomy: Effects of skin flap undermining and superficial musculoaponeurotic system suspension. Arch Otolaryngol Head Neck Surg 1993;119(2):173.

44. Rees TD, Liverett DM, Guy Cl: The effect of cigarette smoking on skin flap survival in the face lift patient. Plast Reconstr Surg 1984;73:911.

45. Adamson PA, Moran ML: Complications of cervicofacial rhytidectomy. Facial Plast Surg Clin North Am 1993;1(2):257.

46. Hamra ST: Discussion. Plast Reconstr Surg 1996;98:1144.

47. Binder WJ: Submalar augmentation: A procedure to enhance rhytidectomy. Ann Plast Surg 1990;24(3):200.

48. Webster RC, Kattner MD, Smith RC: Injectable collagen for augmentation of facial areas. Arch Otolaryngol 1984;110(10):652.

49. Seckel BR: Facial Danger Zones: Avoiding Nerve Injury in Facial Plastic Surgery. St. Louis: Quality Medical Publishing, 1994.

50. Owsley JQ, Zweifler M: Midface lift of the malar fat pad: technical advances. Plast Reconstr Surg 2002;110(2):674.

51. Owsley JQ: Rejuvenation of the midface. Plast Reconstr Surg 2001;108(1):262.

52. Owsley JQ: Face lifting: Problems, solutions, and an outcome study. Plast Reconstr Surg 2000;105(1):302.

53. Owsley JQ, Fiala TG: Update: Lifting the malar fat pad for correction of prominent nasolabial folds. Plast Reconstr Surg 1997;100(3):715.

54. Becker FF, Bassichis BA: Deep-plane vs. superficial musculoaponeurotic system placation face-lift. Arch Facial Plast Surg 2004;6:8.

55. Ivy EJ, Lorenc ZP, Aston SJ: Is there a difference? A prospective study comparing lateral and standard SMAS face lifts with extended SMAS and composite rhytidectomies. Plast Reconstr Surg 1996;98(7):1135.

56. Anderson JR: The tuck-up operation, a new technique of secondary rhytidectomy. Arch Otolaryngol 1975;101(12):739.

57. Kamer FM, Parkes ML: Sequential rhytidectomy. Laryngoscope 1978;88(7 Pt 1):1196.

58. Kamer FM: Sequential rhytidectomy and the two stage concept. Otolaryngol Clin North Am 1980;13(2):305.

59. Yousif NJ, Gosain A, Matloub HS, et al: The nasolabial fold: An anatomic and histologic reappraisal. Plast Reconstr Surg 1994;93:60.

60. Rees TD, Aston SJ: Complications of rhytidectomy. Clin Plast Surg 1978;5:109.

61. Baker DC: Complications of cervicofacial rhytidectomy. Clin Plast Surg 1983;10(3):543.

62. Dedo DD: "How I do it"—Plastic surgery. Practical suggestions on facial plastic surgery. A pre-operative classification of the neck for cervicofacial rhytidectomy. Laryngoscope 1980;90(11 Pt 1):1894.

CHAPTER ELEVEN

Tridimensional Endoscopic Facelift

Oscar M. Ramirez, MD, FACS • *Charles R. Volpe, MD*

HISTORY

The tridimensional endoscopic facelift is based upon the construct of the subperiosteal facelift technique initially described by Tessier.[1] Tessier conceived that this "orthomorphic" subperiosteal facelift would be an innovative way to provide facial rejuvenation in young and middle-age patients.[2] Subsequently, Psillakis published his modifications to the subperiosteal approach, demonstrating that extensive lateral periorbital dissection could provide improved rejuvenation of the cheek region.[3] Soon after, several authors demonstrated their experience with the subperiosteal techniques.[4,5] The extended subperiosteal facelift, described in 1991, introduced several innovative concepts including extensive midface dissection, improved suspension techniques, and a safer method of access across the zygomatic arch.[6] Further refinements in the extended subperiosteal technique[7-9] ushered in the era of endoscopy. In the mid-1990s, techniques adapted from the open subperiosteal rhytidectomy approach proved that endoscopic methods could be developed to perform facial rejuvenation.[10-12]

Over the past decade, the senior author has dedicated his practice to facial rejuvenation using the tridimensional endoscopic facelift technique. The knowledge and experience developed from this approach are presented in this chapter. The authors hope to provide insight into their comprehensive approach to endoscopic facial rejuvenation.

PERSONAL PHILOSOPHY

The aging face is characterized by volumetric change caused by a reduction of the soft tissues and resorption of bone.[13] The volumetric changes affect the central part of the face earlier than the peripheral areas of the face. The central portion of the face comprises the mimetic and sphincteric muscles allowing facial expressions. The peripheral portion of the face is more static and thus more resistant to the aging process. Thus, the face can be broken down into two distinct aesthetic units: the central oval and the peripheral hemicircle.[14] The central oval is composed of the loose, dynamic structures that fall prey to the gravitational forces of nature. Combined with loss of bone volume, it becomes evident that the deflation and gravitational migration of the soft tissues lead to "earlier aging" of the central oval of the face.

The authors favor a comprehensive approach for rejuvenation of both the central oval and peripheral hemicircle of the face. Basic tenets to this approach include (1) a direct approach to the central oval of the face; (2) an interconnected subperiosteal plane of dissection in the upper and midface; (3) use of small hidden slit incisions; (4) absence of visible incisions on the central oval; (5) use of endoscopic techniques; (6) absence of traction with the skin or SMAS (superficial musculoaponeurotic system) from the peripheral hemicircle; (7) ability to modify the skeletal framework in the same operative plane; and (8) ability to correct the deficit of soft tissue volume.

Rejuvenation of the central oval of the face can be accomplished with endoscopic forehead lift,[15] endoscopic midface lift,[16] and mentopexy procedures. The endoscopic forehead lift and midface lift procedures can be used for all degrees of facial rejuvenation. Mentopexy is performed in selective cases. Rejuvenation in the peripheral hemicircle focuses upon the neck and jawline and can be accomplished through a variety of techniques. Younger patients with good skin tone and moderate submandibular fat accumulation benefit from the nonexcisional cervicoplasty.[17] The suture suspension method described is based upon the techniques developed by Giampapa[18] and Guerro-Santos[19] in which important modifications have been made by the senior author. Patients with severe laxity of the skin are treated with a traditional excisional cervicoplasty through submental and periauricular incisions. In select patients, skeletal augmentation of the jawline is necessary to achieve harmony between the aesthetic units of the face. The mandibular matrix system[20] has been developed to correct skeletal deficiencies of the jawline, give more angularity to the jawline, and to provide support for the soft tissues.

Because of the individual nature of the aging process, facial rejuvenation can be provided through the use of soft tissue manipulation, soft tissue augmentation, and alloplastic augmentation (Fig. 11-1). The goal of this chapter is to provide the authors' approach toward the treatment of the aging face. The techniques described form the components of the tridimensional endoscopic facelift procedure.

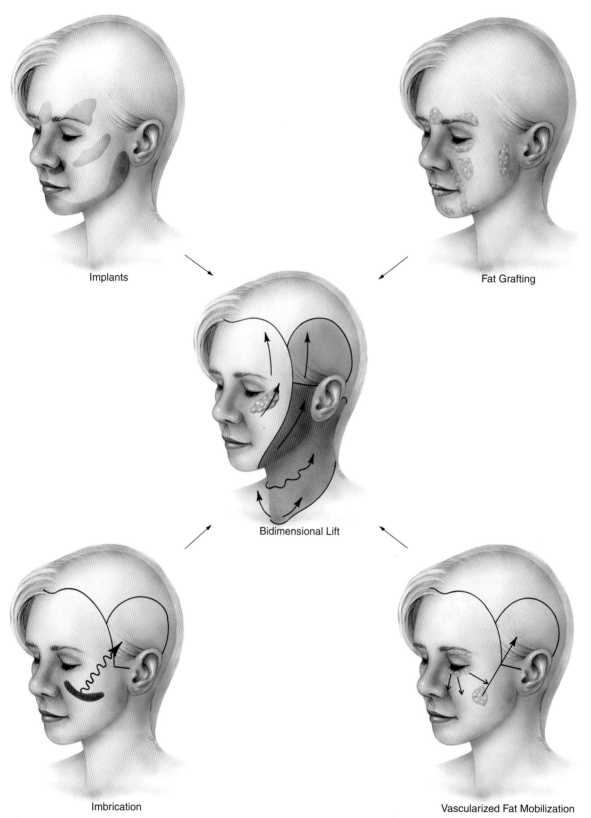

Implants

Fat Grafting

Bidimensional Lift

Imbrication

Vascularized Fat Mobilization

Figure 11-1 This schematic diagram shows the components available for three-dimensional facial rejuvenation. Bidimensional lifting in vertical and lateral planes provides the foundation of the endoscopic facelift. Weak skeletal support can be corrected with alloplastic implants, as shown in the upper left corner of the diagram. Fat grafting, as shown in the upper right corner, is commonly used to enhance areas not corrected by lifting techniques. In addition, fat grafting is used to treat small areas of depression or creases caused by subdermal damage. Imbrication of soft tissues is amenable in the brow, maxillary malar area, and mentum, as shown in the lower left corner. The lower right corner of the diagram shows the areas useful for augmentation by adjacent vascularized fat mobilization, including upper orbital rim augmentation with the upper eyelid fat pads, the infraorbital rim tear-trough area with the lower eyelid fat pads, and cheek augmentation with Bichat's fat pad. (From Ramirez OM: Full face rejuvenation in three dimensions: A "face-lifting" for the new millennium. Aesthet Plast Surg 2001;25:152-164, used with permission from Springer-Verlag, New York.)

ANATOMY OF FACIAL AGING

Successful rejuvenation of the face requires a thorough understanding of the anatomic changes associated with aging. Characteristic features in the frontal region include visible spasm of the corrugator muscles, deep set eyes, and the appearance of deflated brows with hooding and upper eyelid skin excess. The temporal region becomes hollowed. The lower eyelids demonstrate orbital fat herniation, and in advanced stages, exposure of the lower orbital rim leads to creation of a "tear-trough" deformity. The malar area is characterized by loss of thickness and ptosis of Bichat's fat pad. Reduction in mandibular volume through bone resorption results in loss of projection at the mandibular border and hollowness around the jowls. The mandibular bone loss is accentuated in edentulous patients.[21] The chin is subjected to loss of tissue bulk and ptosis leading to the "witch's chin" deformity, as coined by Gonzales-Ulloa.[22] Facial expression lines become accentuated owing to collagen damage and loss of elastic fibers. Significant skin laxity, horizontal neck creases, accumulation of fat in the submental and submandibular regions, platysmal banding, and development of an obtuse cervicomental angle are characteristic.

PREOPERATIVE ASSESSMENT

Patients are all examined in a well-lit room, in a seated position. An initial assessment is performed, noting medical history, surgical history, current medications including herbal supplements, and allergies. Social and family history is noted. A detailed history of previous cosmetic procedures is obtained. Patients are then given the opportunity to express their concerns. We find it extremely helpful to provide the patient with a handheld mirror during this part of the examination. Understanding the patient's desires allows the proper surgical plan to be developed. Finally, a directed physical examination is performed noting the stigmata of the aging process.

Access to photographs of the patient at a younger age can be quite helpful in the creation of a surgical plan. Patients are encouraged to provide them when possible. We keep a book of beautiful faces cut from magazines in each examination room as an aid to explain aesthetic principles and features. If alloplastic implantation is considered, skeletal models and sample implants are available to assist in the explanation of proposed surgical procedures. A comprehensive collection of preoperative and postoperative patient results is available to the patients for perusal. In our opinion, these visual aids are essential to attain the desired aesthetic outcome and patient satisfaction.

PHOTOGRAPHIC DOCUMENTATION

Using a standardized photography studio setup, a series of photographs are compiled prior to surgery. A full-face (anteroposterior, AP) frontal view, right and left three-quarter (oblique) views, right and left lateral views, and a 45-degree down-tilted frontal (AP) view are the minimum images acquired. Ancillary images are acquired based upon the developed surgical plan. The images are printed prior to the operative procedure and are posted in the operating room for intraoperative reference. Similar postoperative photographs are acquired at 3, 6, and 12 months, respectively, and on a yearly basis thereafter. By maintaining a detailed photographic record of the preoperative and postoperative results, careful analysis of the three-dimensional contour changes can be performed.

ADDRESSING THE CENTRAL OVAL OF THE FACE

Heeding the anatomic principles of facial aging, one can see that a comprehensive approach to facial rejuvenation is required to maximize the aesthetic results (see Fig. 11-1). The tridimensional facelift technique embraces this concept. The comprehensive approach developed focuses on both the central oval and peripheral hemicircle of the face. The endoscopic forehead lift and endoscopic midface lift procedures provide the foundation for treating the central oval of the face, bolstered by the mentopexy procedure in select patients.

SURGICAL TECHNIQUE

ENDOSCOPIC FOREHEAD LIFT PROCEDURE

The endoscopic forehead lift procedure begins with careful placement of four incisions in the scalp. The first two incisions are located approximately 2.0 cm on either side of the midline, 1.0 to 2.0 cm posterior to the hairline. For patients with excessively long foreheads (>8 cm) these paramedian incisions are placed directly at the hairline. It is important to keep the forehead incisions as anterior as possible. Otherwise, visualization and dissection in the glabellar region will be compromised. The next set of incisions is located in the temple region, bilaterally, 2.0 cm posterior to the hairline. The incisions should be directed parallel to the hair follicles to prevent unnecessary alopecia postoperatively. Each incision should measure 1.5 cm in length (Fig. 11-2).

Prior to surgical dissection, local anesthesia using 50 mL of 0.5% lidocaine with 1:200,000 epinephrine is diffusely distributed in both the subcutaneous and subperiosteal planes. Early administration of the anesthetic will provide maximal hemostasis, which is required during endoscopic visualization.

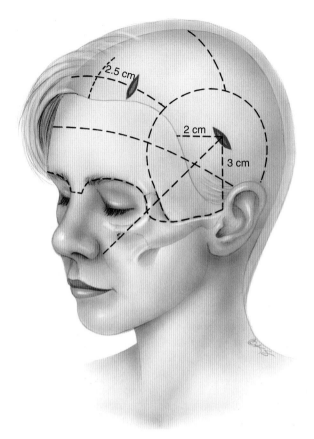

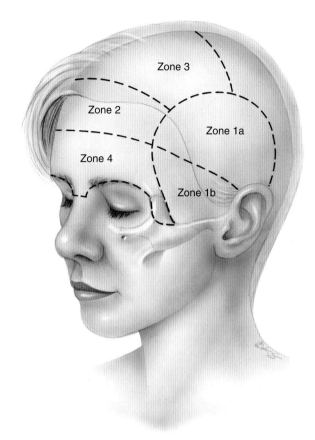

Figure 11-2 Reference lines and measurements for the placement of the endoscopic incisions. Note that an imaginary line drawn on a tangent from the lateral border of the nasal ala through the lateral canthal tendon determines proper placement of the temporal incision.

Figure 11-3 The zone system has been developed to aid safe dissection during the endoscopic forehead and midface procedures. Endoscopic visualization is mandatory when dissecting in zones 1b and 4.

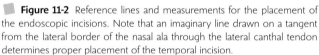

For optimization of the operative procedure, the forehead is methodically divided into four zones that correspond with the sequence of facial dissection (Fig. 11-3). Zone 1 corresponds to the lateral region bounded by the temporalis musculature and zygomatic arch. The upper portion of zone 1 (zone 1A) can be safely dissected in a "blind" fashion. The lower portion of zone 1 (zone 1B) requires dissection under strict endoscopic guidance. Important neurovascular structures, including the frontal branch of the facial nerve, pass through this zone. Zone 2 extends from the hairline to the middle of the forehead. Zone 3 begins at the hairline and extends posteriorly to the vertex of the scalp. Zone 4 corresponds to the area bounded by the superior orbital rims and nasal root inferiorly and the middle of the forehead superiorly. Vital structures, such as the supraorbital and supratrochlear nerves, are located in this zone.

The endoscopic procedure begins with the incision in the temporal area (the upper portion of zone 1). This incision is located perpendicular to a tangent drawn from the nasal ala to the lateral canthal tendon and is 2 cm inside the temporal scalp (see Fig. 11-2). A 1.5- to 1.8-cm incision is made through the skin and subcutaneous tissue, deep through the superficial temporal fascia until

the temporal fascia proper is reached. Dissection is intiated to clear all the soft tissues from the temporal fascia proper. Dissection continues inferiorly remaining above the intermediate temporal fascia. As mentioned previously, the initial dissection (upper portion of zone 1) can be performed blindly in a circumferential fashion for approximately a 2-cm radius. With the tissues elevated, a Silastic port protector is inserted and the remainder of the dissection is performed under endoscopic control.

Elevator No. 8 of the Ramirez endoscopic instrument set (Snowden-Pencer, Inc., Tucker, GA) is used to dissect to the temporal line of fusion superiorly. The elevator is then used to score and elevate the periosteum 1 cm medial to the temporal line of fusion. This is continued superiorly through the lateral portions of zones 4, 2, and 3, respectively.

This dissection will aid in the connection of the temporal and frontal pockets, later in the case. Dissection continues from the temporal incision in an inferior and medial direction around the lateral orbital rim. During the course of this dissection, several temporal veins will come into view. Temporal vein 1, situated in the region of the zygomaticofrontal suture, is usually sacrificed. Temporal vein 2 (also referred to as the "sentinel vein") is encountered while dissecting toward the zygomatic arch. Branches of the zygomaticotemporal nerve may be identified during this dissection. Temporal vein 3 lies just above the zygomatic arch at the junction of its middle and posterior thirds. This is usually not exposed. Temporal vein 2, temporal vein 3, and the branches of the zygomaticotemporal nerve should be preserved when possible. Preservation of these structures is facilitated with a blunt rounded tip elevator. As the procedure progresses inferiorly, the dissection plane moves from temporal fascia proper to the intermediate temporal fascia. The intermediate temporal fat pad will be visualized through the thin intermediate temporal fascia. Dissection along the lateral orbital wall progresses inferiorly to the level of the lateral canthus. This completes the lateral dissection of the endoscopic forehead procedure.

The paramedian incisions are then made as previously described and are carried down through the periosteum. Dissection in zones 2 and 3 can be performed with a blind sweeping technique, as long as the dissection remains in a subperiosteal plane. The endoscope is inserted during dissection in zone 4. In general, zone 4 begins about 3 cm from the superior orbital rims. Endoscopically assisted dissection should always be performed in zone 4 (Fig. 11-4). The initial dissection proceeds toward the lateral aspect of the superior orbital rim. Further dissection laterally toward the temporal line of fusion will allow connection of zones 1 and 4. The dissection then proceeds in a medial direction along the superior orbital rim. Cautious dissection in this area is mandatory. The authors have noted variations in the supraorbital nerve anatomy. Occasionally, an accessory branch of the supraorbital nerve can be identified as far as 3.0 cm superior and lateral to the supraorbital nerve proper. Every effort should be made to preserve any accessory nerve branch. After identification of the supraorbital nerve, dissection continues medially, exposing the origins of the corrugator muscles. The supratrochlear nerve travels in the substance of the corrugator muscles, so careful elevation of the corrugators is required. Typically, three fascicles of the supratrochlear nerve are identified and preserved. Prior to resection of the corrugator muscle, the periosteum of the superior orbital rim is released with a curved elevator. The periosteum should be released from the zygomaticofrontal suture line laterally, moving medially toward the glabella. In patients with heavy tissues, especially males, the periosteum is released by cutting it with endoscopic scissors. With the periosteum cut medially, the supratrochlear nerve and corrugator muscles are clearly delineated.

The corrugator muscle is extensively resected from its point of origin to just beyond the supraorbital nerve (Fig. 11-5). We prefer to resect approximately 80% of the corrugator muscle to assure that glabellar frown lines are eliminated. Once the corrugator has been removed, the depressor supercilii muscle can occasionally be identified.

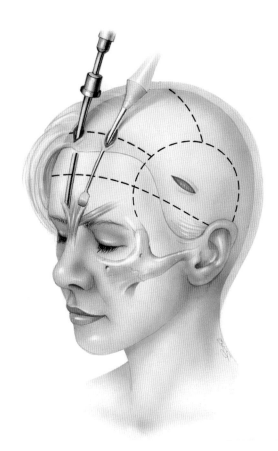

Figure 11-4 Dissection during the endoscopic forehead facelift should extend down along the supraorbital rims and nasal radix to completely elevate the periosteum in the inferior border of zone 4.

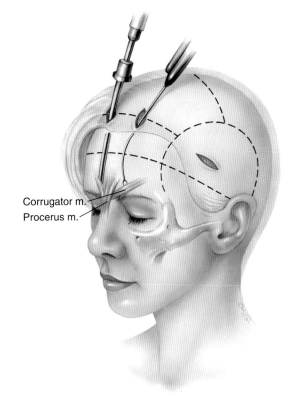

Corrugator m.
Procerus m.

Figure 11-5 The endoscopic grasper is used to resect the corrugator and procerus muscles as shown.

Resection of the depressor supercilii muscle is indicated if medial brow ptosis is present. An endoscopic scissor then is used to divide the periosteum deep to the procerus muscle. The procerus muscle is resected after being thoroughly exposed. Resection of the procerus muscle should proceed down to the level of the nasoglabellar angle. Occasionally, bleeding will occur during procerus resection. Given the superficial location of the dissection, care must be taken when using cautery in this area. Overzealous cauterization in this location can lead to disastrous consequences (burning of the skin). When the muscle resection is complete, the area is packed with epinephrine-soaked pledgets. Attention is then directed back to the temporal region where the endoscopic midface lift is started at this point. Completion of the endoscopic forehead lift procedure with elevation and fixation of the brow typically follows completion of the endoscopic midface suspension. An example of a pure endoscopic forehead lift can be seen in Figures 11-6 through 11-8.

ENDOSCOPIC MIDFACE LIFT PROCEDURE

The endoscopic midface lift procedure begins with the temporal dissection in zone 1, as outlined in the previous section. The temporal vein 2 (sentinel vein), temporal vein 3, and the zygomaticotemporal nerves are preserved

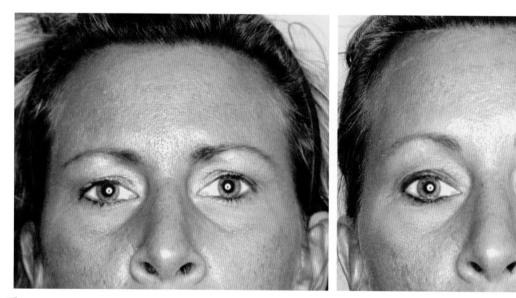

Figure 11-6 Anterior views of a patient who underwent a pure endoscopic forehead procedure. The preoperative view is shown to the left. Improved brow position is shown in the postoperative view on the right.

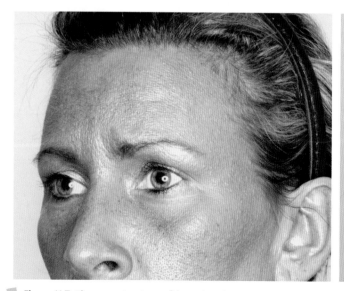
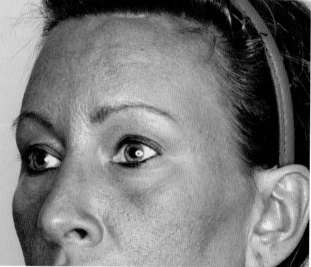

Figure 11-7 Three-quarter views of the patient shown in Figure 11-6. Note the softening of the glabellar creases and more youthful position of the brows in the postoperative view (*right*).

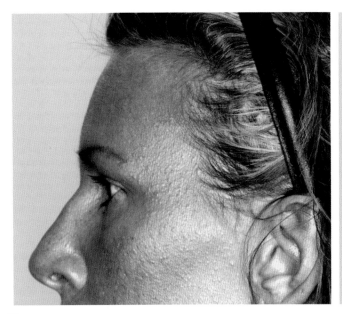 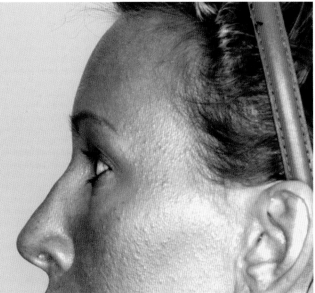

Figure 11-8 Lateral views of the patient in Figures 11-6 and 11-7. Brow ptosis is evident in the preoperative view (*left*). The postoperative image (*right*) shows an aesthetically pleasing brow position.

when possible. The dissection continues in an anterior and inferior direction, remaining above the intermediate temporal fascia. Dissection along the intermediate temporal fascia continues down to the level of the zygomatic arch. The zygomatic arch is entered 2 to 3 mm above the superior border of the arch. This requires division of the intermediate temporal fascia, thus exposing the periosteum of the zygomatic arch. The anterior two thirds of the zygomatic arch periosteum are typically elevated. We find that greater lifting and redistribution of the midface soft tissues occur with this approach. The periosteum of the entire zygomatic arch is elevated only when soft tissues lateral to the cheek need to be lifted.

A word of caution is necessary at this point. Comfort with the endoscopic dissection over the zygomatic arch from the temporal area is associated with a significant learning curve. Moving from the plane of intermediate temporal fascia to zygomatic arch periosteum, although conceptually simple, can be difficult in practice. Therefore, we advocate that surgeons pre-elevate the zygomatic arch or at least elevate to the superior border of the arch from an intraoral approach during the learning process. Pre-elevation in this manner will allow safe communication of both the temporal and lower midface dissection pockets, later in the case. As skill and comfort with the technique increase, dissection can be performed as originally outlined.

The midface dissection at this point continues through an intraoral (upper buccal sulcus) incision. The authors' preferred incision is perpendicular to the alveolar ridge (vertical) at the level of the first premolar. We find that the vertically oriented incision preserves the mucosal integrity at the alveolar ridge, allowing a rapid, watertight

closure that is associated with fewer complications. Under direct visualization, the initial subperiosteal dissection of the maxilla and malar area is performed. The endoscope is used for the upper malar dissection. The use of the endoscope minimizes trauma to the midface structures caused by excessive traction. The endoscope is most useful during periosteal elevation along the lateral half of the zygoma body, its extension underneath the fascia of the masseter muscle, and the anterior two thirds of the zygomatic arch. The fascia covering the upper (medial) portion of the masseter tendon is also elevated from the zygoma. A few longitudinal fibers can be included in the elevated flap as necessary. Endoscopic visualization assists in the preservation of the zygomaticofacial nerve.

Dissection continues along the inferior and lateral orbital rim and continues toward the superior border of the zygomatic arch. Skeletonization of the infraorbital nerve is not necessary under most circumstances.

With the initial midface dissection now complete, the endoscope is returned to the temporal area. An assistant elevates the soft tissue of the midface, thus allowing the surgeon to safely connect the temporal and midface dissection pockets under endoscopic control. Gentle elevation during this step protects the frontal branch of the facial nerve from injury. With wide communication of the temporal and midface pockets, the endoscope is returned through the upper buccal sulcus incision.

The inferior orbital rim is dissected further by elevating the inferior arcus marginalis. A 4-0 PDS (polydioxanone) suture (Ethicon, Somerville, NJ), introduced endoscopically, is used to imbricate the medial suborbicularis oculi fat (SOOF) to the lateral aspect of the inferior arcus marginalis. It is important to check eye globe mobility at this point with a forced duction test because improper placement of this imbricating suture can indirectly trap or place traction upon the inferior rectus muscle.

The lateral aspect of the suborbicularis oculi fat is then grasped with a 3-0 PDS suture, providing the first of three suspension sutures (Fig. 11-9). Both ends of this suture are then passed through the temporal incision, under endoscopic guidance. We find it helpful to tag the suture ends of each suspension suture with a labeled needle driver. This allows the surgeon to keep track of each suspension suture without confusion. The second suspension suture is the lower cheek imbrication, or "modiolus" suture. This suture is placed into the tenuous periosteal/fascia/fat of the inferior maxillary soft tissue near the upper buccal sulcus incision. Both ends of this suture are then directed through the temporal incision and tagged, as previously described.

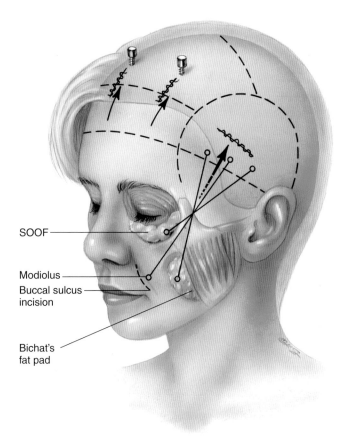

SOOF

Modiolus

Buccal sulcus incision

Bichat's fat pad

Figure 11-9 Treatment of the midface is performed with key suspension sutures that provide lifting in a vertical direction. The sutures are placed from the buccal sulcus incision and directed through the temporal pocket created endoscopically. The orientation of the anchoring and fixation of the corresponding sutures into the temporal fascia proper is indicated. Bichat's fat pad suture is woven through the fat pad and directed in a superomedial direction to add lateral bulk to the cheek over the zygomatic arch. The modiolus suture is directed in a tangential direction to the nasolabial fold and provides lifting of the lower cheek soft tissues. The suborbicularis oculi fat (SOOF) suspension suture is directed most laterally and allows improvement of the tear-trough deformity.

Exposure of Bichat's fat pad follows the placement of the first two suspension sutures. Bichat's fat pad is approached through the superomedial wall of the buccal space. The periosteum and buccinator muscle are spread with the use of a blunt dissector. This allows Bichat's fat pad to herniate through maintaining an intact capsular fascia. The fat pad should be carefully dissected free from the wall of the buccal space. The fat pad should be easily movable for repositioning as a pedicle flap. A 4-0 PDS suture is then woven into the fat pad and the suture ends are delivered to the temporal area, similar to the previous suspension sutures. The endoscope should be used to visualize the delivery of the pedicled fat flap over the zygomatic arch. The endoscope can also assess the trajectory of the suspensions sutures. It is important to avoid criss-crossing the suspension sutures as they are passed temporally.

Each of the suspension sutures is then secured to the temporal fascia proper, in ordered fashion. The sutures should be placed in the temporal fascia proper, below the level of the temporal incision. The first suture, the Bichat's pad fat suspension, should be placed most medially. The inferior malar periosteum/fascia/fat or modiolus suture is placed next, in a more lateral location of the temporal fascia proper. The most lateral suture, the suborbicularis oculi fat suture, is the last to be anchored to the temporal fascia proper. This completes the suspension of the midface.

Butterfly drains are placed bilaterally through separate stab incisions in the temporal scalp. Each drain is carefully directed into the midface and secured to the temporal scalp with a suture. The superficial temporal fascia is then anchored to the temporal fascia proper with two 4-0 PDS sutures, while an assistant provides superomedial traction to the advanced scalp. This maneuver will provide additional support to the suspended soft tissues. The intraoral incisions are then closed with interrupted 4-0 chromic catgut sutures, to provide a watertight closure.

Attention, at this point, is directed back to the forehead region where drain placement, closure of the paramedian incisions, and brow elevation is performed.

Briefly, two suction drains are placed through separate stab incisions in the scalp, adjacent to the paramedian access ports. An endoscopic biter is used to direct the tips of the drains to the level of the glabella and the anterior forehead. Each drain is secured with a heavy drain stitch. The paramedian incisions are closed in two layers. A blunt traction hook is then used to elevate the scalp and to position the brow. When proper brow position is obtained, a small stab incision is made in the scalp, with a No. 11 scalpel. A 1.1-mm drill bit with a 4-mm stop is inserted through the stab incision and a unicortical hole in the calvarium is drilled. A 1.5-mm titanium post (Synthes, Paoli, PA) is then placed in the drill hole. In most cases, two paramedian posts (one on each side) are sufficient to maintain the proper brow

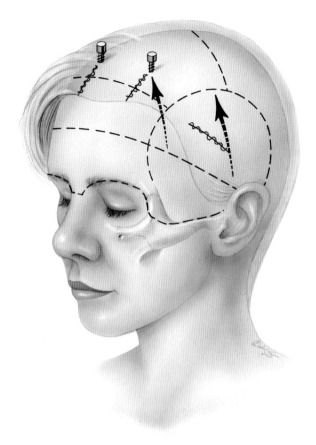

position (Fig. 11-10). Location of the posts will have a significant impact on brow position. Under most circumstances, post placement corresponds to a superomedial axis from the lateral brow. This will provide maximal elevation of the lateral brow. More central post placement is chosen for patients requiring greater elevation of the central and medial brow. Patient examples of full endoscopic forehead and midface procedures are shown in Figures 11-11 through 11-16.

MENTOPEXY

In select cases, addition of the mentopexy procedure is required to provide aesthetic balance to the rejuvenated central oval. The aging chin is a complex entity that frequently is not properly addressed during facial rejuvenation procedures. The "witch's chin" deformity consists of ptosis of the premental soft tissues, a prominent submental crease, and often a loss of bony projection. In an effort to address the complex pathophysiology of the witch's chin deformity, the authors present a multivariate approach toward correction of the ptotic chin. Soft tissue manipulation and the use of alloplastic implants play a role in the treatment of the ptotic chin. A subperiosteal dissection performed through a submental incision is used for each of the procedures described.

The mentopexy procedure begins with a 3-cm submental incision, placed one fingerbreadth posterior to the native submental crease. The skin and subcutaneous tissue are dissected down to the level of the platysma. A skin/subcutaneous tissue flap is then generated, 2 cm in both the anterior and posterior directions. The platysma

Figure 11-10 Arrows depict the vectors of pull to the soft tissues at the completion of the endoscopic forehead/midface procedures. Suture fixation of the temporal scalp to the temporal fascia proper will maintain the soft tissue position. Screw fixation of the forehead will maintain the soft tissue position of the brow in the immediate postoperative period.

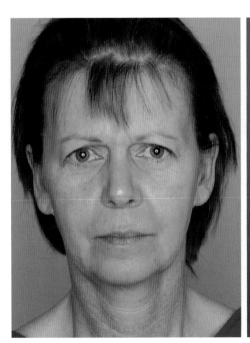
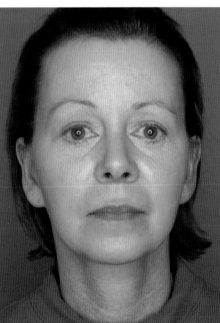

Figure 11-11 This 50-year-old patient had aging changes significant for her chronologic age. She underwent an endoscopic midface lift in conjunction with an endoscopic forehead lift and a mentopexy type I (refer to Figs. 11-19 to 11-21). Note the nasolabial folds and the jowling present in the preoperative (*left*) view. Considerable brow ptosis and lateral hooding are evident. Postoperatively (*right*), the patient demonstrates improved midface fullness and symmetry associated with a more youthful appearance. The improved brow position and absence of lateral hooding are both evident.

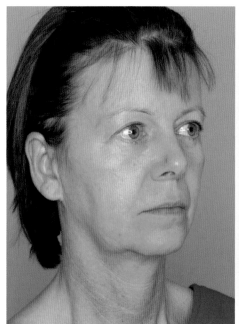
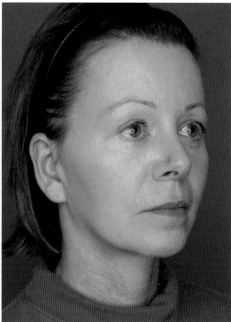

Figure 11-12 Preoperative (*left*) and postoperative (*right*) three-quarter views of the patient shown in Figure 11-11. Improvement in the forehead and midface aesthetic can be clearly seen from the three-quarter view. Support of the cheek mass, transposition of Bichat's fat pad, and elevation of the brow contribute to the more youthful appearance.

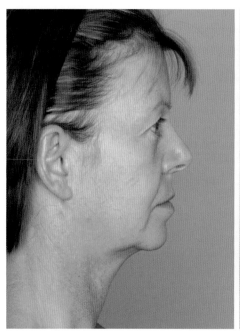
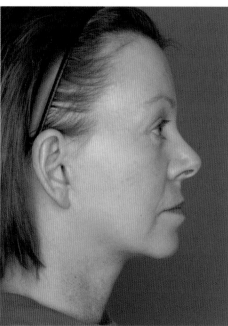

Figure 11-13 Preoperative (*left*) and postoperative (*right*) lateral views of the patient in Figures 11-11 and 11-12. Elevation of the lateral brow eliminates the hooding seen in the preoperative view. Midface rejuvenation provides significant improvement of the lower eyelid to cheek transition. In addition, the degree of jowling is reduced and softening of the nasolabial fold results.

is then incised vertically in the midline up to the level of the inferior border of the mandible.

The periosteum is divided, in a similar fashion, allowing the remainder of the procedure to be performed in a subperiosteal plane. A blunt tip periosteal elevator is then used to elevate the periosteum of the mandible in an anterior and lateral direction. Anterior dissection proceeds to the level of the oral mucosa. Perforation of the

oral mucosa is to be avoided. The periosteal dissection proceeds laterally to the anterior border of the masseter tendon. Care must be taken when dissecting around the mental nerve foramina. We do not skeletonize the mental nerves in an effort to prevent traction-related neuropraxia.

The type I and type II mentopexy procedures utilize suspension of the ptotic soft tissue structures. Suspension is performed with placement of the 3-0 PDS suture at the

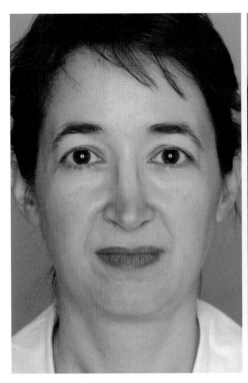
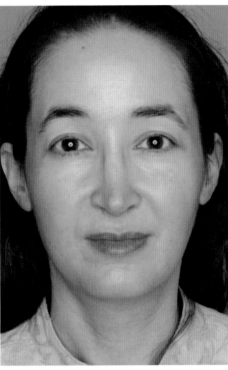

Figure 11-14 This 46-year-old patient underwent an endoscopic midface lift procedure in conjunction with an endoscopic forehead lift and mentopexy type II (refer to Figs. 11-22 to 11-24). Preoperative (*left*) and postoperative (*right*) frontal views are shown, respectively. Note the improved cheek mass position and softening of the nasolabial folds.

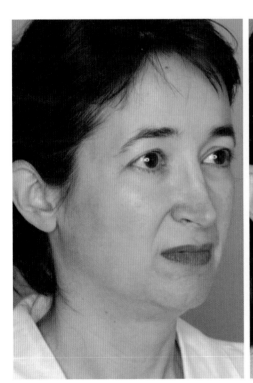
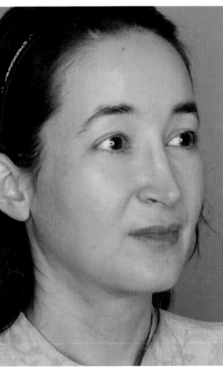

Figure 11-15 Preoperative (*left*) and postoperative (*right*) three-quarter views of the patient shown in Figure 11-14. Slight elevation of the brow and increased fullness of the lateral cheek mass in the postoperative view clearly defines a more youthful appearance.

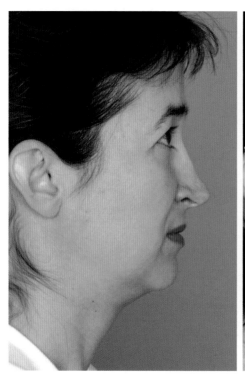
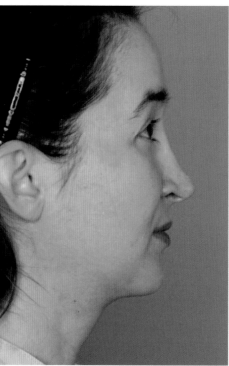

Figure 11-16 Preoperative (*left*) and postoperative (*right*) lateral views of the same patient shown in Figures 11-14 and 11-15. Note the smooth transition from the lower eyelid to cheek in the postoperative (*right*) view.

level of the lowermost aspect of the mentalis muscle/periosteum. A bicortical drill hole is then created in the midline of the mandibular symphysis. The drill hole should be directed in a caudal fashion as shown in Figures 11-17 and 11-18. The suture is then directed through the bone and tied along the posterior border of the mandible. Evaluation of the proper chin position is noted prior to skin closure. Patient examples of the type I and type II mentopexy is shown in Figures 11-19 through 11-21 and Figures 11-22 through 11-24, respectively.

The type III mentopexy procedure follows in a similar fashion. Several caveats should be noted with this technique. Location of the mental nerves should be noted prior to chin augmentation. We routinely measure the

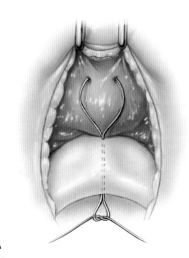
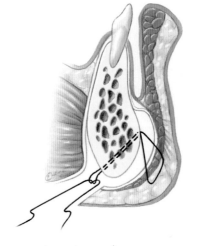
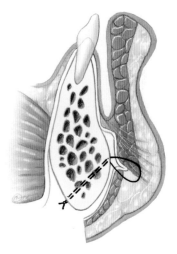

A   **B**   **C**

Figure 11-17 The mentopexy type I. **A** shows the view seen from inferior to superior. The suture is placed in the chin soft tissue at the inferior aspect of the mentalis muscle. **B** and **C** show the effect provided by suture fixation. The chin soft tissue is elevated in a superior and anterior direction. The 3-0 PDS suture is passed through a midline hole drilled through the inferior border of the mandible and is secured to the posterior aspect of the mandible.

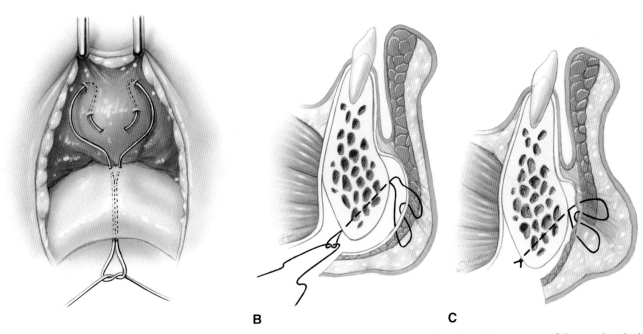

A   **B**   **C**

Figure 11-18 Mentopexy type II. The purse-string 3-0 PDS suture provides elevation and imbrication of the chin soft tissue. Fixation follows as described in Figure 11-17.

distance of each mental nerve from the midline as well as the inferior border of the mandible with the use of calipers. These measurements are then transferred to the chin implant. Any overlap of the implant is removed, leaving a 2- to 3-mm gap around the mental nerve foramina. The implants are secured to the bone with small titanium screws placed in a bicortical fashion. The suspension suture is then driven through the porous polyethylene implant at the desired level. It is not necessary to place the suture through the mandible, as described for the type I and II techniques.

The type IV mentopexy technique, being a redraping technique, does not require suture fixation, but fixation as in a type I mentopexy can be used to centralize the chin. Care must be taken during periosteal scoring to prevent injury to the underlying mentalis musculature. Scoring can be performed with a scalpel or electrocautery placed on a low setting.

Complete mobilization of the periosteum to the level of the anterior masseter tendon is crucial for the success of all types of mentopexy. When the proper aesthetic result is achieved, the dissection pocket is irrigated with

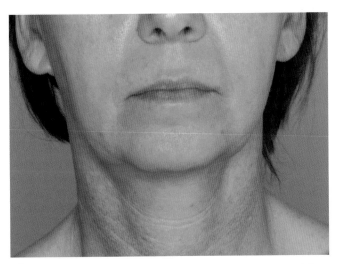
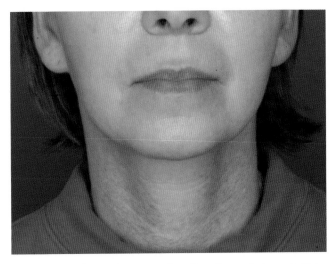

Figure 11-19 Preoperative (*left*) and postoperative (*right*) views following a mentopexy type I procedure as seen from the anteroposterior projection.

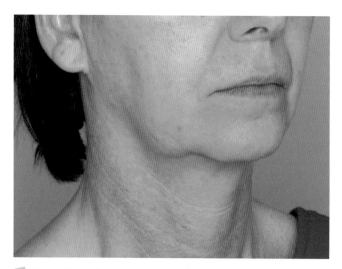
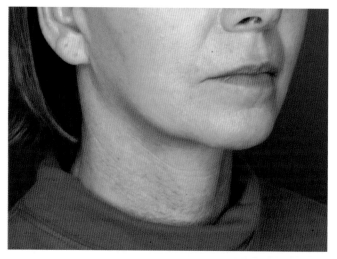

Figure 11-20 Three-quarter views of the patient in Figure 11-19. Preoperative (*left*) and postoperative (*right*) views.

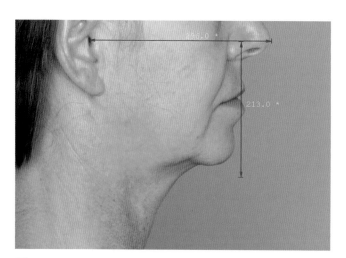
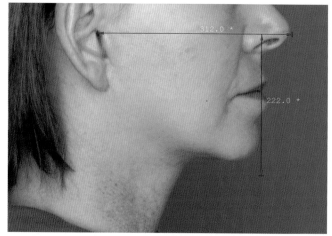

Figure 11-21 Lateral views of the patient in Figures 11-19 and 11-20. Note the chin pad ptosis and poor anterior projection of the chin in the preoperative view (*left*). Postoperatively (*right*), the reference lines demonstrate the improved anterior projection of the chin following the type I mentopexy.

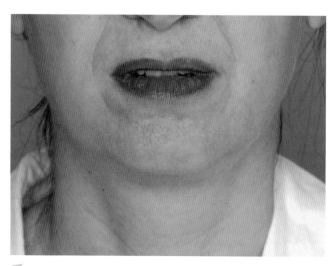
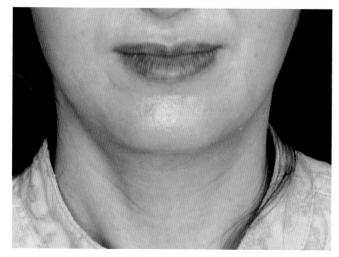

Figure 11-22 Anteroposterior views of a type II mentopexy patient. Preoperative (*left*) view and postoperative (*right*) result are shown.

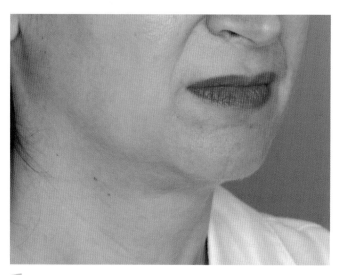

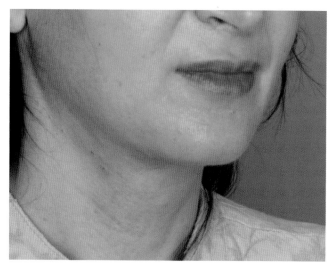

Figure 11-23 Three-quarter views of the patient in Figure 11-22. Preoperative (*left*) and postoperative (*right*) images are shown. The type II mentopexy was performed to address the mild clefting in the chin soft tissue seen in the preoperative view. The purse-string suture of the type II mentopexy obliterated the soft tissue cleft and provided improved chin aesthetics.

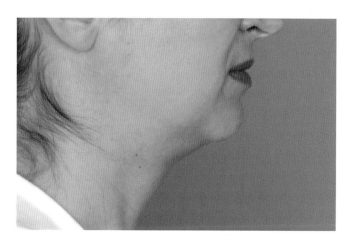

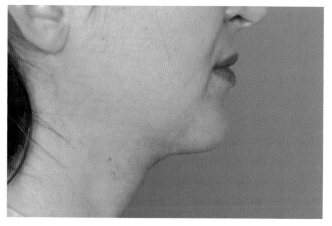

Figure 11-24 Lateal views of the patient in Figures 11-22 and 11-23. Ptosis of the chin in the preoperative (*left*) view is corrected with the mentopexy procedure as shown with the postoperative result (*right*).

antibiotic solution. The platysma is approximated in the midline with interrupted sutures. The skin edges are approximated with 5-0 or 6-0 Prolene sutures. Tape is then applied to the chin for support. If adjunctive aesthetic procedures are to be performed in the neck, the submental incision is covered with a protective bio-occlusive dressing to prevent desiccation. The incision is then closed at the completion of the case.

ADJUNCTIVE PROCEDURES IN THE CENTRAL OVAL OF THE FACE

Skin-Only Blepharoplasty

The endoscopic midface procedure effectively elevates the cheek soft tissues in a superior direction. The recruitment of soft tissue toward the lower eyelid can often be significant. This effect can be exaggerated in patients with lower eyelid skin excess. In situations in which excessive lower eyelid skin exists, we perform a skin-only blepharo-plasty procedure, using a standard subciliary incision. Plication canthopexy or orbicularis muscle suspension can be performed through this skin-only exposure. We find this approach associated with a decreased risk of ectropion and eyelid malposition.

Bichat's Fat Pad Excision

A certain subset of patients who present for facial rejuvenation demonstrate chubby cheeks, significant bulk and pseudoherniation of Bichat's fat pad, and good malar bone support. Augmentation of the cheeks with Bichat's fat pad repositioning is relatively contraindicated in this cohort. These patients benefit from excision of Bichat's fat pad rather than suspension. As previously outlined, the periosteum and buccinator muscle are spread apart in the superomedial wall of the buccal space. This will provide exposure of Bichat's fat pad. The fat pad will readily herniate through the opening in the periosteum/buccinator muscle. With two pairs of blunt forceps, the fat pad can be gently teased out and resected. However, care must be taken during delivery and resection of the fat pad. Undue traction of the fat pad can result in injury to neurovascular structures or Stensen's duct. Bichat's fat pad resection should be performed in a similar fashion to orbital fat pad excision during blepharoplasty procedures. The fat pad is placed on tension during resection and will retract when divided. Bleeding from the retracted Bichat's tissue will be difficult to control safely. Meticulous hemostasis prior to fat pad excision can be facilitated by the use of bipolar cautery.

Fat Grafting

Structural fat grafting as described by Coleman[23] is used as an adjunctive component of the tridimensional facelift in many of our patients. Structural fat grafting provides an excellent means for treating residual facial asymmetries or contour irregularities. Deep residual creases, such as nasolabial and marionette lines, can be improved with this technique. The fat grafts are typically harvested toward the end of the rhytidectomy procedure. We prefer to obtain our fat grafts from the anterior abdomen, through a small infraumbilical incision. If the abdomen has a paucity of fat, grafts should be harvested from alternative locations. Alternative locations for graft harvest include the hips, medial thighs, and posteromedial knee region.

The donor site is infiltrated with 0.5% lidocaine with a 1:200,000 epinephrine solution. We prefer to infiltrate an equivalent amount of anesthetic solution to match the expected fat graft aspirate. All harvesting and graft placement is performed with blunt-tipped cannulas developed specifically for structural fat grafting (Tulip Medical, San Diego, CA). The use of blunt-tipped cannulas for the delivery of the graft material cannot be overstressed. The authors believe that fat embolization is more likely with sharp-tipped needle delivery of the graft material. Inadvertent fat embolization of the middle cerebral artery[24] and right cavernous sinus[25] has been documented following aesthetic fat grafting. The fat grafts are placed in a subcutaneous plane around the face and below the lip vermilion and white roll for lip augmentation. Administered in this fashion, fat grafts can be safely placed in patients undergoing concomitant subperiosteal rhytidectomy. We find this approach advantageous toward the final aesthetic outcome.

ADDRESSING THE PERIPHERAL HEMICIRCLE OF THE FACE

Whereas the endoscopic forehead and midface procedures form the foundation of our comprehensive approach to facial rejuvenation, cervicoplasty techniques form the keystone of success in the peripheral hemicircle of the face. In fact, the most dramatic improvements provided by facial rejuvenation can often be seen in the cervicofacial region. We offer three techniques to achieve success when treating the peripheral hemicircle of the face: the anterior approach cervicoplasty, the excisional cervicofacial lift, and the mandibular matrix system.

Cervicoplasty versus Cervicofacial Rhytidectomy

The nonexcisional anterior approach cervicoplasty provides a means of lower face rejuvenation through minimal access incisions. Considerable aesthetic improvement can be achieved with the technique. However, not all patients are appropriate candidates for this approach. Several points need to be addressed. First, the anterior approach cervicoplasty should be considered an operation designed to postpone a traditional cervicofacial lift. Second, definition around the jawline can be achieved with the nonexcisional cervicoplasty but it is less than that which can be achieved with an excisional approach.

Patients desiring a tight, defined jawline should be offered a traditional cervicofacial procedure. Third, results with the anterior approach cervicoplasty are typically better in female patients. Finally, addition of structural support to the jawline or chin can enhance the final results of a nonexcisional cervicoplasty.[26] The nonexcisional anterior approach cervicoplasty is effective in those with young, elastic skin. Patients with poor skin quality or excessive skin on the neck and jawline should be offered a traditional excisional cervicofacial rhytidectomy.

Anterior Approach Cervicoplasty

Access is obtained through a submental incision measuring 2.5 to 3.0 cm. A subcutaneous dissection plane is developed above the platysma. A uniform 4 mm thickness of subcutaneous tissue is left on the skin flap. Wide subcutaneous dissection is performed in an inferior direction along the midline down to the level of the cricoid cartilage. Laterally, the subcutaneous dissection tapers along the sternocleidomastoid muscles in an oblique direction. We avoid dissection of the upper one third of the sternocleidomastoid muscle in an effort to prevent injury to the greater auricular nerve.

The upper limit of dissection is the mandibular border. The endoscope is used during dissection in the submandibular triangle to avoid injury to branches of the marginal mandibular nerve. Excess fat on the surface of the platysma is removed with scissors or with the aid of a flat suction device applied only on the platysmal surface. Excessive defatting of the skin flap should be avoided to prevent contour irregularities or skeletonized appearance. The fat pad deep to the platysma is then dissected from the anterior bellies of the digastric muscles down to the level of the mylohyoid. The space created from resection of the subplatysmal fat pad is obliterated by plication of the bellies of the anterior digastric muscles. The muscles are plicated with inverted 3-0 nylon sutures. If the digastric muscles are bulky or the hyoid bone is low, we perform a tangential excision of the superficial fibers of the digastric bellies.

Dissection under the platysma then proceeds from medial to lateral. The lateral aspect of the dissection extends beyond the submandibular salivary glands. It is important to free the platysma from the capsule of the submandibular salivary gland.

Failure to do so will result in pseudoherniation of the submandibular gland when the platysma is advanced medially. With the subplatysmal plane complete, the medial borders of the platysma muscles are approximated in the midline. Redundant muscle is trimmed from the medial borders, which are plicated with inverted 3-0 nylon sutures.

The next step is to place a 3- to 4-cm backcut in the platysma muscle below the level of the thyroid cartilage. The lateral jugular vein should be preserved. If further definition of the neck is required, a suture suspension with a double armed 3-0 Gore-Tex (W.L. Gore, Flagstaff, AZ) suture is performed. The suture suspension starts with the placement of bilateral 1-cm incisions in the occipital scalp, approximately 2 cm posterior to the mastoid process. The incisions are carried down to the level of the mastoid fascia. The Gore-Tex suture is placed beneath the medial edge of the platysma muscle at the level of the hyoid bone. The suture is directed superficially 1.5 cm from the medial edge and is directed toward the occipital incision using an endoscopic needle holder. After being retrieved, the suture is placed through the deep mastoid fascia-periosteum and delivered back through the occipital incision. Again, the suture is brought over the surface of the platysma muscle back toward the midline. As the midline is approached, the suture is driven through the platysma 1.5 cm from the midline and is directed to the medial border of the platysma. The suture is placed in a parallel fashion approximately 1 cm superior to the first course of the suture. The same steps are then performed on the contralateral side. The two free ends of the suture are then tied together under moderate tension. Appropriate tension can be gauged by the ability to place a finger beneath the sutures. Where ptosis of the submandibular glands exists, we weave the sutures on the superficial fascia overlying the gland similar to that described by Feldman.[27] If further definition is required, Z-platysmaplasty or a limited corset platysmaplasty can be performed.

MANDIBULAR MATRIX SYSTEM

Size and shape of the mandible affects the harmonious relationship of the skeletal support and the soft tissue envelope that defines a beautiful face. The mandible is the framework of the lower face. Deficiencies in mandibular volume and shape can negatively affect the aesthetics of the mouth, chin, and neck. The mandibular matrix system was developed to address the absence of an inadequate mandibular contour. The mandibular matrix system allows a method of skeletal support restoration that can be applied to the entire mandible. The system provides an excellent construct to redefine the jawline, especially when combined with standard cervicoplasty procedures.

The system is composed of a series of implants made from porous polyethylene. The excellent biocompatibility characteristics make porous polyethylene the authors' choice for alloplastic augmentation of the mandibular framework. The implants allow for rapid vascularization and tissue ingrowth. The rapid integration of the implant material makes porous polyethylene the ideal alloplast for a mobile and dynamic structure such as the mandible. The mandibular matrix system can be fashioned to mimic the normal contour of the jawline. The multiple components of the implant system allow augmentation of the entire mandible or individual segments that may be deficient.

The implants have been designed to provide tridimensional restoration of the mandible. The implants wrap around the inferior border of the mandible. Owing to this shape, the implants are self-stabilizing and require minimal or no screw fixation. This is a significant advantage as compared to two-dimensional onlay implants. In addition, the component system allows the restoration of the entire mandibular contour through minimal access incisions. The system is composed of a two-piece extended wraparound chin implant and gonial angle implants specifically designed for the right and left mandibular angles, respectively. A prejowl implant can be included in this system when necessary.

THE IMPLANT SYSTEM

Extended Wrap-Around Chin Implant

These implants are available as square or round implants, as viewed anteriorly. The implants are available in three sizes: small, medium, and large. These sizes correspond to 3, 5, and 7 mm of anterior projection, respectively. Each implant is composed of right and left sides that are joined in the center by an alignment tab. The alignment tab is designed to allow stabilization of the two halves of the implant. Use of the alignment tab becomes optional when proper alignment of the implant along the inferior mandibular border is jeopardized.

Mandibular Angle Implant

These implants are designed to wrap around the inferior and posterior borders of the mandibular or gonial angle. The implants are specifically manufactured in right and left sides and are available in small, medium, and large sizes. These sizes correspond to 3, 7, and 11 mm of lateral projection, respectively. The greatest projection of the implant is at the level of the new gonial angle.

Prejowl Implant

The prejowl implant is designed for patients who demonstrate a significant geniomandibular groove but do not require chin augmentation. The implant is supplied in two parts, divided medially. The implant has a 4.0-mm maximal projection that corresponds with the level of the prejowl depression.

Button Chin Implant

The button chin implant is a small tridimensional implant designed for patients who require improved anterior projection of the chin but do not require lateral augmentation along the mandible. The implant is available in 3.0-mm thickness. The implant is designed to comfortably wrap around the symphysis of the mandible. The wraparound feature provides stability to the implant, making rotation or migration of the implant virtually impossible.

IMPLANT PLACEMENT

The surgical technique employed with the insertion of the mandibular matrix system has been refined since the early description in 2000. General anesthesia is recommended for all cases. When combined with adjunctive aesthetic procedures, the matrix system should be placed as early as possible. Access incisions should be closed immediately, in order to prevent possible contamination. Retromolar and lower buccal sulcus incisions can be used for the insertion of the mandibular angle implants and extended chin implants, respectively. The authors, however, now place both the mandibular angle and extended chin implants through a 3-cm submental incision and the assistance of the 4-mm endoscope, whenever possible. The mandibular angle implants are secured with a 2-0 PDS suture and the extended chin implants are secured with small titanium self-drilling or self-taping screws, in bicortical fashion.

Careful planning is necessary for the placement of the submental incision. Augmentation of the bony symphysis will advance the soft tissue envelope. This tends to rotate the submental incision anteriorly. Therefore, we typically place the incision 1 cm posterior to the submental crease. By doing this, the incision remains hidden in the submental area.

The dissection is carried down through the subcutaneous adipose tissue to the level of the platysma. A thick subcutaneous dissection is then performed 2 cm anterior and 2 cm posterior to the incision. The platysma, mentalis muscle, and periosteum are then divided in the midline, perpendicular to the direction of the submental skin incision. A subperiosteal dissection is then performed in an anterior direction, to the level of the mentolabial fold. This can be performed under direct visualization, with the aid of a lighted Aufricht retractor. Care must be taken to avoid perforation of the oral mucosa.

The dissection continues laterally to expose the entire anterior and inferior surface of the mandible. This dissection is facilitated with the use of a No. 4 Ramirez elevator (Snowden-Pencer, USA). The mental nerves must be identified and carefully dissected free from the surrounding structures. Nerve injury can be prevented by early identification of the structures and avoidance of excessive retraction. The lateral dissection proceeds to level of the anterior border of the masseter muscle. This can be accomplished with the assistance of the 4-mm endoscope or small fiberoptic lighted retractor. At this point, dissection is complete for the insertion of the extended chin implant Silastic sizers.

Insertion of the mandibular angle implants requires careful dissection of the pterygomasseteric sling. The 4-mm endoscope is inserted and a subperiosteal dissection continues with an angle periosteal retractor (Snowden-Pencer, USA). The pterygomaxillary sling is elevated in continuity (Fig. 11-25). Under direct visualization, the inferior aspect of the mandibular angle is freed from the tendinous and periosteal attachments. The posterior border of the ascending ramus is cleared in a similar fashion. The bony surface of the mandibular angle is then exposed sufficiently in anterior, inferior, and posterior directions to allow the insertion of Silastic mandibular angle implant sizers.

With the dissection complete, the cavity is irrigated with antibiotic solution followed by packing with neurosurgical pledgets soaked in diluted Betadine and epinephrine solution (1:30,000). The pledgets are left for several minutes to provide hemostasis and improve endoscopic visualization during implant placement.

As stated previously, oral incisions can be used for the placement of the implant system. However, the authors feel that this approach may increase the incidence of

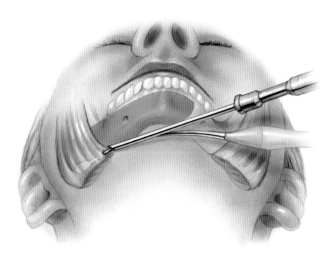

Figure 11-25 The endoscopic dissection of the pterygomasseteric sling. Note the pink area highlighted on the mandible. This represents the area of subperiosteal dissection required for placement of the mandibular matrix system.

bacterial seeding of the implant and development of early postoperative infection.

Comfort with the endoscopic approach and access to the appropriate instrumentation should act as a guide to the method of implant introduction.

The extended chin and mandibular angle implants have been developed with corresponding Silastic sizers. Each sizer has a similar projection, length, and depth at the groove of the implant. The mandibular implant sizers are introduced followed by the extended chin implant sizers. The endoscope is then introduced to assess the fit of the sizers and the adequacy of the soft tissue dissection. The external contour of the jawline is then assessed. The appropriate size implants are chosen based upon fit and desired aesthetic contour. Calipers are then used to measure the distance of the mental nerves from the midline and the lower border of the mandible. These measurements are recorded and transferred to the chosen extended chin implant. Grooves in the extended chin implant can then be carved with the use of a No. 10 scalpel and a cutting board. Adequate space (2–3 mm) around the mental nerve foramina should be created. Further carving of the extended chin and mandibular angle implants can be performed with a scalpel or a high-speed burr. All carving should be done on a back table away from the patient. The prepared implants are then washed of debris and soaked in antibiotic solution.

The sizers are removed and the endoscope is inserted to assure that hemostasis has been achieved. A smooth sterile plastic sleeve is then rolled into a conical shape and inserted into the incision. This sleeve isolates the implant from the skin surface and creates a smooth, protected surface for the rough porous polyethylene to slide against. Without the sleeve, insertion of the implant can be a humbling experience. The mandibular implants are then directed to the proper anatomic location under endoscopic guidance or with a small fiberoptic lighted retractor. The implants can be manipulated with the assistance of two periosteal elevators.

The mandibular angle implant is then fixed into position with either a small titanium screw or 2-0 PDS (Ethicon, Somerville, NJ) suture passed through a predrilled bicortical hole through the body of the mandible. The wraparound design of the mandibular angle implant prevents rocking of the implant when properly placed and allows fixation of the implant along its anterior border. If screw fixation is chosen, trajectory of the infra-alveolar (mental) nerve must be noted prior to drilling.

With the angle implants secured, the extended chin implants are inserted in a similar fashion. Use of the smooth plastic sleeve during implant insertion cannot be overstressed. Smooth insertion with minimal retraction will reduce the incidence of injury to the mental nerves. The extended chin implant is then positioned along the inferior border of the mandible. The location of the

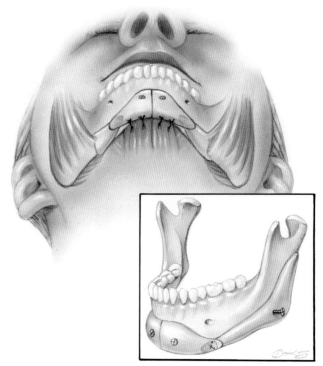

Figure 11-26 Final placement of the entire mandibular matrix system. The gonial angle implants are positioned along the mandible beneath the pterygomasseteric sling. Note that the implants are secured with titanium screws. The authors secure the chin implants with titanium screws as depicted. The lateral wings of the chin implant should overlap the gonial angle implants. This maintains a smooth contour to the augmented mandible. Though screw fixation of the gonial angle implants can be used, the authors prefer to secure the angle implants with a single 2-0 PDS suture placed through a drill hole in the inferior portion of the mandible. Significant support provided by the pterygomasseteric sling makes suture fixation of the gonial implants possible.

mental nerve is checked prior to screw fixation of the implant. Each side of the chin implant is fixed with a single small titanium screw in bicortical fashion, after predrilling. The lateral aspect of the extended chin implant should overlap the anterior border of the mandibular angle implant when attempting to achieve a wide profile. The lateral wings of the extended chin implant can be trimmed (no overlap with the angle implant) to maintain a narrow profile (Fig. 11-26).

Should the use of prejowl implants or a button chin implant be indicated, the implants can be placed through the same submental exposure. Fixation can be achieved with small titanium screws in either a unicortical or bicortical fashion. Aesthetic outcome will dictate the role these alternative implants play.

Prior to closure, the surgical cavity is irrigated with antibiotic solution. The platysma is sutured in the midline with interrupted sutures. If other aesthetic procedures are to be performed at the level of the neck, the skin incision is covered with a bio-occlusive dressing. This prevents tissue desiccation prior to skin closure. Skin closure, when appropriate, is performed with 5-0 or 6-0 Prolene

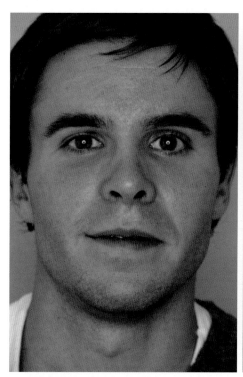
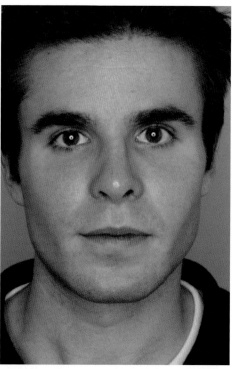

Figure 11-27 Anteroposterior preoperative (*left*) and postoperative (*right*) views of a 20-year old patient who underwent placement of the mandibular matrix system. The patient's preoperative concerns centered around the relative mandibular asymmetry and the narrow, pointed chin. Improved definition of the mandibular angles and balanced chin width are shown in the postoperative view.

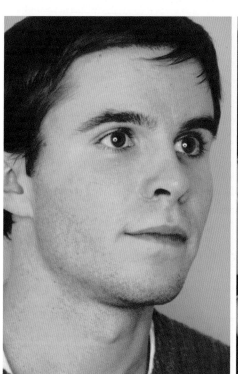
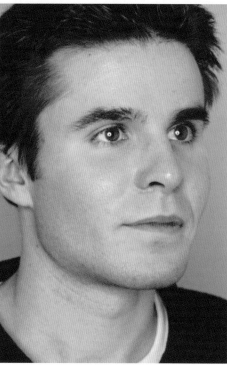

Figure 11-28 Three-quarter views of the patient in Figure 11-27. Preoperative (*left*) and postoperative (*right*) views are shown. The mandibular matrix system improves the definition of the entire mandible. Aesthetic balance of the mandible is achieved postoperatively with greater definition of the mandibular angle and chin width.

(Ethicon, Somerville, NJ) interrupted sutures. A bio-occlusive dressing is applied over the incision after closure. A tight facelift dressing is applied at the end of all procedures to reduce swelling and dead space fluid accumulation. Patient examples are shown in Figures 11-27 through 11-32.

POSTOPERATIVE CARE

After extensive facial procedures, patients are monitored for 23 hours and discharged home under the care of a well-informed relative or practical nurse. The butterfly drains are attached to vacuum tubes and changed periodically during the next 48 hours. We find that

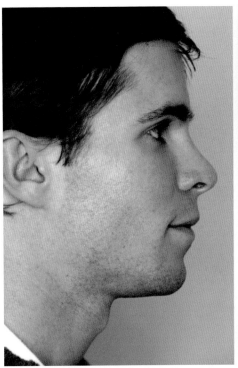

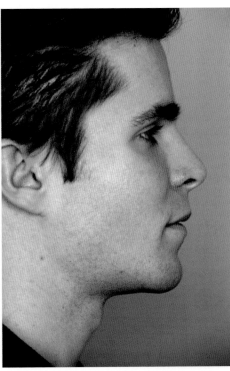

Figure 11-29 Lateral views of the patient in Figures 11-27 and 11-28, preoperative (*left*) and postoperative (*right*). Note the improvement of chin projection and shape with the extended wraparound chin implant of the manibular matrix system.

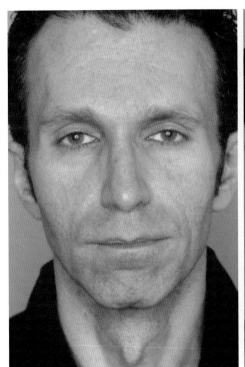

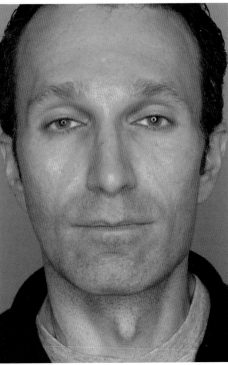

Figure 11-30 This 42-year-old patient demonstrates relative asymmetry of the upper and lower face. Preoperative antero-posterior view (*left*) shows a sharp, pointed chin and poor projection of the mandibular angles. Postoperative anteroposterior view (*right*) after placement of the mandibular matrix system. Note the improved balance of the upper and lower face. The wrap-around chin implant improves lower facial shape and the increased biangular distance provided by the gonial angle implants improves the overall manibular width.

evacuation of this fluid minimizes the amount of facial edema postoperatively. Drain output of 10 to 20 mL should be expected, on average. Drain removal occurs typically on the second postoperative day. Antibiotics, started prior to surgery, are continued for 5 days, postoperatively. Steroids have not provided reduced postoperative edema in our patients and are not routinely given. Supportive taping of the forehead and midface begins at the end of the operative procedure and continues for approximately 7 to 10 days. A snug-fitting cervical collar dressing is placed postoperatively for patients undergoing cervicofacial procedures. This dressing is kept in place for 24 to 48 hours and then is changed daily. Loose-fitting dressings and patient

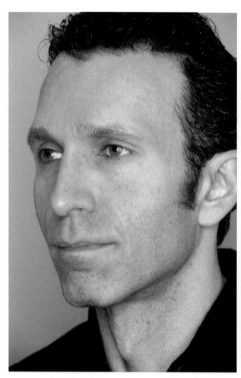

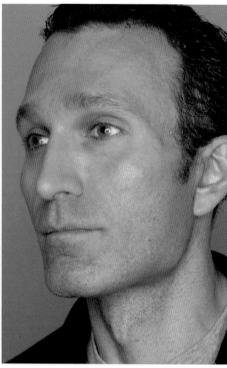

Figure 11-31 Three-quarter views of the patient in Figure 11-30. The preoperative view (*left*) shows the asymmetry of the broad upper face and narrow lower face. Postoperatively (*right*), improved definition of the mandibular angle and projection of the chin creates a more balanced aesthetic result. Harmony between the upper and lower face has been achieved.

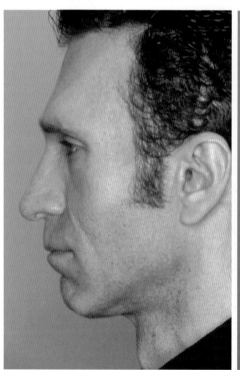

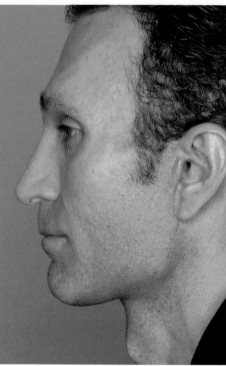

Figure 11-32 Lateral views of the patient in Figures 11-30 and 11-31, preoperative (*left*) and postoperative (*right*). Note the improved projection of the chin and definition of the mandibular angle.

noncompliance can lead to seroma formation in the cervicofacial region. Fluid collections in this region should be promptly evacuated to minimize postoperative scarring. Sutures are removed by day 7, in most cases. The titanium forehead posts are removed between days 10 and 14.

COMPLICATIONS

Complications related to the endoscopic subperiosteal facelift procedures include nerve injury, hematoma, infection, alopecia, and skin flap necrosis. Nerve injury, perhaps the most devastating complication, is typically seen with excessive traction during endoscopic manipulation. In an effort to decrease traction-related nerve injury, we prefer to use a 4-mm endoscope and a blunt cobra-tip sleeve to elevate the tissues. Retraction is avoided where possible and slender retractors are implemented when retraction is necessary. Minaturized instruments for dissection and manipulation have also been employed. With implementation of these steps, neuropraxia of the frontal branch of the facial nerve occurred in 0.4% of patients. Neuropraxia of the zygomaticus branch of the facial nerve and the infraorbital nerve occurred in 0.2% and 0.4% of patients, respectively.[28] No permanent injury to motor nerves has been seen to date.

Hematoma and infection can be minimized with meticulous operative technique and adequate irrigation of the subperiosteal pockets with antibiotic solution prior to closure. Subcutaneous hematoma under the cervicofacial flaps has been seen in 1.2% of patients. These hematomas have typically occurred secondary to acute hypertensive episodes in the immediate postoperative period. Immediate drainage of collections prevented any adverse sequelae.

Late infection has been observed in one patient undergoing an endoscopic forehead lift and midface lift procedure. The patient complained of severe pain in the right cheek region 10 days after operation. Fluctuance and tenderness of the cheek mound was noted. Incision and drainage of the collection resulted in resolution of the infection without further sequelae. Permanent alopecia is rarely seen following the endoscopic facelift procedure.

Adequate infiltration of local anesthetic, preoperatively, and the judicious use of electrocautery can prevent unnecessary permanent alopecia. With the current method of forehead fixation, temporary alopecia is seen in 0.2% of patients. Treatment with a 50:50 topical mixture of 0.1% tretinoin and 5% minoxidil, applied twice daily, is prescribed. Necrosis of the retroauricular skin flaps following cervicofacial rhytidectomy tends to occur iatrogenically or associated with a history of smoking. Treatment involves débridement and local wound care. Readvancement of the flap may be necessary in severe cases. Avoiding excessive tension of the cervicofacial flaps provides a more prudent answer.

For smokers, we recommend a 12-week course of Trental (Aventis Pharmaceuticals, Bridewater, NJ) and smoking cessation aided by a 10-week course of Zyban (GlaxoSmithKline, Greenville, NC) to prevent skin flap necrosis.

Future Considerations

Aesthetic surgery has benefited from great technologic advances over the past two decades. Advances in endoscopic technology and instrumentation have allowed pioneering surgical techniques to be developed. This is especially true in the field of facial rejuvenation.

The tridimensional endoscopic facelift technique, born from these technologic advances, provides a comprehensive approach to treat facial aging.

As with any surgical innovation, camps are divided as to the effectiveness of the endoscopic approach.[29-32] Both positive and negative reports should be evaluated and interpreted with a critical eye. The endoscopic methods put forth in this chapter are associated with a significant learning curve. Success with these techniques requires sound knowledge of the anatomic principles, surgical skill, and critical appraisal of the aesthetic outcomes. With time, refinement of the skills required will allow predictable and lasting results. Proper patient selection will further guarantee success with this approach. Patient satisfaction has been tremendous among our patient population.

We believe that the tridimensional endoscopic facelift technique will undergo further refinement and benefit from future technologic advances. However, this advancement will only come from those who embrace the approach. Innovation can only be delivered from experience.

REFERENCES

1. Tessier P: Face lifting and frontal rhytidectomy. In Ely JF (ed): Transactions of the 7th International Congress on Plastic Reconstructive Surgery, Rio de Janeiro, 1980, p 393.
2. Tessier P: Lifting facial sous-perioste. Ann Chir Plast Esthet 1989;34:1993.
3. Psillakis JM, Rumley TO, Camargo A: Subperiosteal approach as an improved concept for correction of the aging face. Plast Reconstr Surg 1988;82:383-392.
4. Tapia A, Ferreria B, Blanch A: Subperiostic lifting. Aesthet Plast Surg 1991;15(2):155-160.
5. Fuente del Campo A: Facelift without preauricular scars. Plast Reconstr Surg 1993;92(4):642-653.
6. Ramirez OM, Maillard GF, Musolas A: The extended subperiosteal facelift: A definitive soft tissue remodeling for facial rejuvenation. Plast Reconst Surg 1991:88:227.
7. Ramirez OM, Fuente del Campo A: Facial rejuvenation: Subperiosteal brow and facelift. In Rees RS (ed): Plastic Surgery Educational Foundation: Instructional Courses, Vol. 6. St. Louis: CV Mosby, 1993.
8. Ramirez OM: Extended subperisoteal facelift. Plast Surg Tech 1995;1:223.
9. Krastinova-Lolov D: Mask lift and facial aesthetic sculpturing. Plast Reconstr Surg 1995;95(1):31-36.
10. Core GB, Vaconez LO, Askren C, et al: Coronal facelift with endoscopic techniques. Plast Surg Forum 1992;XV:227.
11. Ramirez OM: Endoscopic full facelift. Aesthet Plast Surg 1994;18:363-371.
12. Ramirez OM: Endoscopic techniques in facial rejuvenation: an overview. I. Aesthet Plast Surg 1994;18:141-147.
13. Delmar H: Anatomy of the superficial parts of the face and neck [In French]. Ann Chir Plast Esthet 1994;39(5):527-555.
14. Ramirez OM: The central oval of the face: Tridimensional endoscopic rejuvenation. Facial Plast Surg 2000;16(3):283-298.

15. Ramirez OM, Robertson KM: Update in endoscopic forehead rejuvenation. Facial Plast Surg 2002;10(1):37-51.

16. Ramirez OM: Three-dimensional endoscopic midface enhancement: A personal quest for the ideal cheek rejuvenation. Plast Reconstr Surg 2002;109(1):329-340.

17. Ramirez OM: Cervicoplasty: Non-excisional anterior approach. Plast Reconstr Surg 1997;99(6):1576-1585.

18. Giampapa VC, DiBernardo BE: Neck recontouring with suture suspension and liposuction: An alternative for the early rhytidectomy candidate. Aesthet Plast Surg 1995;19(3):217-223.

19. Guerro-Santos J: The neck lift. In Vistnes LM (ed): Procedures in Plastic and Reconstructive Surgery: How They Do It. Boston: Little, Brown, 1991, p 153.

20. Ramirez OM: Mandibular matrix implant system: A method to restore skeletal support to the lower face. Plast Reconstr Surg 2000;106(1):176-189.

21. Bartlett SP, Grossman R, Whitaker LA: Age-related changes in the craniofacial skeleton: An anthropometric and histologic analysis. Plast Reconstr Surg 1992;90(4):592-600.

22. Gonzales-Ulloa M: Ptosis of the chin: The witch's chin. Plast Reconstr Surg 1972;50:54.

23. Coleman SR: Facial recontouring with lipostructure. Clin Plast Surg 1997;24(2):347-367.

24. Feinendegen DL, Baumgartner RW, Schroth G, et al: Middle cerebral artery occlusion and ocular fat embolism after autologous injection in the face. J Neurol 1998;245(1):53-54.

25. Moon SY, Chang GY: Images in clinical medicine. A complication of cosmetic surgery. N Engl J Med 2004;350(15):1549.

26. Ramirez OM: Cervicoplasty: A nonexcisional anterior approach. A 10-year follow-up. Plast Reconstr Surg 2003;111(3):1342-1345.

27. Feldman JJ: Corset platysmaplasty. Plast Reconstr Surg 1990;85(3):333-343.

28. Ramirez OM, Heller L: Facial rejuvenation. In Peled IJ, Manders EK (eds): Esthetic Surgery of the Face. London: Taylor & Francis, 2004, pp 73-90.

29. Sozer O, Biggs TM: Our experience with endoscopic brow lifts. Aesth Plast Surg 2000;24(2):90-96.

30. De Cordier BC, de la Torre JI, Al-Hakeem MS, et al: Endoscopic forehead lift: Review of technique, cases, and complications. Plast Reconstr Surg 2002;110(6):1558-1568.

31. Knize DM: Reassessment of the coronal incision and subgaleal dissection for foreheadplasty. Plast Reconstr Surg 1998;102(2):478-489.

32. Chiu ES, Baker DC: Endoscopic brow lift: A retrospective review of 628 consecutive cases over 5 years. Plast Reconstr Surg 2003;112(2):628-633.

CHAPTER TWELVE

Aesthetic Midface Implants

William J. Binder, MD, FACS • Brian P. Kim, MD • Babak Azizzadeh, MD, FACS

HISTORY

Tessier was one of the earliest surgeons to utilize autogenous bone grafts in the 1960s to correct congenital and traumatic deformities of the facial skeleton.[1] Donor site morbidity, prolonged operative time, and resorption of tissue grafts limited the widespread use of these techniques. Alloplastic implants were first introduced in the late 1960s when Spadafora and Hinderer pioneered the use of synthetic implants for aesthetic facial enhancement.[2,3] Since that time, many other prominent surgeons have advocated the use of alloplastic implants for facial aesthetic surgery.[4-9]

The use of facial implants continued to grow beyond its indication for *malar* augmentation. As early as the 1970s, Gonzalez-Ulloa recognized the ability of midface implants to rejuvenate the midface when performed with standard rhytidectomy.[4] Most of his work focused on improving facial appearance by altering cheek shape and contour. This "profileplasty" was a natural progression from the earlier craniofacial techniques popularized by Tessier and others. Many realized that midface augmentation could produce fuller cheeks and a more youthful appearance. However, the emphasis of this early work was more on improving the overall shape of the face, rather than reversing the effects of aging on the midface.

After extensive modification of early implant prototypes, Binder advocated the use of midface augmentation as an independent and powerful method for midface rejuvenation in the 1980s.[10] An important innovation in Binder's work was the increased emphasis on *submalar* "soft tissue" augmentation, which he showed could have a significant impact on midface aesthetics by restoring the volume lost because of atrophy associated with the aging process. In the 1990s, Terino further promoted alloplastic facial contouring as a way of improving the overall facial aesthetics.[11]

PERSONAL PHILOSOPHY

The last two decades have seen rapid advances in the understanding and treatment of midface aging.[10,12-16] Midface rejuvenation has evolved far beyond the rhytidectomy procedure to involve deeper and more fundamental levels of dissection with attempts at elevating and replacing lost midface volume. The pathophysiology of the aging process is a key factor in determining the correct surgical treatment. It is now well understood that the aging process results not only in the descent of the midface but also in the atrophy of the soft tissue in multiple facial planes. Midface rejuvenation can therefore be achieved not only through suspension techniques but also by the augmentation of the soft tissue and skeletal foundation. As a result, we have found that alloplastic implants are an effective way to alter the midface appearance in appropriate candidates. Midface augmentation is a straightforward, long-lasting, and relatively low-risk surgical option that can consistently and predictably improve midface aesthetics. It has the ability to replace lost facial soft tissue volume and to increase the anterolateral projection of the area, thereby reducing midface laxity and decreasing the depth of the nasolabial folds (Fig. 12-1). Implants are readily reversible and can be combined with standard rhytidectomy procedures. The net effect is a softening of the sharp angles and depressions of the aged face, resulting in a natural "unoperated" look. In appropriate candidates, moderate facial rejuvenation can be achieved simply with the placement of submalar midface implants without concomitant rhytidectomy (Fig. 12-2). This technique is particularly applicable to middle-aged patients (ages 35 to 45 years) who show early signs of facial aging and atrophy without significant soft tissue laxity of jowls or deep neck rhytids.

In patients who require rhytidectomy because of significant lower facial laxity, alloplastic implants can also augment the bony scaffold of the malar region, thereby improving the fundamental base upon which facial tissues are suspended. This midface recontouring allows for dramatic results that are not possible with soft tissue techniques alone. The benefit is especially apparent in patients who have a combined deficiency of the facial skeleton and soft tissues, and in those patients who have a prominent malar skeleton but lack adequate submalar soft tissue. Midface implant augmentation facilitates rhytidectomy in several ways. The skin and soft tissue can be draped over a broader, more convex midface region

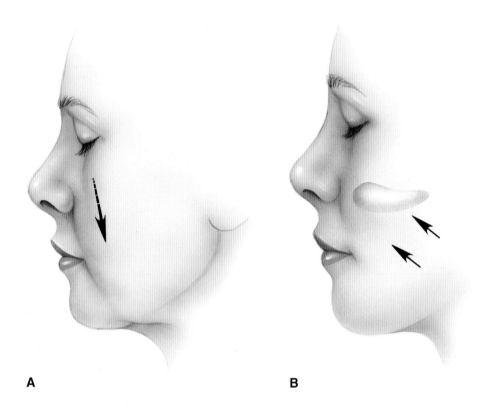

A   **B**

Figure 12-1 Suspension effect of midface implants. Midface implants augment the facial skeleton and restore soft tissue volume. The combined effect is to relocate the soft tissue to a more anterosuperior location and restore the hollow regions of the midface.

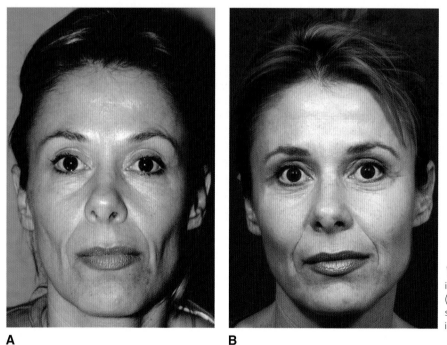

A   **B**

Figure 12-2 Facial rejuvenation with submalar implant. Preoperative (**A**) and 3-year postoperative (**B**) views of a 45-year-old woman with type II submalar atrophy who underwent three-submalar implant placement.

after implant augmentation (Fig. 12-3). There is also minimal traction on the perioral tissues and lateral commissure if placed prior to the rhytidectomy, which can help to avoid an "overoperated" appearance. Similarly, the subperiosteal dissection of the midface during the implant placement also releases the deep attachments of the superficial musculoaponeurotic system (SMAS) to the facial skeleton, allowing greater mobilization and suspension of ptotic soft tissues, which greatly enhances the results of sub-SMAS and deep plane rhytidectomy.[12]

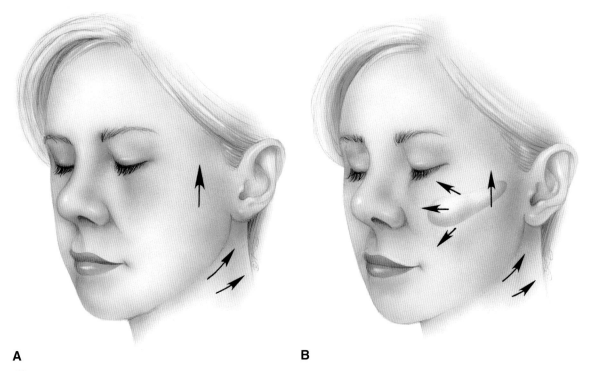

A   **B**

Figure 12-3 Convexity effect of midface implants. Facelifts generally stretch skin over a flat midface structure in a two-dimensional pattern (*arrows* in **A**). Malar and submalar implants create a more convex midface region allowing for a more natural skin draping and resulting in a third dimension for facial rejuvenation (*arrows* in **B**).

Many patients who present for revision rhytidectomy and require volume restoration can also be improved by expanding the midface region while decreasing downward vertical traction forces on the lower eyelid.

The deep plane facelift, subperiosteal facelift, and fat grafting have become popular methods for improving the aesthetics of the midface.[12-18] These techniques can be useful alternatives to alloplastic implants in appropriate candidates; however, they do have limitations in addressing the underlying pathophysiology of midface aging. The subperiosteal midface lift and deep plane rhytidectomy can have a tremendous impact on the midface by suspending the existing soft tissue but cannot replace the deeper or superficial soft tissue that is lost with aging. Furthermore, subperiosteal midface lifts cause significant edema and distortion to the periorbital region that can last for several months. Facelift surgery may even worsen the overall appearance by "skeletonizing" the face in patients with significant midfacial volume loss or extremely prominent bone structure.

Injectable soft tissue fillers such as hyaluronic acids, calcium hydroxylapatite, and collagen can efface the nasolabial fold, but they seldom yield permanent results or produce significant volume enhancement. They may serve as a valuable option in treating early stage nasolabial fold and facial atrophy in younger individuals. Injectable poly-L-lactic acid (Sculptra, Dermik Aesthetics, Bridgewater, NJ) may be able to produce more dramatic volume enhancement than other fillers but generally requires yearly maintenance. Free fat transfer can also produce moderate volume augmentation, but long-term results and longevity are not predictable.

Midface implants not only help reverse the effects of aging, but they are also useful in a variety of other conditions. Midface contouring can mask post-traumatic and congenital deficiencies while avoiding lengthy reconstructive surgeries and graft donor site morbidity.[19] Implants can improve the facial atrophy that results from anorexia nervosa or the effects of protease inhibitors in treating conditions such as human immunodeficiency virus (HIV) lipodystrophy (Fig. 12-4).[20] We have also successfully used facial implants for patients with longstanding facial paralysis and Bell's palsy who have significant unilateral facial and muscle atrophy.

ANATOMY

Youth is marked by an abundance of facial soft tissue, allowing for full cheeks and smooth, pleasant contours without sharp irregularities or indentations.[21] The aging process begins to appear in persons who are in their 30s and 40s and significantly progresses by the time individuals reach their 50s and 60s. The effects of the midface aging process are a result of volume loss, the gradual descent of soft tissue, and decreased skin elasticity.

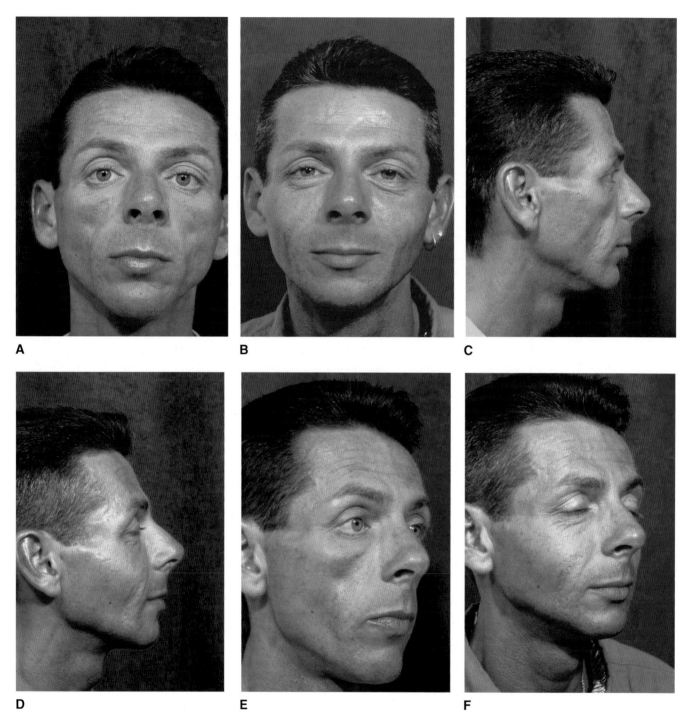

A   B   C

D   E   F

Figure 12-4 Submalar midface implants for treatment of HIV lipodystrophy. Preoperative (**A**, **C**, and **E**) and 1-year postoperative (**B**, **D**, and **F**) views of a 34-year-old man who underwent customized submalar implant placement.

The malar, buccal, temporal, and infraorbital fat pads atrophy and lose their fascial support, becoming progressively ptotic secondary to gravity. The malar fat pad, suborbicularis oculi fat (SOOF), and orbicularis oculi muscle descend inferiorly, causing an exaggeration of the nasolabial folds and exposure of the infraorbital rim. Cavitary depressions and submalar hollowness may develop in addition to the deepening nasolabial and nasojugal folds. The end result is flattening of the midface with an aged and fatigued appearance, often unmasking underlying bony anatomy.

Surgical treatment of the aging face requires a keen understanding of the soft tissue and bony landmarks of the midface. The *malar eminence* is a key element that is localized to the anterior one third of the zygomatic arch, and is a common area of implant augmentation.

Placement of implants in individuals who have a normally developed malar region can lateralize the apex of the cheek and result in a high and angular malar eminence. The *submalar triangle* is bound superiorly by the zygomatic prominence, medially by the nasolabial fold, and laterally by the masseter muscle. It is another vital region of the midface that can be contoured, resulting in the correction of midface volume loss (Fig. 12-5). The submalar triangle is the most common site of midface deficiency in the aging face and can be easily rejuvenated with alloplastic implants.

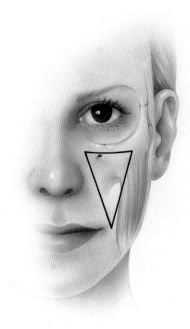

Figure 12-5 Submalar triangle. The submalar triangle is bordered superiorly by the zygomatic prominence, laterally by the masseter muscle, and medially by the nasolabial fold. It is the most common area of deficiency with aging.

PREOPERATIVE ANALYSIS

All patients who present for facial rejuvenation undergo a complete history and physical examination. Photographs and digital imaging aid in determining the exact nature of the patient's concerns. Photographs taken from the basal and apical bird's eye view can help determine the degree of midface volume loss and asymmetry and aid in the selection of appropriate implants. When evaluating a patient for midface rejuvenation, it is important to determine the relative contributions of soft tissue inadequacy and skeletal deficiency. Skeletal and soft tissue asymmetry is also an important consideration in the preoperative consultation. Asymmetries may become exaggerated postoperatively if not diagnosed and accounted for by modifying the implants at the time of surgery. In addition to assessing the midface, it is also important to analyze and address the upper and lower face. Many patients who are candidates for midface augmentation will also require other surgical procedures to enhance the overall facial aesthetics. Midface implants can be performed in conjunction with standard rhytidectomy and blepharoplasty with excellent outcome.

To assist in determining the appropriate facial implant, it is best to recognize the characteristic patterns of midface deformity (Table 12-1).[22,23] It is very important to separately evaluate the bony malar region and the soft tissue component in the submalar area. Patients with type I deformity have primary malar hypoplasia with ample midface soft tissue. This deformity is best addressed with malar shell implants that cover the bony midface, resulting in a high arched, laterally projected cheek (Fig. 12-6). The newer shell implants are more stable and less prone to migration when compared to traditional malar "button" implants.

Type II submalar deficiency occurs in patients who have normal malar skeleton associated with soft tissue

Table 12-1   Patterns of Midface Deformity

Types	Description of Deformity	Augmentation Required	Implant
Type I	Primary *malar* deficiency and hypoplasia Inadequate malar bony prominence Adequate submalar soft-tissue	*Lateral* malar projection and augmentation	*Malar* shell implant with slight extension into the submalar space to create a soft transition
Type II	Primary *submalar* deficiency Normal malar projection Flattened and deficient submalar soft-tissue	Restore midface volume with *anterior* projection of the submalar space	*Submalar* implant placed over the anterior maxilla and messeteric tendon with slight extension onto the malar eminence to create a soft transition
Type III	Combined *malar* and *submalar* deficiency Malar hypoplasia Submalar volume deficiency	Restore complete midfacial volume by both *anterior* and *lateral* projection of submalar and malar regions	*Combined* malar and submalar implant

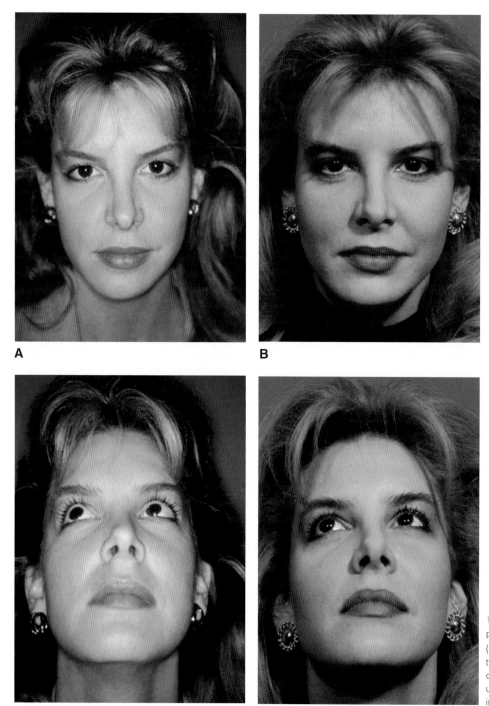

A

B

C

D

Figure 12-6 Type I midface deformity. Preoperative (**A** and **C**) and postoperative (**B** and **D**) photographs of a patient with type I *malar* hypoplasia who has relative deficiency of the midface skeleton and underwent placement of malar shell implants.

atrophy of the midface. This is the most common deficiency found in the aging face as the soft tissue components of the midface start to atrophy and lose luster. Soft tissue atrophy and inferior descent leave a hollowed-out appearance, resulting in a flat and dull-appearing midface. Type II deficiency is best treated with submalar implants that fill in the midface depressions and give greater anterior projection to the flattened face (Figs. 12-2, 12-7, and 12-8).

Type III deformity occurs when there is a combined bony malar hypoplasia and soft tissue deficiency. These patients have the propensity to suffer exaggerated effects of aging because ptotic soft tissues have little bony support and readily descend along the nasolabial folds and oral commissure. Type III patients can greatly benefit from the placement of combined malar-submalar implants (Fig. 12-9). Many of these patients would be poor candidates for rhytidectomy alone, because there is

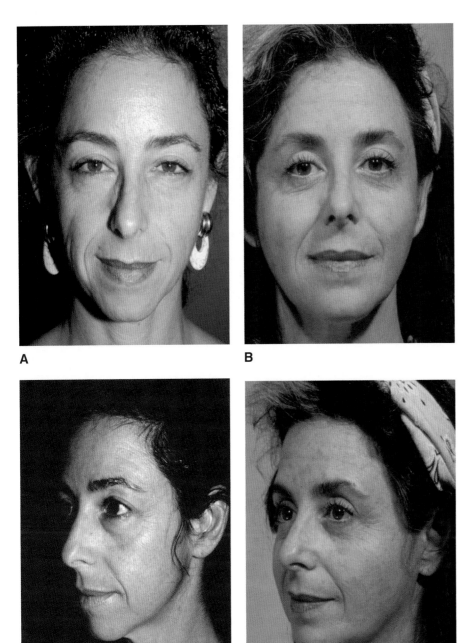

Figure 12-7 Type II midface deformity. Preoperative photographs (**A** and **C**) of a patient with type II *submalar* deficiency. The patient had adequate facial skeleton but deficiency of the submalar soft tissues. Seven-year postoperative photographs (**B** and **D**) after placement of submalar and chin implants demonstrating the long-term enhancement of facial rejuvenation.

limited underlying skeletal support with which to resuspend the skin and soft tissue. The surgical results are often suboptimal and short-lasting.

SURGICAL TECHNIQUE

GENERAL GUIDELINES

Biomaterials such as silicone, polytetrafluoroethylene (Medpor, Porex Surgical Products, Newnan, GA), and expanded polytetrafluoroethylene (Gore-Tex, W.L. Gore & Associates, Inc., Flagstaff, AZ) can be used for midface augmentation. We prefer silicone because it is flexible, has a low incidence of infection, and can be easily inserted and removed.[6-11] The transoral approach is utilized to place the implant in a subperiosteal pocket. This approach allows easy insertion of the implant and direct visualization of all midface anatomic structures (especially the infraorbital nerve). There are no external skin scars and the inferior dissection helps avoid postoperative traction on the lower eyelid. In the

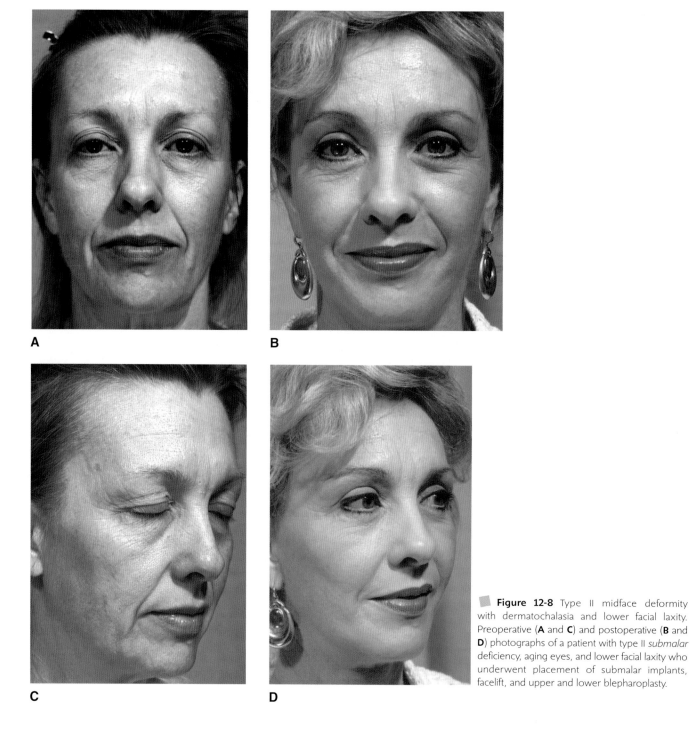

A

B

C

D

Figure 12-8 Type II midface deformity with dermatochalasia and lower facial laxity. Preoperative (**A** and **C**) and postoperative (**B** and **D**) photographs of a patient with type II *submalar* deficiency, aging eyes, and lower facial laxity who underwent placement of submalar implants, facelift, and upper and lower blepharoplasty.

subperiosteal plane, silicone implants become firmly attached to the facial skeleton by capsular fibrosis, which helps ensure against implant migration during the postoperative period.[23] A potential disadvantage of this approach is the increased risk of wound infection; the implant could be contaminated by oral microbes because it is placed through the mouth. Fastidious surgical technique can help to reduce this risk. Occasionally, other approaches such as the subciliary and lateral facelift approaches are utilized.

When performing concomitant rhytidectomy, the surgeon can insert the implants before or after the facelift surgery. Type I and III patients, who have a malar component to the midface augmentation procedure, should have the implants placed prior to the rhytidectomy so that the surgeon can compensate for the structural changes that may not be obvious after swelling occurs. When implants are placed prior to the facelift procedure, it is prudent to place a Penrose drain into the oral incisions to prevent seroma and hematoma formation.

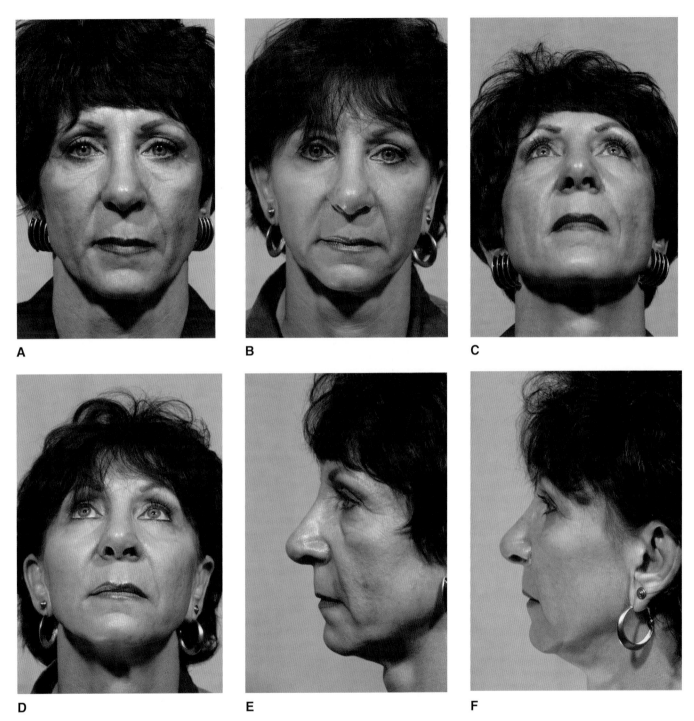

Figure 12-9 Type III midface deformity. Preoperative (**A**, **C**, and **E**) and postoperative (**B**, **D**, and **E**) photographs of a patient with type III volume-deficient face who lacks adequate facial skeletal structure and soft tissue bulk who underwent placement of combined *malar-submalar* implants with enhanced midface volume and overall improvement of facial aesthetics.

Type II patients who will require only submalar soft tissue augmentation can undergo the rhytidectomy procedure prior to the implantation. The advantages of placing the alloplastic implant at the end of the procedure include maintaining a dry implant pocket, reducing subperiosteal bleeding, and closing the intraoral wound immediately following the augmentation, thereby reducing the risk of infection.

PREPARATION FOR SURGERY

Patients are started on a broad-spectrum oral antibiotic the day before the procedure. In the preoperative holding area, crucial areas of the midface are marked on the face while the patient is sitting upright (Fig. 12-10). The markings include the midface volume deficit, areas of depression, infraorbital nerve axis, and the malar

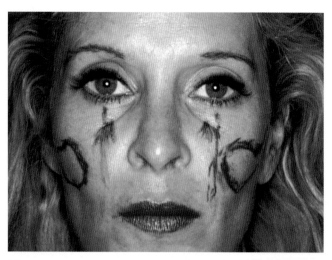

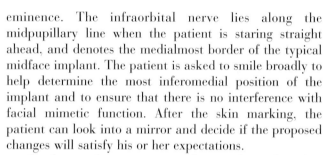

Figure 12-10 Preoperative markings. With the patient sitting upright, the areas of midface deficiency requiring augmentation are marked. The infraorbital nerve axis along the midpupillary line designates the medial border of dissection.

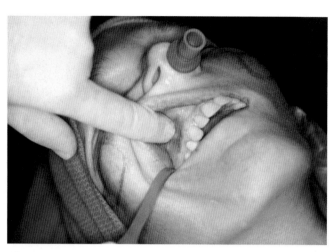

Figure 12-11 Oral incision. The gingival-buccal incision is made over the lateral canine fossa. Only 5 mm is required as the initial incision, because the mucosa will stretch and provide adequate exposure of the midface skeleton. A 1- to 1.5-cm cuff of gingiva is maintained inferiorly.

eminence. The infraorbital nerve lies along the midpupillary line when the patient is staring straight ahead, and denotes the medialmost border of the typical midface implant. The patient is asked to smile broadly to help determine the most inferomedial position of the implant and to ensure that there is no interference with facial mimetic function. After the skin marking, the patient can look into a mirror and decide if the proposed changes will satisfy his or her expectations.

Implant placement can be performed using intravenous sedation or general anesthesia. Intravenous antibiotic and steroids are routinely utilized. After an adequate anesthetic state is reached, 1% lidocaine with epinephrine is injected into the gingival-buccal sulcus and the midface in a subperiosteal plane. Hyaluronidase (Wydase, Wyeth-Ayerst, Philadelphia, PA) is added to the anesthetic solution to help disperse the local anesthetic evenly and minimize contour irregularities from the accumulation of fluid. The face is then massaged in order to disperse the solution evenly. The operative site is prepared with povidone-iodine (Betadine, Purdue Frederick, Norwalk, CT) from soaked gauze sponges placed into the gingival-buccal sulcus at the level of the canine fossa for 10 minutes.

INCISION AND DISSECTION OF MALAR EMINENCE

A 5-mm stab incision is made in the gingival-buccal sulcus over the lateral canine fossa and maxillary buttress (Fig. 12-11). It is unnecessary to make a large incision, because the mucosa can stretch to accommodate larger implants. The incision is made in an upward oblique direction and is carried immediately and directly onto the maxillary bone. Compression of the mucosa against bone

during incision will help minimize bleeding. At least a 1-cm cuff of gingival mucosa is left to facilitate closure at the end of the procedure. Dentures can remain in place during the operation, as they will not interfere with implant insertion and actually direct the placement of the incision to the correct location.

The periosteum of the anterior maxilla is elevated superiorly and laterally (Figs. 12-12 and 12-13). The surgeon's external free hand is crucial in guiding the direction and extent of dissection using the preoperative markings. The subperiosteal elevation is started with the Joseph elevator but is quickly changed to a broader 10-mm Tessier elevator (Fig. 12-14). Extensive dissection, stretching, and traction around the infraorbital foramen are avoided. If the proposed implant is large or has a significant medial component, the infraorbital nerve is carefully identified in order to avoid placement of the implant over the foramen.

Dissection is extended laterally to the malar-zygomatic junction and zygomatic arch. The subperiosteal plane is utilized for dissection particularly over the lateral zygomatic arch where branches of the facial nerve traverse just superficial to this plane (Fig. 12-15). Gentle blunt dissection over the midzygomatic arch will help avoid injury to the temporal branch of the facial nerve. A broad instrument is far safer than a delicate thin elevator. Thin elevators can more easily puncture the periosteum laterally, where there is limited visibility during the dissection.

EXPOSURE OF THE SUBMALAR TRIANGLE AND CREATION OF AN IMPLANT POCKET

The submalar space requires exposure in patients with types II and III midface deficiencies. The submalar space

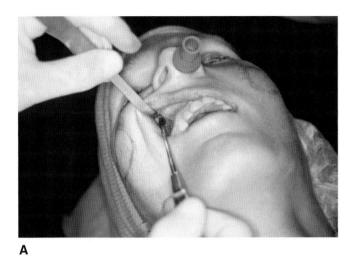

A

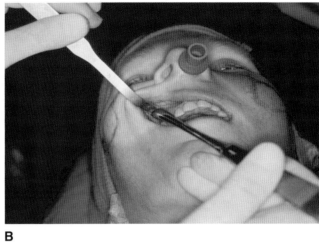

B

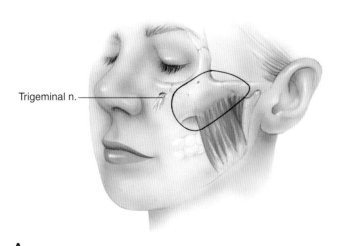

C

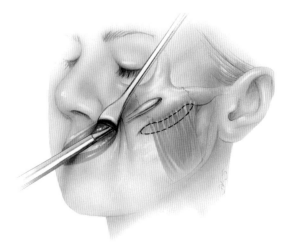

Figure 12-12 Periosteal elevation. The periosteum is elevated over the maxilla superiorly and laterally. The borders of dissection are the masseteric tendon and infraorbital rim.

Trigeminal n.

A

B

Figure 12-13 Midface dissection. The outlined area in **A** represents the extent of the malar and submalar dissection. The dashed area in **B** represents the submalar dissection over the superior tendinous origin of the masseter muscle.

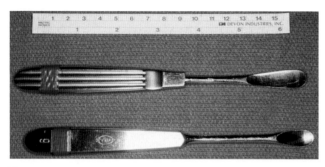

Figure 12-14 Periosteal elevators. Periosteal elevation begins with the narrow elevator to gain initial access, but most of the dissection should be performed with the broad 10-mm Tessier elevator (shown in this figure).

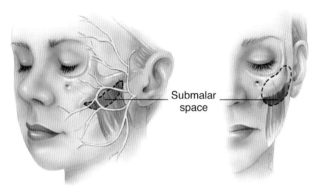

Submalar space

Figure 12-15 Facial nerve branches in the region of dissection. It is crucial to dissect in the subperiosteal plane over the zygomatic arch in order to avoid injury to the temporal branch of the facial nerve. The use of a broad elevator will help prevent perforation of the periosteum in this region. The buccal branches are also at risk if the masseteric dissection is not performed carefully.

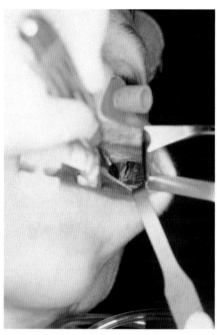

Figure 12-16 Submalar triangle and masseteric tendon. The lateral aspect of the dissection will be over the masseteric tendon, inferior to the lateral zygomatic arch. In this region, the soft tissues are gently elevated over the glistening white fibers of the tendon, allowing placement of the tail of the submalar implant.

is an anatomic hollow that extends about 3 cm below the zygoma. To expose this region, the subperiosteal dissection is continued inferiorly below the zygoma and over the superior tendinous origin of the masseter muscle. The glistening white tendinous attachment of the masseter can be visualized by gentle elevation of the overlying soft tissue from the deeper plane of the tendon (Fig. 12-16). The muscle attachments are not divided because they are a crucial platform for the lateral portion of the submalar implant. Posteriorly the submalar space becomes much narrower and is not easily accessed. The posterior limit is carefully dissected by advancing a blunt elevator along the inferior border of the zygomatic arch. Masseter contraction at its superior border tends to be limited, thereby preventing postoperative implant displacement.

A pocket is created over the malar-zygomatic complex and submalar triangle that is large enough to accommodate the appropriate implant. The implant should easily fit into this dissected space, which should always be larger than the implant without any compression by the surrounding tissues, especially in the posterior region. An implant that is forced into an inadequately sized pocket will become displaced. If the posterolateral portion of the pocket is inadequately exposed, constriction of this area will push the implant anteriorly and cause migration or extrusion. One should be able to move the implant at least 3 to 5 mm in all directions. In general, the periosteum and soft tissues reapproximate immediately after surgery and obliterate the dead space within 24 to 48 hours.[22]

INSERTION OF IMPLANT

The location and size of the implants are typically determined preoperatively depending on the facial analysis, type of deformity, and patient desires. When choosing the appropriate midface implant, it is best to use an implant that is slightly smaller than the desired volume changes, in order to account for the bulk of the overlying soft tissue and fibrous capsule formation. *Malar* shell implants for type I deformity rest on top of the malar and zygomatic bone in a more superior and lateral position (Fig. 12-17). *Submalar* implants for type II deformity generally lie over the anterior face of the maxilla. Combined *malar-submalar* implants for type III deformity will cover both the malar bony eminence and the submalar triangle. Positioning an implant in the submalar triangle is more subjective than placement over the malar eminence requiring a greater judgment to effect the desired facial contour changes.

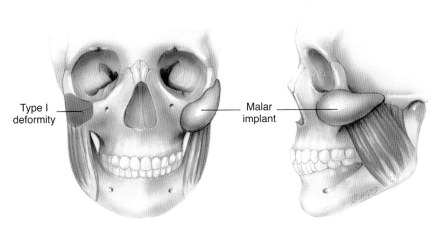

A

Figure 12-17 Implant placement. *Malar* shell implants for type I deformity rest on top of the malar and zygomatic bone in a more superior and lateral position (**A**). *Submalar* implants for type II deformity generally lie over the anterior face of the maxilla (**B**). Combined *malar-submalar* implants for type III deformity will cover both the malar bony eminence and the submalar triangle (**C**).

Type I deformity

Malar implant

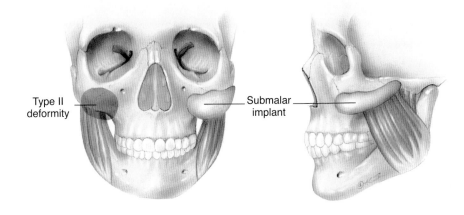

B

Type II deformity

Submalar implant

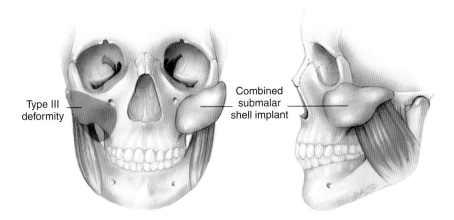

C

Type III deformity

Combined submalar shell implant

Sizers should be used to determine and confirm the appropriate implant shape and size. The actual implants should be placed in antibiotic solution (Bacitracin 50,000 U/L) at the beginning of the procedure and allowed to soak until insertion. A variety of implant sizes and shapes should be available in the operating room, and the surgeon must be ready to customize these implants (Fig. 12-18). Shaving an implant by even 1 mm can have

a significant impact on the final result, especially in patients with thin facial skin.

It is very important to assess for facial symmetry following the insertion of the implants. A ruler can be used to measure the distances from the medial border of the implants to the midline. Preexisting facial asymmetry can be very challenging, requiring exquisite attention to the bony and soft tissue topography (Fig. 12-19). As a

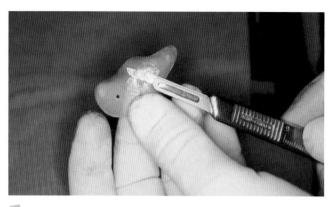

Figure 12-18 Intraoperative carving of implant.

result, each implant may need to be asymmetrically contoured and positioned. Standing at the head of the table helps in evaluating for contour symmetry after both implants have been placed. This is particularly evident in patients who have particularly thin skin or prominent facial skeleton. In these patients, the edges and contours of larger, thicker implants tend to be palpable with visible irregularities if not addressed during the initial procedure.

SECURING THE IMPLANT

After final placement, the implant will need to be secured. Larger implants that are not prone to migration within a

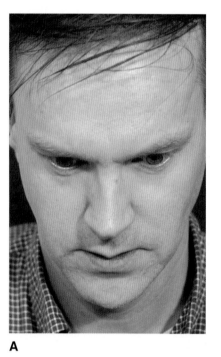

A

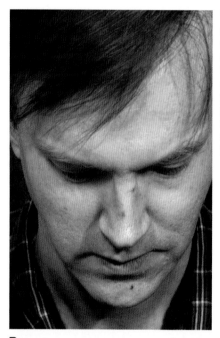

B

Figure 12-19 Facial asymmetry. This patient has a very common pattern of facial asymmetry (**A** and **C**). The patient's right side is narrower with malar eminence in a higher position and more projected. The left side is wider, flatter, and more posteriorly displaced. Postoperative photographs (**B** and **D**) after placement of asymmetrical midface implant placement. A medium malar shell implant was placed in the right side, whereas a large combined malar-submalar implant was placed in the left side of the face.

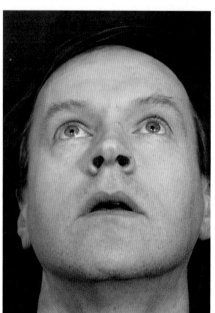

C

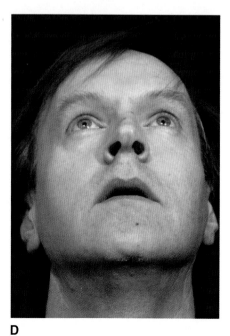

D

relatively tight pocket may not require fixation. Several methods can be used to fix the implant in order to avoid postoperative migration. We prefer to use external suture fixation using one of two techniques.[23] The first technique is an *indirect lateral suture fixation*. Long (10-inch) double-armed Keith needles on 0-0 silk suture are passed through the lateral end of the implant (Fig. 12-20). These needles are then placed into the wound and are directed posterolaterally, exiting the temporal region behind the hairline. The implant is then placed into the final position and the sutures are tied over a cotton roll bolster. This method is best for malar shell implants (type I deformity) by applying a superolateral tension on the implants and maintaining their position over the bony malar-zygomatic eminence.

The second suture technique is a *direct external fixation* (Fig. 12-21). This method is better for submalar and combined malar-submalar facial implants (type II and III deformities). It is also the preferred technique when the implants have excessive mobility within the wound pocket. Midface implants usually have two preformed fenestrations. The position of the medial fenestration should be marked on the external skin while the implant is inside the subperiosteal pocket. Locating these holes can be achieved with a right-angle clamp that pushes the implant upward, underneath the fenestration, causing an external protuberance that can be marked on the external skin. Symmetry is confirmed by measuring and comparing the distance of each marking to the midline. After marking the medial fenestrations, the implants are removed and placed on top of the midface. The implants are positioned to coincide with the desired contour and preoperative markings; the second mark is then made on the skin to coincide with the location of the lateral fenestration of the implant. Double-armed 3-0 silk sutures are used to go through the medial and lateral fenestrations with the loop around the deep surface of the implant. The needles are then placed into the wound pocket and passed perpendicularly through the skin markings corresponding to each fenestration. The implant is then brought into the pocket, ensuring proper position and symmetry. The sutures are gently tied over cotton roll bolsters overlying the anterior cheek. These bolsters help compress the midface and reduce any potential dead space and prevent fluid from collecting in the subperiosteal pockets. External sutures and bolsters are removed 24 to 48 hours after operation.

If implants are placed prior to a concurrent rhytidectomy procedure, they can be secured with internal suture fixation, which allows the oral incision to be completely closed. If external suture fixation is desired, the implant should be left in place with the oral incision temporarily or loosely closed. When the rhytidectomy is completed, the oral incision is reopened in order to fix the implant with external sutures. Intraoral Penrose drains can be placed if required.

WOUND CLOSURE AND DRESSING

The intraoral incisions are copiously irrigated with antibiotic solution and closed in one layer with chromic sutures. Bandages are then placed over the external suture bolsters and an elastic facial dressing is applied. We prefer a full elastic garment dressing that applies even midface compression (CaroMed International, Tucson, AZ) and remains in place for 24 hours (Fig. 12-22). The suture bolster closes the midface pocket anterior to the implant while the elastic dressing applies adequate pressure to obliterate the pocket posterior to the implant. The patients are encouraged to use this elastic dressing after the bolsters are taken out for an additional 24 to 48 hours. If performed with rhytidectomy, a lighter neck and facial compression dressing composed of cotton and cling is also used.

POSTOPERATIVE CARE

Postoperatively, the patients can recover at home or an aftercare facility. They are encouraged to use ice packs for 3 to 4 days and sleep with the head elevated. All patients are prescribed antibiotics, analgesics, and antinausea medication. The first follow-up appointment is on post-operative day 1 or 2 when facial dressings and external sutures are removed. At this time, any drains placed

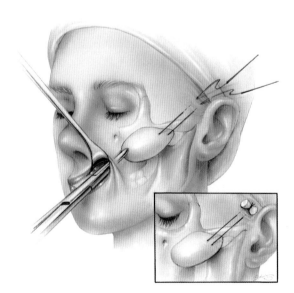

Figure 12-20 Indirect lateral suture fixation. This method is best used for malar shell implants (type I deformity) by applying a superolateral tension on the implants and maintaining their position over the bony malar-zygomatic eminence. Long (10-inch) double-armed Keith needles on 0-0 silk sutures are passed through the lateral end of the implant and directed posterolaterally, exiting the temporal region behind the hairline. The implant is then placed into the final position and the sutures are tied over a cotton roll bolster.

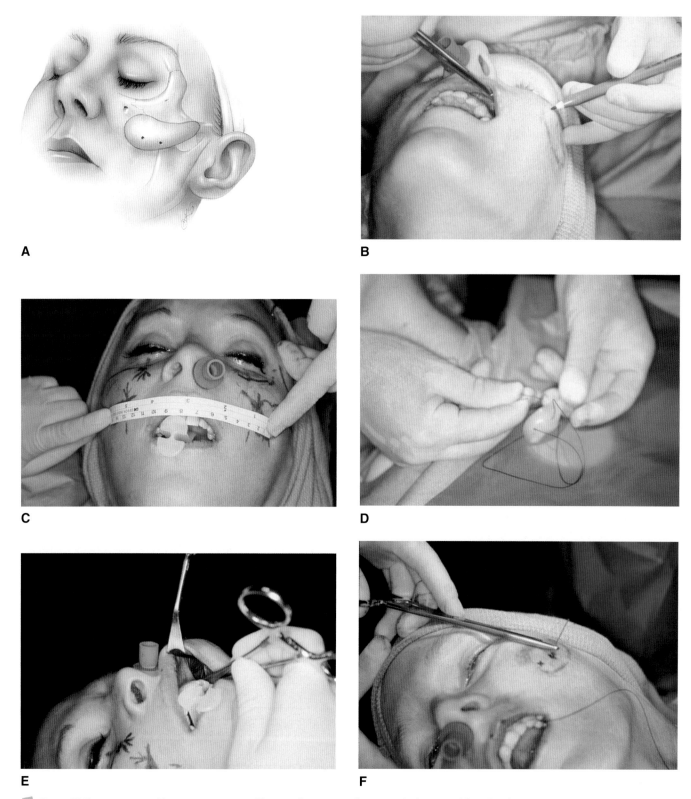

Figure 12-21 Direct external fixation. Direct external fixation allows precise fixation and is best suited for submalar and combined implants in type II and III patients. The implant is adjusted in the pocket to obtain the exact desired location (**A**). A right-angle clamp is utilized to mark the location of the implant fenestrations by pressing behind the fenestration outward through the facial skin and marking the area of protuberance (**B**). A second fenestration mark is placed to ensure adequate orientation. Symmetrical placement of markings is checked (**C**). The suture needles are passed perpendicularly through the skin markings corresponding to each fenestration (**D–H**).

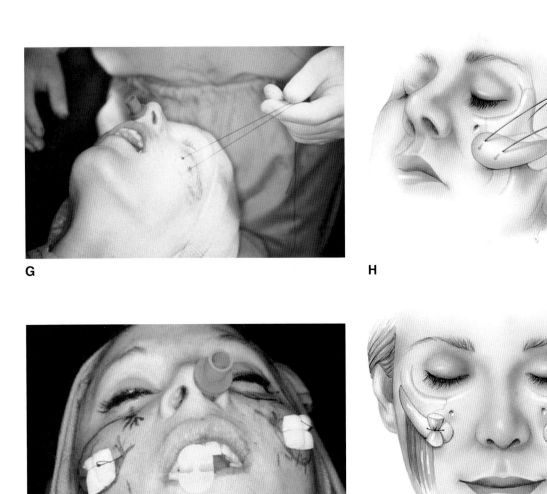

G

H

I

J

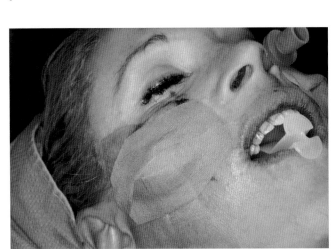

K

Figure 12-21 *Continued.* After ensuring precise location and adequate fixation of the midface implants, the sutures are tied over a cotton roll bolster (**I–J**). Benzoin and a flexible bandage can then be placed over the bolster (**K**).

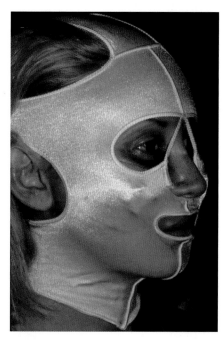

Figure 12-22 Elastic facial dressing. A full face compression garment can help reduce postoperative edema and fluid collection.

during rhytidectomy are also removed. Patients are then seen on a regular basis until facial edema resolves. The patients are generally able to return to routine activity 5 to 7 days following the procedure. About 80% to 85% of the edema will resolve within 3 to 4 weeks. The remaining 15% to 20% of facial edema will gradually resolve over the ensuing 6 months.

COMPLICATIONS

The most frequent complications of facial implants include malposition and choosing an incorrect implant.[6,24] Postoperative displacement may result from incorrect positioning, insufficient pocket size, or inadequate fixation of the implant. Other complications include bleeding, hematoma, and seroma. It is important to assess the patients within 48 to 72 hours after surgery to ensure against significant facial asymmetry. The placement of drains can help prevent fluid collection, especially when a concurrent rhytidectomy is performed or when there has been excessive bleeding during the procedure.

The rate of infection for alloplastic silicone implants is about 1%.[24] Soaking the implant in antibiotic solution, irrigating the wound pocket, and preventing the accumulation of fluid and blood in the surgical pocket can all help to minimize the risk of infection. Implant extrusion is extremely rare and usually occurs through the intraoral incision due to an inadequate dissection of the posterolateral pocket. Other complications include infraorbital and facial nerve injury. Infraorbital numbness

can persist from days to weeks postoperatively but is rarely permanent. Damage to the frontal branch of the facial nerve can occur during dissection of the zygomatic arch, and the buccal branch could be injured with aggressive masseter dissection.

Future Directions

Alloplastic implants will continue to gain a more prominent role in facial aesthetic surgery. Currently, computer technology allows for more precise facial implants that can be customized for correcting complex facial defects.[19,20] Computer-aided design (CAD) and manufacturing (CAM) of implants starts with a high-resolution computed tomographic (CT) scan of the face. A precise life-size three-dimensional model is then computer-generated via stereolithography. The surgeon then creates a custom silicone implant template using this model along with direct analysis of the patient's face that can also be facilitated with a moulage. This template is then used to produce a mold and ultimately a silicone implant that precisely fits the topography of the bony skeleton with the desired surface contour. These custom-designed prostheses are especially useful for cases of severe facial asymmetry seen in patients with longstanding facial paralysis as well as congenital and post-traumatic defects. The late stage sequelae of facial trauma can be especially difficult to treat with conventional open reduction and internal fixation. In this setting, camouflage with custom implants can be an effective and straightforward way to achieve facial symmetry and normalcy, while avoiding lengthy, extensive reconstructive surgery and donor site morbidity.

REFERENCES

1. Tessier P: The definitive plastic surgical treatment of the severe facial deformities of craniofacial dysostosis: Crouzon's and Apert's diseases. Plast Reconstr Surg 1971;48(5):419-442.
2. Spadafora A, De los Rios E, Toledo Rios R: Pomulos planos (platizigion): Endoprotesis de polietileno insertadas por via sub periostica de arco cigomatico [Flat cheeks: Polyethylene endoprostheses inserted subperiosteally along the zygomatic arch]. Prensa Med Argent 1971;58(40):1946-1950.
3. Hinderer UT: Malar implants for improvement of the facial appearance. Plast Reconstr Surg 1975;56(2):157-165.
4. Gonzalez-Ulloa M: Building out the malar prominences as an addition to rhytidectomy. Plast Reconstr Surg 1974;53(3):293-296.
5. Brennan HG: Augmentation malarplasty. Arch Otolaryngol 1982;108(7):441-444.
6. Wilkinson TS: Complications in aesthetic malar augmentation. Plast Reconstr Surg 1983;71(5):643-649.
7. Silver WE: The use of alloplast material in contouring the face. Facial Plast Surg 1986;3:81-98.
8. Whitaker LA: Aesthetic augmentation of the malar-midface structures. Plast Reconstr Surg 1987;80(3):337-346.

9. Prendergast M, Schoenrock LD: Malar augmentation. Patient classification and placement. Arch Otolaryngol Head Neck Surg 1989;115(8):964-969.

10. Binder WJ: Submalar augmentation. An alternative to face-lift surgery. Arch Otolaryngol Head Neck Surg 1989;115(7):797-801.

11. Terino EO: Alloplastic facial contouring by zonal principles of skeletal anatomy. Clin Plast Surg 1992;19(2):487-510.

12. Psillakis JM, Rumley TO, Carmargos A: Subperiosteal approach as an improved concept for correction of the aging face. Plast Reconstr Surg 1988;82:383.

13. Tessier P: Lifting facial sous-perioste. Ann Chir Plast Esthet 1989;34:193.

14. Ramirez OM: The subperiosteal rhytidectomy: The third-generation face-lift. Ann Plast Surg 1992;28(3):218-232.

15. Hamra ST: The deep plane rhytidectomy. Plast Reconstr Surg 1990;86:53.

16. Kamer FM: One hundred consecutive deep plane face lifts. Arch Otolaryngol Head Neck Surg 1996,122:17-22.

17. Chajchir A, Benzaquen I: Liposuction fat grafts in face wrinkles and hemifacial atrophy. Aesthet Plast Surg. 1986;10(2):115-117.

18. Coleman SR: Facial recontouring with lipostructure. Clin Plast Surg. 1997;24(2):347-367.

19. Binder WJ, Kaye A: Reconstruction of posttraumatic and congenital facial deformities with three-dimensional computer-assisted custom-designed implants. Plast Reconstr Surg 1994;94(6):775-787.

20. Binder WJ, Bloom DC: The use of custom-designed midfacial and submalar implants in the treatment of facial wasting syndrome. Arch Facial Plast Surg 2004;6(6):394-397.

21. Broadbent TR, Mathews VL: Artistic relationships in surface anatomy of the face: Application to reconstructive surgery. Plast Reconstr Surg 1957;20(1):1-17.

22. Binder WJ: A comprehensive approach for aesthetic contouring of the midface in rhytidectomy. Facial Plast Surg Clin North Am 1993;1(2):231-255.

23. Binder WJ, Schoenrock LD, Terino EO: Augmentation of the malar-submalar/midface. Facial Plast Surg Clinic North Am 1994;2(3):265-283.

24. Rubin JP, Yaremchuk MJ: Complications and toxicities of implantable biomaterials used in facial reconstructive and aesthetic surgery: A comprehensive review of the literature. Plast Reconstr Surg 1997;100(5):1336-1353.

CHAPTER THIRTEEN

Mentoplasty

Robert A. Glasgold, MD • Mark J. Glasgold, MD • Alvin I. Glasgold, MD

HISTORY

Chin augmentation has been performed using autografts, alloplastic materials, and mandibular advancement procedures.[1] Autografts are complicated by the need for a donor site, difficulty with shaping the grafts, and their unpredictable pattern of resorption.[1] In contrast, alloplastic implants have proved to be an easy and reliable means of augmentation. The most common method of augmentation is with alloplastic implants, including Silastic, Gore-Tex, Mersilene mesh, and Medpore implants.[2-4] Silastic chin implants have the longest history of continuous use of any of the alloplastic implants. They have been safely used since the 1960s with a high degree of satisfaction. Mandibular advancement procedures require specialized equipment and add significant morbidity to the procedure with little advantage.

The most significant evolution in mentoplasty has been in implant design. The earliest Silastic implants were carved individually by the surgeon. In 1966, Safian and Dow Corning introduced the first preformed Silastic implants.[1] These implants were equivalent to what is now referred to as a curvilinear implant or a central implant without a lateral component. Augmentation was isolated to the central mentum and provided only an anterior projection. The most significant advance in implant design was the introduction of the anatomic style of implant by Toranto in 1982.[5] These types of implants have lateral tapering extensions, which wrap around the mandible, providing anterior projection of the mentum, filling of the prejowl sulcus, and an overall recontouring of the mandible. The result is a more natural augmentation of the chin-jawline complex. These implants are available as either anatomic implants (McGhan Medical, Santa Barbara, CA) or extended anatomic implants (Implantech, Ventura, CA). Realizing the importance of isolated prejowl augmentation in certain patients, Mittleman introduced his prejowl implant, which has a thin central portion and bulk only in the lateral arms.[6]

The surgical technique for mentoplasty using alloplastic implants has not significantly changed in recent years. The two common surgical approaches are an external technique through a submental incision and an intraoral technique through a gingivolabial sulcus incision. Both approaches are commonly used today, generally determined by the preference of the individual surgeon.

PERSONAL PHILOSOPHY

An optimal facial skeletal structure serves as the foundation for rhytidectomy and other facial rejuvenation procedures. Patients with poor skeletal foundations, as seen with microgenia, will not only tend to show certain stigmata of aging earlier, such as poor necklines and jowling, but will also obtain less than ideal results from a facelift. In the appropriate patients, correction of microgenia is a critical technique for facial rejuvenation, either as a stand-alone procedure or in conjunction with facelifting (Fig. 13-1).

Alloplastic implantation provides a safe, reliable, and relatively simple means for chin augmentation. The ideal implant material should have a very low incidence of infection or rejection. It should also provide predictable long-term results and be easy to remove if necessary. In our practice we use preformed Silastic extended anatomic implants for augmentation mentoplasty. Silastic implants meet all the preceding criteria. Silastic implants are flexible enough to allow for easy insertion and provide a natural feel and appearance. Silastic is a nonporous material around which a fibrous capsule forms, allowing easy removal.[7]

An extended anatomic implant fills the central mentum and has lateral arms with sufficient bulk and extension to fill the prejowl sulcus that taper off laterally to give a natural jawline. These implants have a lower incidence of shifting than the central implants. The extended anatomic implants are usually available in four sizes, providing between 5 and 9 mm of anterior projection. As the implant size increases, so does the length and bulk of the implant's lateral arms. Several companies produce this type of implant, but sizing is not consistent among the different manufacturers.

Central implants do not have a lateral extension to fill the prejowl sulcus. In patients with preexisting jowls, the

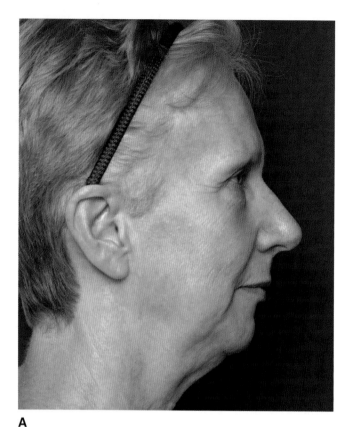

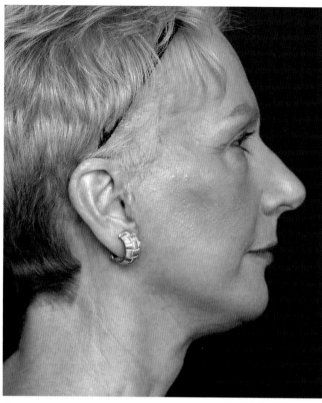

A

B

Figure 13-1 Preoperative (**A**) and 6-month postoperative (**B**) views of a patient who underwent mentoplasty with a medium extended anatomic implant and facelift.

central implant will accentuate the prejowl sulcus, often making the jowl appear more prominent. This is the opposite effect of the extended anatomic implant, which, by filling the prejowl sulcus, will reduce or camouflage the appearance of a jowl. In patients without jowling, central implants tend to make the chin appear pointy, again not producing as attractive an augmentation as the extended anatomic implant.

When performing a mentoplasty we routinely have a 2-mm Silastic extension wafer available.[8] The wafer provides a degree of intraoperative flexibility in terms of implant sizing. On intraoperative assessment, if the patient would benefit from further anterior projection, a wafer can be placed under the central portion of the chin implant, increasing anterior central mentum projection by 2 mm. This allows for an increase in anterior projection while avoiding the added cost and surgical trauma of replacing the implant with a larger one.

We perform all mentoplasties with an extraoral approach through a submental incision. In our experience the submental incision heals very well and allows easier and more accurate placement of the implant. This is particularly true when using extended anatomic implants, which require a lateral subperiosteal pocket along the inferior mandibular border. This dissection is difficult

through an intraoral approach because of the location of the mental nerves. The submental approach also allows for suture fixation of the inferior aspect of the implant to the periosteum of the inferior border of the mandible, thereby preventing implant shifting and vertical migration. Suture fixation ensures the implant is properly aligned, with no palpable or visible step-off deformity from implant to mandible. Implants placed through an intraoral approach are exposed to oral contaminants and have a greater potential for infection.

ANATOMY

The chin is composed of the overlying skin, subcutaneous tissues, muscles, and the mandible. Each component affects the overall appearance of the chin-jawline complex and its appearance with aging. The muscle components of the chin are the mentalis, depressor labii inferioris, and depressor anguli oris muscles, all of which are innervated by the marginal mandibular branch of the facial nerve. The mentalis muscle arises from the incisive fossa on the mandible and inserts inferiorly into the dermis of the chin. The mentalis muscle acts to elevate the chin. The depressor labii inferioris and depressor anguli oris muscles arise from the oblique line of the mandible and insert into the lip. Together they act to depress the lower lip and corners of the mouth, respectively.

The portions of the mandible relevant to mentoplasty are the symphysis, parasymphysis, and the body of the mandible. Understanding the location of the mental foramen and mental nerve, which provides sensation to the chin and lower lip, is crucial. The mental foramen is generally located inferior to the second premolar.[9] If measured, the foramen is found approximately 2.5 cm lateral to the midline. The location of the mental foramen is midway between the alveolar ridge superiorly and the inferior edge of the mandible. The foramen is found approximately 1 cm above the inferior border of the mandible.

The anatomy of this chin-jawline complex changes with age. Soft tissue and bone atrophy in the central mentum can lead to or exaggerate the appearance of a receding chin. Development or exaggeration of a prejowl sulcus is also due to soft tissue and bone atrophy. Age-related atrophy of the anterior mandibular groove, located inferior to the mental foramen, contributes to the prejowl sulcus.[6] Jowling, which also exaggerates the prejowl sulcus, results from ptosis of skin, muscle, subcutaneous fat, and buccal fat pad.

PREOPERATIVE ASSESSMENT

Patient evaluation begins with an understanding of what problems can be corrected with a mentoplasty. These issues are important for both the older patient seeking facial rejuvenation and the younger patient desiring an improved facial appearance. A receding chin produces an imbalance of the lower third of the face and can be corrected with a chin implant. Increasing chin projection will also improve the patient's appearance on front view, whereas a weak lower third can give a rounded, less angular facial appearance. Prominent overprojected lower lips can be camouflaged by increasing a patient's chin projection, thereby creating a more balanced appearance. Mentoplasty can also aid in creating a stronger jawline by filling the prejowl suclus.

The most common abnormality of the chin is microgenia (retrogenia), which refers to an underprojection of the chin with normal occlusion. Patients with a receding chin have a short hyoid-to-mentum distance, which is usually associated with an obtuse cervicomental angle. Chin augmentation will improve this relationship by increasing the distance from hyoid to mentum, giving the appearance of a more acute cervicomental angle (Fig. 13-2). In the younger patient with submental fullness and

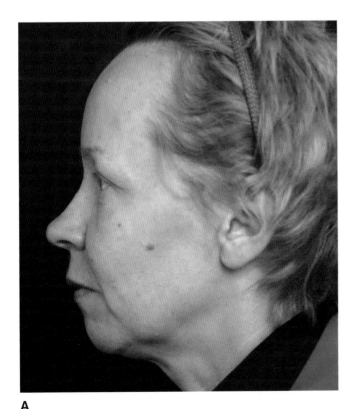
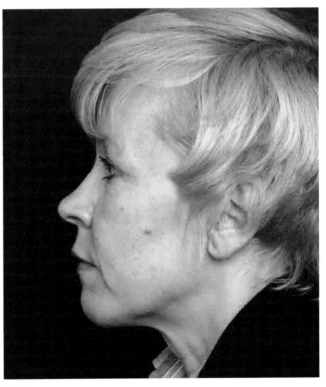

A   **B**

Figure 13-2 Preoperative view of a patient with microgenia, displaying a short hyoid-to-mentum distance and a deep prejowl sulcus (**A**) and six-month postoperative view following mentoplasty with a medium extended anatomic implant (**B**).

good skin tone, the addition of submental liposuction can significantly enhance the result of chin implantation, creating a more acute cervicomental angle (Fig. 13-3).

The simplest and most practical means to determine appropriate chin projection on profile is by dropping a perpendicular line down from the Frankfurt horizontal which should touch both the lower vermilion and the pogonion (the anteriormost projection of the chin). Patients whose projection falls behind this line should be considered for augmentation mentoplasty. Patients should also be evaluated while smiling. In a patient with borderline microgenia, smiling may increase projection to a degree that augmentation would be inappropriate. The ideal anterior projection is gender-specific. In women, 1 to 2 mm of underprojection is acceptable, whereas men can tolerate a slight overprojection, providing a stronger chin. Malocclusions should be noted and, if present, referred for orthognathic evaluation.

Development of a prejowl sulcus is a characteristic sign of aging. In a patient with minimal jowling, filling the prejowl sulcus with an implant may give a jawline comparable to that achieved with a facelift. When the jowl and prejowl sulcus are more prominent, filling the prejowl sulcus alone will usually be inadequate and a facelift becomes the primary means of restoring a strong jawline.

In patients undergoing rhytidectomy for correction of the jowl, it is important to evaluate whether the prejowl sulcus will be completely effaced through correction of the jowl alone. In some patients, the degree of atrophy in the prejowl sulcus is so significant that rhytidectomy alone cannot produce the desired jawline. These patients should be considered for prejowl sulcus augmentation with or without central mentum projection, depending on their chin projection on profile (Fig. 13-4).

Patients undergoing mentoplasty should be evaluated for certain preexisting conditions, any of which, if present, should be reviewed with the patient so that the patient is aware of these preoperatively. These conditions include hypesthesia of the chin and lip region, marginal mandibular nerve weakness, asymmetries of the chin and jawline, and contour irregularities of the chin.

Digital photography with computer imaging is helpful in the evaluation and consultation. Reviewing a patient's photograph, particularly on profile, will often help the patient understand the importance of chin augmentation for obtaining an optimal result. Computer imaging allows patients to visualize the effect of augmenting the chin and filling the prejowl sulcus.

SURGICAL TECHNIQUE

Preoperatively all patients receive intravenous prophylactic cefazolin or clindamycin, if penicillin allergic. The implant is prepared by placing a guide suture through each end of the implant to facilitate its placement and prevent the tail of the implant from folding upon itself (Fig. 13-5). A 2-0 silk suture threaded onto a Keith needle is passed through the lateral end of the implant, approximately 3 mm from the distal edge. This is then repeated with a second 2-0 silk suture and Keith needle for the contralateral side. Each of the free ends of the 2-0 silk are rethreaded onto the Keith needle. The implant is then soaked in clindamycin solution until its placement.

A submental incision, approximately 2 cm in length, is designed with its medial portion just anterior to the submental crease and gently curving posteriorly to the crease at the lateral aspects. The superior skin edge is retracted upward while dissection is carried down through the soft tissue and muscle. The periosteum is incised at the inferior portion of the anterior surface of the mandible. A cuff of periosteum is preserved at the inferior border of the mandible, to which the implant is eventually sutured. A subperiosteal pocket is elevated centrally, creating a pocket that is large enough to accommodate the implant. We prefer to elevate the central subperiosteal pocket using electrocautery.

The lateral subperiosteal pocket is initiated with electrocautery, hugging the inferior border of the mandible. A Joseph elevator is introduced to elevate the subperiosteal pocket (Fig. 13-6). External palpation with the contralateral hand will help guide the subperiosteal dissection, ensuring that the pocket remains along the inferior border of the mandible to avoid trauma to the mental nerve. Once the pocket is elevated, an Aufricht retractor (8 × 45 mm) is placed into the pocket (Fig. 13-7). A Joseph elevator is then inserted into the pocket under the Aufricht retractor and the subperiosteal pocket is gently stretched to ensure the implant will fit comfortably into the pocket. The subperiosteal pocket is then elevated on the contralateral side prior to placing the implant.

After bilateral subperiosteal dissection is completed, the Aufricht retractor is used to hold open the pocket. The Keith needle with guide suture is passed through the subperiosteal pocket under the retractor, aiming toward the angle of the mandible, and is passed out through the skin (Fig. 13-8). The guide suture is grasped by an assistant and gentle traction is provided to guide insertion of the implant as it is fed into the pocket with a straight clamp. The guide suture ensures proper placement of the lateral tail of the implant, and prevents the thin tail from folding on itself. Once the implant is inserted and the Aufricht retractor removed, continued traction is placed on the guide suture to maintain its position during insertion of the contralateral side (Fig. 13-9). The Aufricht is now placed in the contralateral side and the implant inserted in the same manner as the first side (Fig. 13-10).

Once the implant is inserted its position should be evaluated both by manual palpation and visual inspection. Central placement is confirmed by aligning the

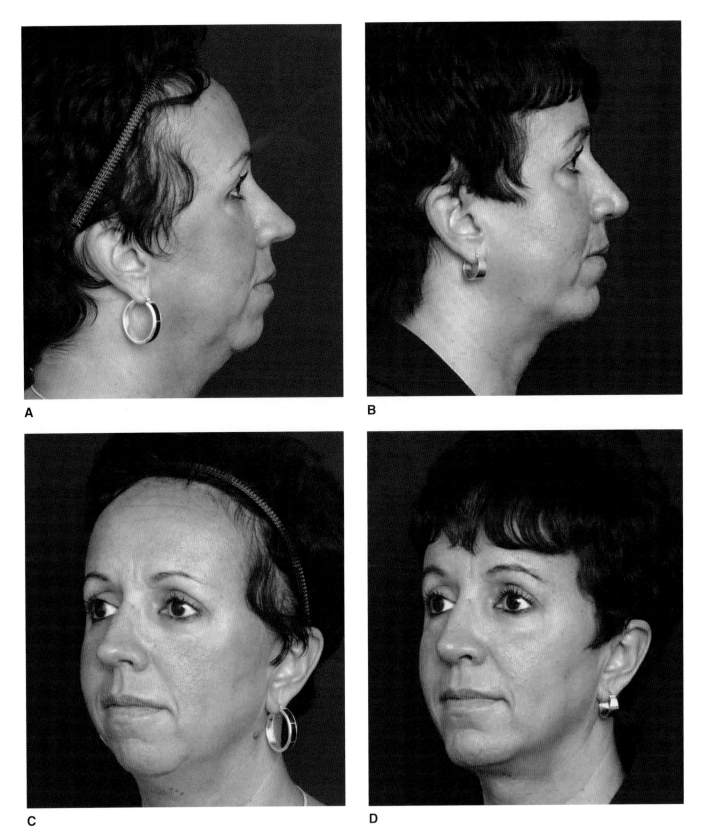

Figure 13-3 Preoperative profile (**A**) and oblique (**C**) views of a patient with microgenia, a poorly defined jawline, and a prejowl sulcus. One-year postoperative profile (**B**) and oblique (**D**) views after correction with mentoplasty with an extra-large extended anatomic implant and submental liposuction.

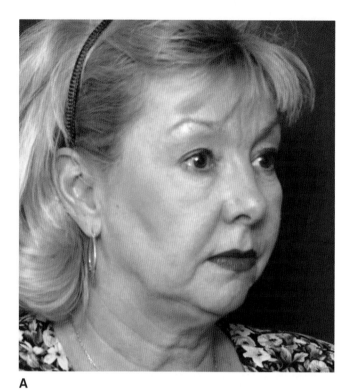

A

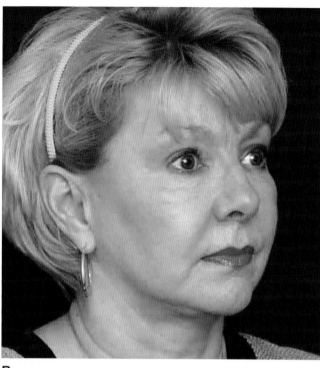

B

Figure 13-4 Preoperative view of a patient with microgenia, heavy jowls, and a deep prejowl sulcus (**A**): In this patient, mentoplasty provided anterior chin projection and filling of the prejowl sulcus, the latter of which would have been suboptimally corrected with a facelift alone. One-year postoperative view following mentoplasty with a medium extended anatomic implant and facelift (**B**).

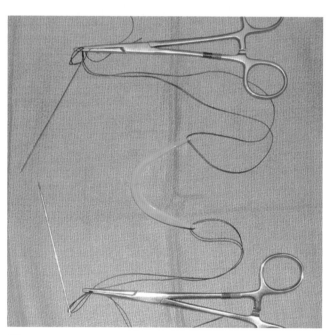

Figure 13-5 Extended anatomic implant prepared for placement with a 2-0 silk suture threaded through each of its lateral ends and onto Keith needles.

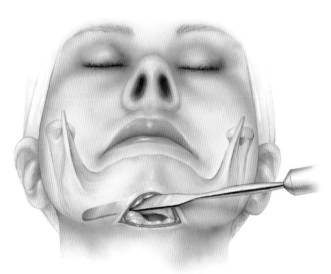

Figure 13-6 The lateral subperiosteal pocket is elevated along the inferior border of the mandible with a Joseph elevator.

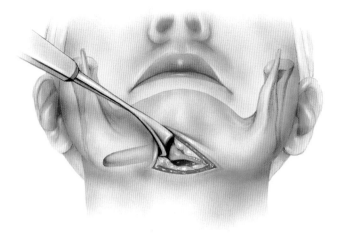

Figure 13-7 The lateral subperiosteal pocket is exposed with the Aufricht retractor.

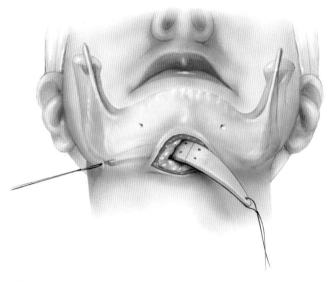

Figure 13-9 After the implant is fed into the pocket on the right, traction is maintained on the guide suture to prevent displacement while inserting the contralateral side.

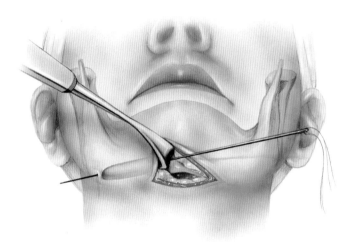

Figure 13-8 Keith needle, with guide suture, being passed through lateral pocket and out through the skin at the angle of the mandible.

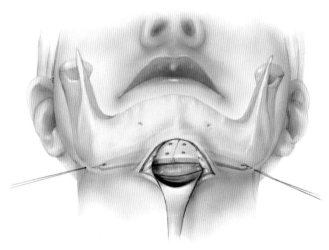

Figure 13-10 Chin implant placed within the subperiosteal pockets.

central blue mark on the implant with the junction of the upper two central incisors. Manual palpation should ensure that the implant lies flat against the mandible and that it is sitting along the inferior border of the mandible. The degree of anterior projection should be evaluated. It is important to remember that the intraoperative appearance can be affected by the swelling from the local anesthetic and surgical manipulation, as well as the mandibular recession due to the patient's supine position. Positional recession is the more significant concern in evaluation and is compensated for by holding the jaw in its proper anatomic position for evaluation.

If further augmentation is deemed necessary after implant placement, an extension wafer (Glasgold Wafer, Implantech, Ventura, CA) can be placed to provide 2 mm

of additional anterior projection (Fig. 13-11). The extension wafer does not have a central mark; making a nick at its central point on the inferior edge will help ensure proper alignment. The wafer is then simply inserted under the central portion of the implant (Fig. 13-12). Once correctly positioned it is sutured to the chin implant with two 4-0 polydioxanone (PDS) sutures, each placed approximately 1 cm lateral to midline.

After it has been confirmed that the implant is appropriately placed, the implant is sutured to the inferiorly based cuff of the periosteum with two 4-0 PDS sutures (Fig. 13-13). These sutures are placed as laterally as possible. If an extension wafer is used, the 4-0 PDS suture is placed through the periosteal cuff and then through both the wafer and overlying implant (Fig. 13-14).

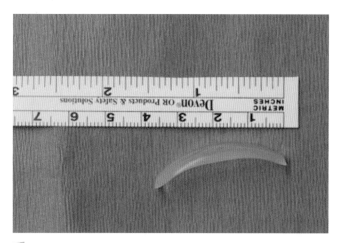

Figure 13-11 Extension wafer (Glasgold Wafer) for use with anatomic or extended anatomic chin implants to provide an additional 2 mm of central anterior projection.

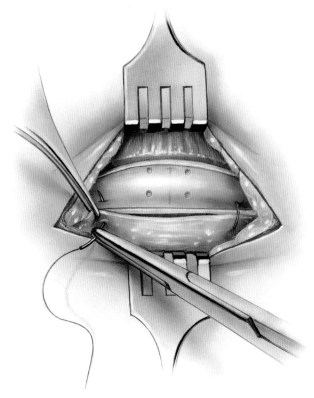

Figure 13-13 The implant is secured inferiorly to the mandibular periosteum with two 4-0 PDS sutures.

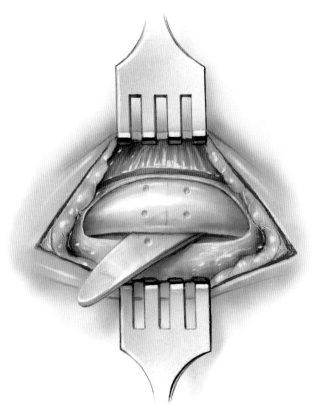

Figure 13-12 In cases in which the need for further projection is determined intraoperatively after implant placement, an extension wafer can be placed under the central portion of the implant to provide an additional 2 mm of projection.

If chin implantation is performed in conjunction with a facelift, the mentoplasty is performed first. Once the chin implant is placed and sutured in, the muscle is closed prior to proceeding with the subcutaneous submental dissection to address the submental fat and platysma. If liposuction is performed, it is done first through a small incision in the center of the planned submental incision before extending the incision for the mentoplasty.

In some patients, isolated prejowl augmentation is needed to achieve a straight jawline. Although preformed implants for prejowl augmentation are available, we prefer injection augmentation with either autologous fat or a synthetic filling material. When patients undergoing a facelift need prejowl augmentation, the fat is harvested and injected into the prejowl sulcus prior to proceeding with the facelift at the same setting. For patients who are having prejowl augmentation as a stand-alone procedure, this can be done in the office using a local anesthetic.

POSTOPERATIVE CARE

All patients are placed on a 10-day postoperative course of oral cefadroxil or, if penicillin allergic, clindamycin. No dressing is used for patients who undergo only mentoplasty. Patients are instructed to apply ice to the surgical site. It is not uncommon for patients to complain of

The muscle is reapproximated over the implant with interrupted 4-0 PDS sutures. The subcutaneous tissues are reapproximated with several interrupted 4-0 PDS sutures. The skin incision is closed with a running 6-0 Prolene suture.

12 months should pass before reimplantation. This allows sufficient time for swelling to resolve and scar to form so that sizing for another implant will be accurate.

If the chin appears overprojected during the postoperative period, the patient should be observed and reassured over a period of at least 3 months to allow swelling to subside before deciding to downsize the implant. In the case of undercorrection, an extension wafer can be placed under the existing implant as described previously; alternatively, the implant can be replaced with a larger one.

Asymmetries following augmentation are generally from a preexisting asymmetrical mandible, which should have been reviewed with the patient preoperatively. Implant shifting can occur, and would most commonly be in the cephalad direction. Shifting is prevented by using the submental approach, which allows suture fixation of the implant to the mandibular periosteum.

Numbness and paresthesias in the distribution of the mental nerve are secondary to traction on the nerve during surgery and are almost universally self-limited, lasting from weeks to months. Marginal mandibular weakness is a very rare temporary complication secondary to traction on the nerve while the implant pocket is being created.

Bone resorption of the central mandible following alloplastic chin implants has been described. In practice this has not been a significant issue.[5,10,11] To minimize resorption, the implant should be placed on the more firm cortical bone of the lower border of the mandible.[10] Placement of the implant in a sub- or superperiosteal position has not been shown to significantly affect the incidence of bone resorption.[12]

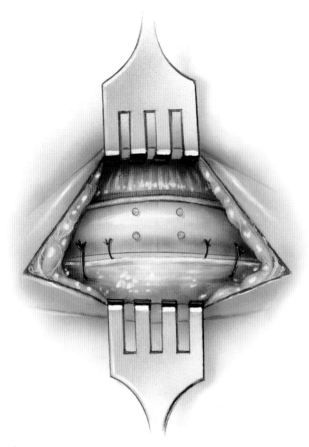

Figure 13-14 When an extension wafer is used, the wafer and implant are first sutured together (the medial sutures). Then the implant and wafer are secured as a single unit to the mandibular periosteum inferiorly with two 4-0 PDS sutures.

postoperative pain; the larger the implant the greater the tendency for patients to experience discomfort. Patients are seen on postoperative day 7, at which time the skin sutures are removed.

COMPLICATIONS

Complications following mentoplasty with alloplastic implants include infection, over- or undercorrection, asymmetry, numbness in the distribution of the mental nerve, marginal mandibular nerve weakness, and mandibular resorption. Infection is very rare, especially with a submental approach. It can occur in the immediate postoperative period as well as months to years later. Infection usually presents as increasing pain, tenderness, or swelling. Once the infection is identified, treatment includes a course of oral antibiotics (amoxicillin-clavulonic acid or clindamycin). If infection is not resolving with antibiotics, the implant should be removed. In over 30 years of experience we have had to remove an implant secondary to infection on only a few occasions. If an implant is removed because of infection, a period of 6 to

Future Considerations

The implants presently available provide a wide range of options for augmentation, and will likely be used for many years to come. Autologous fat transfers have been performed to augment the chin. This technique minimizes implant-related problems, but provides a less predictable outcome in terms of anterior projection with a longer recovery period. Ongoing advances in the field of injectable filling materials provide a possible alternative means of chin augmentation. Currently we use these materials for isolated filling of the prejowl sulcus, but the possibility exists that improvements may lead to the ability to achieve a long-term complete chin augmentation with an injectable material.

REFERENCES

1. Safian J: Progress in nasal and chin augmentation. Plast Reconst Surg 1966;37:446-452.
2. Adams J: Facial augmentation with solid alloplastic implants. In Glasgold AI, Silver FH (eds): Applications of Biomaterials in Facial Plastic Surgery. Boca Raton: CRC Press, 1991.

3. Binder W, Kamer F, Parkes M: Mentoplasty—A clinical analysis of alloplastic implants. Laryngoscope 1981;91: 383-391.

4. McCollough EG, Hom DB, Weigel MT, et al: Augmentation mentoplasty using mersilene mesh. Arch Otolaryngol Head Neck Surg 1990;116:1154-1158.

5. Toranto I: Mentoplasty: A new approach. Plast Reconst Surg 1982;69:875-878.

6. Mittleman H: The anatomy of the aging mandible and its importance to facelift surgery. Facial Plast Surg Clin North Am 1994;2:301-309.

7. Silver FH, Maas CS: Biology of synthetic facial implant materials. Facial Plast Surg Clin North Am 1994;2:241-253.

8. Glasgold A, Glasgold M: Intraoperative custom contouring of the mandible. Arch Otolaryngol Head Neck Surg 1994;120:180-184.

9. Mittelman H: Augmentation of the chin and pre-jowl sulcus. In Terino EO, Flowers RS (eds): The Art of Alloplastic Facial Contouring. St. Louis: CV Mosby, 2000.

10. Friedland JA, Coccaro PJ, Converse JM: Retrospective cephalometric analysis of mandibular bone resorption under silicone rubber chin implants. Plast Reconstr Surg 1976;57:144-151.

11. Vuyk HD: Augmentation mentoplasty with solid silicone. Clin Otolaryngol 1996;21:106-118.

12. Pearson DC, Sherris DA: Resorption beneath silastic mandibular implants. Effects of placement and pressure. Arch Facial Plast Surg 1999;1:261-264.

CHAPTER FOURTEEN

Facial Suction Lipectomy

Jeannie H. Chung, MD • Edwin F. Williams III, MD, FACS

HISTORY OF THE TECHNIQUE

Since its introduction into the United States in the early 1980s, liposuction has become the most commonly performed aesthetic procedure.[1] Liposuction has been used from head to toe with reproducible results and minimal complications. Though the initial experience stemmed from its applications in body sculpting, suction lipectomy has become a powerful method to remove undesirable adipose tissue and to contour the cervicofacial region. There is currently a wealth of literature documenting advances in techniques and instrumentation used in liposuction, and a review of the history of this technique is important to establish its fundamental principles and provide a context for evolving applications.[2-8]

The earliest references to adipose tissue removal date to the 1920s in France.[9] In 1921, Dujarrier removed fatty tissue from a ballerina's leg using a uterine curette; this resulted in amputation secondary to vascular injury and gangrene. Initial catastrophic results such as this discouraged further attempts at lipoextraction for several decades. In the early 1970s, Schrudde removed fat for aesthetic purposes using a uterine curette through a buttonhole technique, which he called "lipoexeresis."[10] This technique was prone to complications, however, as large subcutaneous cavities were created, predisposing patients to seroma formation and irregular skin contours. Furthermore, as a suction device was not used, constant irrigation was necessary to remove large segments of adipose tissue. A more practical approach to lipoextraction was developed in the mid-1970s by Fischer and Fischer, who designed a cannula attached to a suction device to facilitate tissue removal.[11,12] A similar approach was independently developed by Kesselring, who built upon the work of Schrudde and advocated suction-assisted lipectomy.[13]

Although the addition of a suction device proved to be a major advance, problems with sharp-edged curettage instruments and large cavities created by wide tissue undermining persisted. Most of these problems were solved with the advent of the blunt technique, still in use today. Inspired by the Fischers' work, Illouz in Paris reported his 5-year, 3000-case experience with suction-assisted lipolysis using a new blunt-tipped suction cannula.[14] His "wet technique" included injection of the aspiration site with a hypotonic saline solution, theoretically to rupture the adipocytes. The blunt-tipped cannulas were connected to a high-power suction machine and were used to created tunnels in a fan-shaped manner to aspirate fat.

Fournier made further technical refinements on Illouz's technique. He advocated a "dry" technique without pre-infiltration of hypotonic solution. He did not believe that infiltration with hypotonic solution was necessary, and his histologic analysis of aspirated adipose cells treated with the "wet technique" demonstrated that there was, in fact, no cellular disruption. Furthermore, Fournier proposed taping the suctioned areas to collapse the aspiration tunnels and advocated the idea of syringe liposuction as an alternative to suction pumps.[15]

American surgeons visited France and learned the techniques of liposuction. In 1977, the first American to visit France was Field, a dermatologic surgeon.[16] Other American surgeons followed, and in 1980, Martin, an otolaryngologist, visited Illouz and began to perform liposuction in Los Angeles in 1981. Soon, symposia and training courses were held to disseminate the techniques of liposuction. The American Society of Plastic and Reconstructive Surgeons was primarily under the tutelage of Illouz, whereas Fournier was largely responsible for encouraging participation and teaching physicians from all specialties. The first American course in liposuction was given by Newman, an otolaryngologist and cosmetic surgeon, and Dolsky, a plastic surgeon, in Philadelphia in 1982. Since that time, there has been great intellectual dialogue and innovation, leading to significant advances in cannula instrumentation, aspiration methods, lipo-shaving, and anesthetic techniques.

PERSONAL PHILOSOPHY

Facial liposuction has revolutionized facial aesthetic surgery by allowing surgeons to contour and improve anatomic regions that were not adequately addressed previously; indeed, liposuction has become an integral technique in the successful rejuvenation of the face. The authors recognize that many excellent aesthetic surgeons differ in the nuances of their liposuction techniques. This chapter does not attempt to provide an impartial treatise on facial suction lipectomy, but rather provides a practical strategy born of significant clinical experience to produce optimal results.

Of the overall population undergoing facial liposuction, the authors find that only a select group of patients benefit from primary facial liposuction alone. Such primary liposuction procedures are reserved for younger patients with localized adipose tissue and good skin tone, which allow for adequate skin contracture and redraping. In the authors' experience, facial suction lipectomy is frequently used in conjunction with other facial rejuvenation procedures (e.g., mentoplasty, platysmaplasty, or rhytidectomy) and is most effective in recreating an acute cervicomental angle.

Although the tunneling technique is frequently used to remove adipose collections in the submental region, the authors prefer the "layer technique" in which a skin flap is elevated prior to aspiration (Fig. 14-1). The authors find that this technique facilitates excellent skin redraping

without the risk of dimpling and skin irregularities from septal attachments inherent in the tunneling technique.

Liposuction has traditionally been described as being performed by the "open" versus "closed" technique. In the open technique, skin is elevated to expose the fatty tissue layer, which is then removed under direct vision with the cannula. In the closed technique, multiple tunnels are created with the cannula, through which fat is suctioned blindly. While the distinction between these different methods is important academically, the authors find that these differences are often blurred in practice.

In all surgical endeavors, the authors strive for straightforward and safe techniques. For many aesthetic procedures, new instruments, equipment, and technology are being introduced to facilitate use, improve results, and minimize complications. However, these advancements need to be evaluated with a critical eye. At its most fundamental level, suction lipectomy involves a rigid cannula connected to a suction device. New technology, such as the liposhaver and ultrasound-assisted liposuction

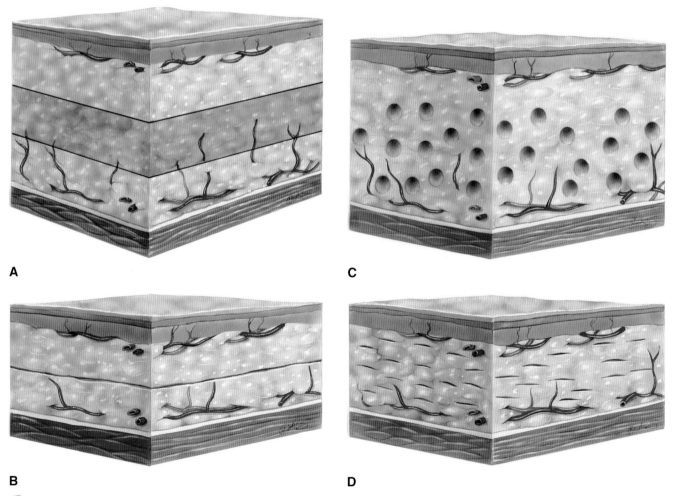

A

C

B

D

Figure 14-1 Schematic representation of the layer technique for liposuction. The skin is widely undermined in the subcutaneous plane (**A**), which allows for uniform retraction of the skin after liposuction (**B**). With the tunneling method, random passes are created with the aspiration cannula (**C**), creating a greater risk of dimpling and uneven skin contours as the skin retracts (**D**).

(UAL), has been used in efforts to improve on the removal of undesirable adipose tissue. Although these techniques are reviewed in this chapter, the authors have had success with "traditional" time-tested techniques and feel encumbered with unneeded gadgetry. One does not need to engage in the newest technique or purchase the most modern equipment to have excellent results.

Although liposuction techniques in the face and neck have been used for other indications such as lipomas and defatting of skin and myocutaneous flaps, this chapter focuses specifically on its cosmetic applications. This chapter provides preoperative guidelines for proper patient selection, reviews options for anesthesia, highlights necessary equipment, and outlines salient technical points.

ANATOMY

A thorough understanding of facial anatomy is critical to the successful application of lipectomy techniques. A comprehensive review of the head and neck is beyond the scope of this chapter, but it is important to highlight the anatomic structures and landmarks relevant to facial liposuction. Although various regions have been addressed with liposuction (Fig. 14-2), the most common area of concern for patients remains the neck. Cervical anatomy has many variations, and the specific anatomic features pertinent to aesthetic appearance merit special attention. These considerations are critical in performing appropriate preoperative evaluation and tailoring the ultimate surgical approach.

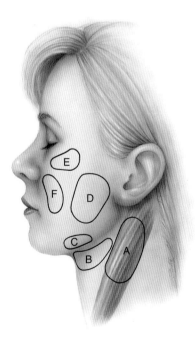

Figure 14-2 Common cervicofacial regions for liposuction include the lateral neck (*A*), submandibular and submental triangles (*B*), jowl pad (*C*), parotid, buccal, and malar areas (*D, E*), and preantrum (*F*).

The portion of the neck that is best addressed by liposuction is the central subunit, which is bounded superiorly by the inferior border of the mandible, posteriorly by the anterior border of the sternocleidomastoid muscle, and inferiorly by the thyroid cartilage. Beneath the skin lies a variable amount of fat. The quality of this fat varies from patient to patient as well as from one anatomic region to another. The adipose layer lies superficial to the platysma, a thin broad-based muscle that originates from the superficial fascia over the pectoral and deltoid muscles, ascends over the clavicle, and inserts on the mandible below the oblique line and the skin at the lateral angle of the mouth. The posterior and superior borders extend in continuity with the superficial musculoaponeurotic system (SMAS). Significant variation may exist in the midline of the platysma, from the mentum to the hyoid bone. In some patients, the muscle fibers decussate across the midline, creating a muscular sling. In others, the absence of decussation may lead to a diastasis that worsens over time. Rejuvenation of the neck requires manipulation of one or more of these structures. It is important to note that optimal results following liposuction depend as much upon the resiliency and elasticity of the overlying skin as the amount of fat removed.

Liposuction is usually performed in the adipose layer superficial to the platysma, an extremely safe region devoid of vital neurovascular structures. However, the surgeon will occasionally need to remove deeper layers of adipose tissue or dissect deep to the platysma to mobilize its medial ends (i.e., platysmaplasty). These maneuvers warrant extreme caution given the risk of injury to the deep neurovascular structures. The anterior jugular veins and perforating branches of the submental vascular plexus lie deep to the platysma, near its midline. If violated, they may be difficult to control, particularly with limited exposure and visualization. The marginal mandibular branch of the facial nerve is also at risk when liposuction is directed over the mandible. The marginal mandibular nerve courses inferiorly, anterior to the angle of the mandible, 1 to 2 cm below the inferior margin of the mandible into the submandibular triangle. The nerve then ascends over the mandible to innervate the depressor muscles of the mouth 2 cm lateral to the oral commissure. Although the marginal mandibular nerve lies under the cover of the platysma, some patients may have attenuated muscle fibers; aggressive suctioning for jowls and mandibular contouring may place this nerve at risk of inadvertent injury.

In 1980, Ellenbogen described five visual criteria that create the appearance of a youthful neck.[17] These criteria are (1) a distinct mandibular border without jowl overhang, (2) a subhyoid depression, which gives the appearance of a long and thin neck, (3) a visible thyroid cartilage contour, (4) a visible anterior border of the sternocleidomastoid muscle, and (5) a cervicomental angle measuring between 105 and 120 degrees (Fig. 14-3). These criteria were

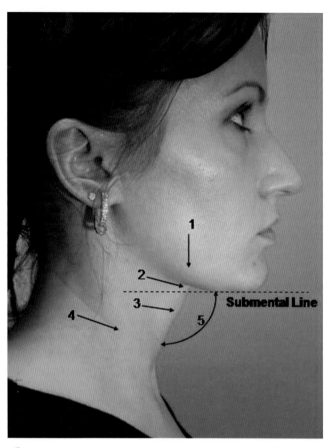

Figure 14-3 Five visual criteria for a youthful neck as described by Ellenbogen: distinct mandibular line (*1*), subhyoid depression (*2*), thyroid cartilage bulge (*3*), anterior border of the sternocleidomastoid muscle (*4*), and a cervicomental angle between 105 and 120 degrees (*5*). (From Ellenbogen R, Karlin JV: Visual criteria for success in restoring the youthful neck. Plast Reconstr Surg 1980; 66(6):826-837.)

initially used to assess the results of platysma cervical lifts, but they are also applicable in the more global assessment of the neck. Not all of these criteria may be attainable with liposuction, but they serve as useful guidelines for the goals of surgical treatment.

PREOPERATIVE ASSESSMENT

As with any cosmetic procedure, success depends on patient selection and careful preoperative evaluation. At the first consultation, the surgeon should investigate the patient's motivation for surgery and expectations regarding its outcomes. Patients who believe that a change in their appearance will dramatically alter their personal or professional lives are bound for disappointment. The psychological profiles of these patients make them poor candidates for surgical intervention. It is imperative that the surgeon and patient be in accord regarding the goals of treatment.

A full medical history should also be assessed to evaluate the appropriateness of surgical intervention and

to identify risk factors for suboptimal results. Comorbidities such as hypertension, coagulopathies, diabetes, and smoking may complicate healing in the postoperative period. Patients with significant weight gain are not good candidates for local liposuction, as it is not a cure for overall obesity. However, liposuction is effective for patients who are plagued with unwanted local deposits of fat, which may be a result of hereditary predisposition, poor dietary and exercise habits, age, medications, hormones, or weight gain. Even when weight loss regimens are implemented, facial areas such as the submental region are difficult to change. Though exercise programs help to tone muscles throughout the body, it is difficult to strengthen muscles of the face and neck; in addition, toned muscles do not necessarily reduce the amount of superficial adipose tissue. Hereditary predispositions of local fat accumulations are especially difficult to address. Although the mechanism of adipocyte hyperplasia is unknown, it has been previously assumed that a stable number of adipocyte cells existed after puberty. Newer evidence suggests that new adipocytes may be formed with excessive weight gain to store excess lipids.[18] Although most weight gain is handled by the enlargement of existing adipocytes, excessive gain strains adipocytes to a critical mass and stimulates the formation of new fat cells.[19] With diet and weight loss, lipid content of cells may be reduced, but the number of adipocyte cells remains constant.[20] Liposuction is the only medical approach known to decrease the number of adipocytes.

A critical anatomic and aesthetic evaluation is essential for proper patient selection. A systematic approach will prevent the surgeon from overlooking any critical anatomic features and from making an erroneous assessment of the locus of concern. Evaluation should start with an assessment of the patient's overall body habitus. Patients of short and stocky stature with wide necks will not achieve a thin, contoured neck even with significant liposuction (Fig. 14-4).

The surgeon must then assess the following:

1. **Skin condition.** Skin should be evaluated for flexibility, elasticity, firmness, and adherence to the underlying tissues, all of which play a critical role in predicting outcomes.[21,22] Skin with elastic integrity will more effectively redrape over the underlying liposuctioned contour. Dedo suggested that skin contractility may be suboptimal in patients older than 40 years old and Gryskiewicz found that a crepe paper appearance of the skin was the best preoperative predictor of failure from isolated liposuction without rhytidectomy.[2,22]

2. **Amount and location of fat.** The surgeon should assess the location and amount of fat by palpation. This is best accomplished with the pinch and roll technique.[2,3] The skin should be palpated or rolled between two fingers to determine the thickness of the skin and fat. In the cervical region, the presence

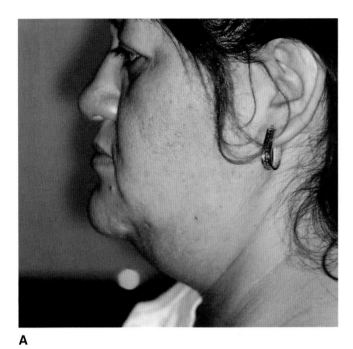

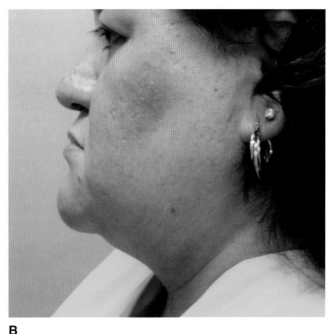

A   **B**

Figure 14-4 Preoperative lateral view of a 42-year-old woman with a short, wide neck, low-lying hyoid bone, and thick, heavy skin (**A**). She has excess adipose tissue in her central neck with significant blunting of the cervicomental angle. Postoperative view at 6 months following liposuction through submental and infra-auricular incisions (**B**). Although the patient has some improvement in her neck, her intrinsic neck anatomy, skin texture, and the presence of substantial subplatysmal fat prevent an optimal result from liposuction alone

of preplatysmal fat should be differentiated from subplatysmal fat. With palpation, subplatysmal fat is generally firmer owing to its connective tissue and fibrous content.[2]

3. **Integrity of the platysma.** The surgeon should evaluate the thickness and laxity of the platysma. The presence of platysmal bands at rest indicate that some form of platysmaplaty should be performed for proper rejuvenation of the neck.[3,8] Furthermore, cervical liposuction may expose occult bands.[23] This may be assessed by having patients strain their neck with their teeth clenched while making a grimace; with this provocative test, platysmal bands due to laxity of the muscular anterior borders may be revealed.

4. **Condition of the surrounding skeletal framework.** Deficiencies in the surrounding skeletal framework of the cervicofacial region may significantly affect the results of liposuction. Both Dedo and Kamer devised classification systems evaluating cervical abnormalities to guide preoperative evaluation and selection of the most appropriate surgical option.[22,24] Dedo proposed that patients with either a short mandible-to-hyoid distance or low-lying hyoid have an obtuse cervicomental angle, limiting the effects of submental surgery (Fig. 14-5). Correct projection of the mentum will give the impression of an acute cervicomental angle. To better assess this, the surgeon may drop a plumb-line

down from the lower lip. In women, the mentum should be at or slightly behind this line when viewed from the lateral aspect. In men, the mentum should be on or slightly anterior to this line.

5. **Prominence of surrounding soft tissue structures.** The surgeon should assess for ptotic submandibular or large parotid glands. Liposuction in the submandibular region may enhance the appearance of the submandibular glands.[2,23] Similarly, liposuction of cheek fat may enhance the anterior border of an enlarged parotid gland. Furthermore, patients with heavy masseter musculature may not benefit from facial liposuction.

After a thorough physical evaluation has been performed, the surgeon determines if a patient is an appropriate candidate for isolated liposuction. The ideal patient for isolated liposuction has good skin elasticity, is of stable and average weight, and has a localized adipose collection out of proportion to the rest of the body.

Some patients are not good candidates for isolated liposuction and would benefit from adjunctive procedures. Without offending patient sensibilities, the surgeon must recommend the procedure(s) likely to provide the most benefit. Obviously, the surgeon should make recommendations in light of the patient's area of concern. For example, augmentation mentoplasty is a wonderful adjunct to cervical liposuction in creating the appearance of an acute cervicomental angle. However, most patients

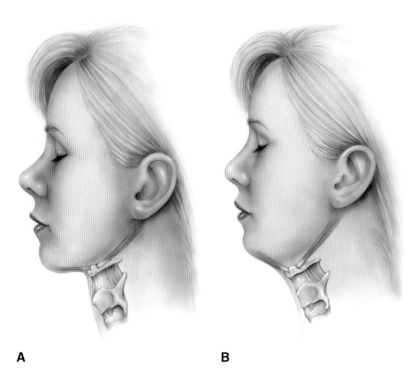

Figure 14-5 The hyoid bone should ideally rest cephalad and posterior to the mentum for a youthful neckline (**A**). A low-lying anterior hyoid bone limits the results of submental liposuction and cervical rejuvenation (**B**).

A   **B**

do not seek consultation with a surgeon for a chin implant; rather, they ask for improvement in their neck contour, and it is only when the advantage of an implant is pointed out that patients realize the benefits. Older patients need to be counseled that liposuction alone will not improve the appearance of aging skin or facial wrinkles. These patients may benefit from other rejuvenative procedures such as rhytidectomy or skin resurfacing.

Preoperative clinical photographs and documentation are essential. Frontal, oblique, and lateral views should be taken in the Frankfurt plane against a solid background. Photographs are critical for preoperative planning and equally important for documentation. Some patients may not fully appreciate the postsurgical results until they are reminded of their preoperative appearance. Computer imaging may also be useful during initial consultation and preoperative assessment. It allows the surgeon to communicate through a tangible medium and illustrate the benefits of adjunctive procedures such as augmentation mentoplasty. Furthermore, computer imaging may confirm that the patient's vision of the postoperative result coincides with that of the surgeon. In all things, it is the responsibility of the surgeon to use computer imaging in a judicious and forthcoming manner.

At the conclusion of the consultation, the surgeon offers his or her opinion on the aesthetic procedure(s) that would best address the patient's area of concern. The surgeon then counsels the patient on realistic outcomes to prevent postsurgical disappointment and provides a detailed review of the expected postoperative course to allay apprehension and anxiety. Such communication and open dialogue will facilitate a smooth perioperative course.

SURGICAL TECHNIQUE

The goals of facial suction lipectomy are to remove unwanted deposits of fat and to create a smooth contour. Although these goals seem straightforward, several technical nuances need to be appreciated to avoid complications and to provide optimal surgical results. Although the techniques are similar to those used in body contouring, the surgeon needs to be cognizant of the anatomic and aesthetic considerations specific to the facial region. The thin nature of facial skin and the close proximity of the marginal mandibular nerve leave little room for error in the aggressive reduction of fat. With meticulous attention to technique and adherence to the fundamental principles mentioned previously, facial liposuction may achieve successful results with a low rate of morbidity.

EQUIPMENT

A reliable aspiration device is inherent to successful liposuction. Multiple suction devices are commercially available, but the most effective and efficient machines share several characteristic features. Although perfect vacuums (1 atm, 760 mm Hg, 29.92 inches Hg) are difficult to achieve in the clinical setting, suction devices that are able to achieve vacuums close to 29 inches Hg are the most desirable. Low noise output (<55 DbA scale) and high flow rate (>100 L/min) are also desired features.[21] In the cervicofacial region, vacuum pressures of 22 to 23 inches Hg are usually adequate for smooth and continuous suction. The surgeon should check the suction pressure prior to the start of any procedure to ensure that the pressure is within the desired range.

Handheld syringe liposuction, popularized by Fournier, is also a safe and efficient alternative to suction pump fat removal.[15] Fournier believed this method minimized blood loss and provided the surgeon with accurate measurements of the amount of fat removed. Furthermore, the potential for cross-contamination is eliminated because a common suction device is not employed. Syringe liposuction is also an excellent backup should there be mechanical or electrical problems with a suction pump.

Other features of suction devices that facilitate ease of use include operator control of the vacuum pressure, whether by foot switch or finger-controlled release. This allows the surgeon to prevent unintentional removal of fat as the cannula is withdrawn. Current suction models also have filters between the disposable canister and pump to prevent biohazardous contamination.

In addition to a reliable suction source, appropriate cannulas should be chosen. An abundance of cannulas are currently available (Fig. 14-6). The surgeon will typically become familiar with three or four cannulas that he or she will use routinely, depending on the location and phase of liposuction (e.g., active fat removal, sculpting, or feathering). In the cervicofacial region, most frequently used cannulas range in size from 1 mm (microcannulas) to 6 mm in diameter. Larger cannulas have the capacity to remove greater volumes of fat and are appropriate for areas such as the submental triangle. However, microcannulas are useful for fine sculpting and contouring, particularly in areas near vital neurovascular structures, such as the marginal mandibular nerve. Microcannulas are frequently used to contour the jowls, cheeks, and nasolabial folds.

Cannulas with blunt tips are preferable in the cervicofacial region. Blunt cannulas have openings located a few millimeters away from the tip and are gentler on the tissues than those designed with end openings. Cannulas with the opening at the tip may act as a shaver when passed over tissue and may function more as a curette than a gentle suction device. The spatula-shaped tip is useful for undermining skin flaps in the preplatysmal and

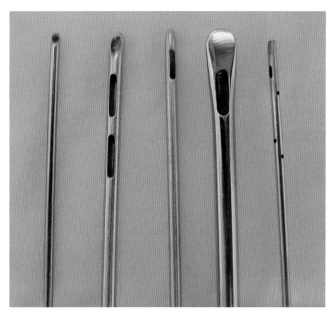

Figure 14-7 Aspiration cannulas with different tip shapes, aperture sizes, and numbers allow versatility in their function and in the areas to receive suction lipectomy. The cannula on the far right is suitable for infiltration whereas the spatula tip cannula (second from right) is useful on the adipose tissue overlying the parotid and buccal regions. The cannula on the far left has its opening at the tip of the cannula rather than the side which allows it to remove fat through a shaving mechanism.

preparotid fat, as their shape allows the surgeon to stay superficial to the platysma and parotid fasciae. The flat shape also creates a better seal on the tissue. However, these cannulas may become easily obstructed.

Cannulas are manufactured with varying numbers of apertures (Fig. 14-7). Those with more openings allow fat to be suctioned more rapidly. We prefer a cannula with a single suction aperture for active fat removal, though multiple apertures are useful on the microcannulas to facilitate fat removal through a smaller diameter lumen. There are also cannulas that may be attached to the handle via a Luer-Lok connection, which are more economical than those permanently attached to handles (Fig. 14-8). The Luer-Lok system also allows cannulas to be attached to aspiration syringes for syringe liposuction. Finally, Luer-Lok microcannulas may be attached to small syringes and are useful in autologous fat injection.

MARKINGS

It is prudent in the preoperative holding area to mark the patient while in the upright position, as the soft tissue contours may become distorted when the patient lies supine. Important anatomic structures, such as the inferior border of the mandible, anterior and posterior borders of the sternocleidomastoid muscle, superior border of the thyroid cartilage, course of the marginal mandibular nerve, and external jugular veins, are marked

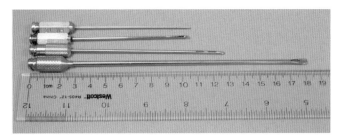

Figure 14-6 Liposuction cannulas are available in a variety of lengths, diameters, and tip specifications.

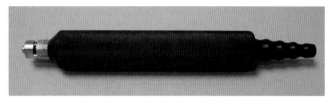

A

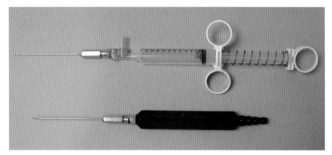

B

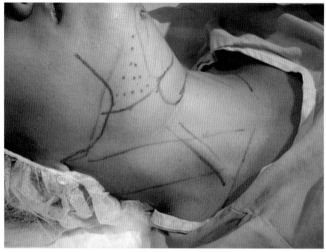

A

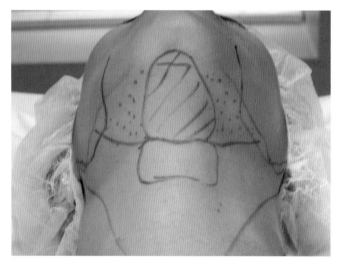

B

Figure 14-8 The Luer-Lok mechanism allows an interchangeable system whereby various aspiration cannulas may be used with a single handle. With a typical Luer-Lok handle (**A**), the cannulas attach at one end (*left*) and the suction tubing at the other (*right*). The same Luer-Lok cannulas may be attached to a syringe for syringe liposuction (**B**).

(Fig. 14-9). Furthermore, submental fat, jowl pads, and other fat deposits are also marked. One approach utilized alternating cross-hatches to distinguish between the main areas to be treated versus the adjacent areas to be feathered. Markings for any planned adjunctive procedures may be placed at this time. Even with careful preoperative marking, tissues may become distorted on the operating table with changes in position, edema, and local infiltration; for this reason, it may be useful to have preoperative photographs available during the procedure.

ANESTHESIA

Several options for anesthesia are available, depending on physician and patient preference. Traditionally, facial plastic surgeons and plastic surgeons have been trained to perform surgical procedures in the operating room with general anesthesia or intravenous (IV) sedation. For isolated facial suction lipectomy, IV sedation usually suffices. When adjunctive procedures are performed, general anesthesia may be used. Local nerve blocks to the infraorbital, mental, and transverse cervical nerves may also be used to provide peri- and postoperative anesthesia.

Our dermatology colleagues have advanced the frontier of office-based procedures using local anesthetic techniques. In 1987, Klein introduced the tumescent technique, allowing the safe administration of larger doses of lidocaine.[25] The recommended maximum dose of lidocaine was 7 mg per kilogram of body weight when given with epinephrine. Klein showed that lidocaine could be safely given up to 35 mg/kg if diluted in large volumes of hypotonic

Figure 14-9 Preoperative markings on a three-quarters view of the important neurovascular structures (marginal mandibular nerve and external jugular vein) and landmarks (sternocleidomastoid muscle, mandibular border, and thyroid notch) (**A**). A system of different markings helps delineate areas of greatest fat accumulation (*diagonal lines*) and areas to be feathered (*stippling* in **B**).

fluid (Table 14-1), as decreasing the concentration of lidocaine resulted in slower peak plasma levels. Another advantage with tumescence is decreased blood loss.[26,27] The tissue bed is bathed in the tumescent fluid for at least 15 minutes, allowing prolonged vascular exposure to epinephrine.

For office-based liposuction with tumescence, patients may be given 1 mg of oral diazepam and 25 mg of intramuscular meperidine prior to the procedure. Proper monitoring is necessary if additional IV sedation is given. The entry site for the liposuction cannula is then infiltrated with 1% lidocaine mixed with 1:100,000 epinephrine, and a microcannula used for infiltration is placed through a small incision. The microcannula is sub-

Table 14-1   Klein's Tumescent Formula for Liposuction*

Component	Amount
Lidocaine	50 mL of 1% lidocaine solution (500 mg)
Epinephrine	1 mL of 1:1000 solution of epinephrine solution (1 mg)
Sodium bicarbonate	12.5 mL of 8.4% NaH_2CO_3 solution
Normal saline	1 L of 0.9% NaCl solution

*For cervical liposuction, a 500 mL bag of normal saline suffices. The amount of the components must be adjusted accordingly.
From Klein JA: Tumescent technique for liposuction surgery. Am J Cosmet Surg 1987;4:263-267.

sequently connected to an IV bag containing the tumescent fluid (Fig. 14-10). In this fashion, the micro-cannula may be used to simultaneously create tunnels in the adipose tissue and deliver the tumescent fluid. Once the requisite 15 minutes has passed to allow for adequate vasoconstriction and anesthesia, liposuction may be performed.

Although tumescent anesthesia has a strong following among those with office-based practices, the authors prefer IV sedation for facial contouring. Tumescence offers a significant advantage when used for body contouring, as volumes up to 2000 mL of adipose tissue may be removed; however, typical volumes of fat removed in the cervicofacial region do not usually exceed 150 mL. Even though some proponents feel that tumescence facilitates dissection in the proper tissue planes, the authors find that the resultant tissue distortion makes assessment difficult and hinders precise facial contouring.

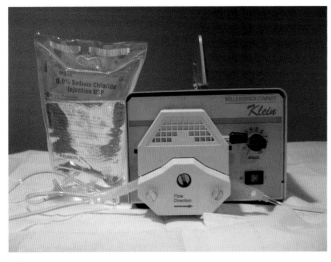

Figure 14-10 A model of a tumescent infusion pump with adjustable flow rates and a foot pedal (not shown), which allows the surgeon to control infiltration.

TECHNIQUE

Most areas of the face and neck can be accessed during primary liposuction through a combination of small incisions. The most common approaches are submental, pretragal, infralobular, postauricular, and intranasal. These incisions are well hidden and well tolerated by the patient. The choice of incisions depends on the site(s) to be treated.

Primary liposuction has been used to contour the submentum, lateral neck, jawline, melolabial folds, and midface. In our experience, the majority of patients who benefit from isolated liposuction seek improvement in the appearance of their necks. The ideal patient for submental liposuction is the younger patient with localized fat and resilient skin, devoid of platysmal pathology (Fig. 14-11). Optimal results depend as much on the ability of the skin to rebound and redrape as on the amount of fat that is removed.

The tunneling method initially developed by the Fischers is used by many facial plastic surgeons. Although the authors do not routinely utilize the tunneling technique in the submental region, it does incorporate fundamental techniques applicable in many parts of the face and neck. This technique is useful in areas of minimal fat where skin flap elevation would not be beneficial (e.g., the melolabial folds, facial lipomas). The tunneling technique for the submental region is outlined here.

Submental liposuction begins with an incision that is made 1 mm posterior to the submental crease. Proper incision placement is essential to prevent deepening of this crease with subsequent scar contracture, a deformity that is likened to a "witch's chin." The incision is typically 1 cm in length to accommodate a 4- to 6-mm cannula. The incision should be large enough to accommodate the cannula with additional space to prevent friction burn on the wound edges from the back-and-forth motion of the cannula. The incision is carried through the skin and subcutaneous adipose tissue, and 1 to 2 cm of the surrounding skin is elevated sharply using small Iris or tenotomy scissors. This creates a tissue pocket, which facilitates placement of the cannula tip in the appropriate subdermal plane. The cannula is then introduced with the aperture directed toward the adipose tissue and away from the skin flap. During cannula insertion, the suction should be off to prevent inadvertent injury to the adjacent skin.

Once the cannula tip has been safely introduced beneath the skin, interconnecting tunnels are created radially from the mentum to the anterior borders of the sternocleidomastoid muscle laterally and the thyroid notch inferiorly, similar to spokes radiating from the center of a bicycle wheel (Fig. 14-12). Some surgeons advocate pretunneling without suction to facilitate dissection in the proper plane. After the tunnels are created in the region of the planned liposuction, suction is

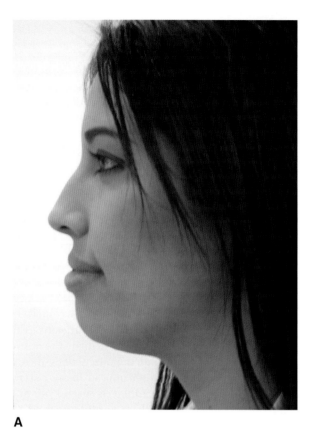

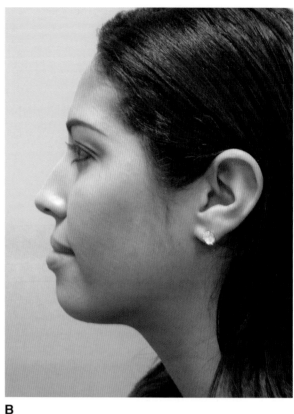

A   B

Figure 14-11 An ideal candidate for isolated submental liposuction with localized fat and resilient, elastic skin (**A**). Notable improvement could be seen in her neck contour, 6 months following submental liposuction (**B**).

applied and multiple passes are re-executed in the same spoke-like fashion. The right-handed surgeon should control the cannula with the right hand while the left hand constantly folds the skin over the cannula. This maneuver will help to assess the depth of the cannula tip as well as the thickness of the adipose layer. Throughout the procedure, the surgeon pauses and palpates the neck and target areas to ensure a smooth, even contour. Bulges and irregularities indicate uneven liposuction; dimpling connotes tethering of the septal attachments, which should be released. As the submentum lies in the center of the "spokes," care should be taken to ensure even aspiration. Hollowing and a submental depression may occur if too much liposuction is performed in this region. The tunnels created by this method allow the superficial tissues to compress into the newly created dead space.

Another proposed advantage of this technique is the preservation of septal attachments from the subcutaneous tissue to the dermis above. These septa contain blood vessels and nerves, and their preservation ensures continued vascular and nervous supply to the skin.[28] Furthermore, these attachments are believed to aid in the contracture of overlying skin.

Although many surgeons espouse the tunneling technique, contracture of the septal attachments between the tunnels may result in dimpling and skin irregularities.

The authors currently use the layer technique for the submental region to minimize the possibility of uneven skin contours.[29] The initial steps are identical to those outlined previously. Once the area around the submental incision is dissected in the proper plane, wide double-hook retractors are used to retract the superior and inferior skin flaps for proper tensioning. The right-handed surgeon typically stands at the head of the bed and holds the inferior retractor with the left hand. The assistant stands on the right side of the bed while holding the inferior retractor. Rather than creating dry tunnels with a cannula, the surgeon widely undermines the submental region to the anatomic borders mentioned above with Metzenbaum scissors (Fig. 14-13). Undermining should not proceed over the mandible in efforts to prevent injury to the marginal mandibular nerve. At least 3 to 4 mm of adipose tissue should be left on the underside of the skin flap to prevent an uneven contour and to preserve the skin's vascularity. Wide undermining also allows excellent redraping of skin without tethering from septal attachments and the consequent skin irregularities. The authors have not had any problems with long-term dysesthesias or vascular compromise of skin flaps in their patients.

Once the skin flaps have been widely elevated, the liposuction cannula is passed evenly across the expanse of

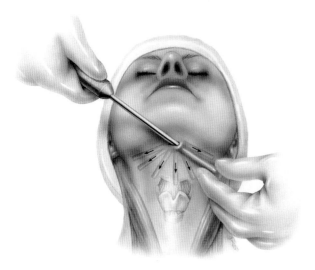

A

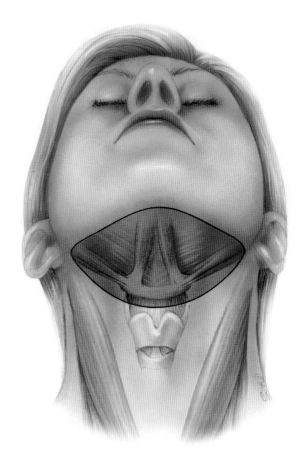

Figure 14-12 Submental liposuction is performed in a systematic fashion from a submental incision (**A** and **B**). The submentum serves as a fulcrum from which the cannula is advanced in a radial fashion, like the spokes of a wheel, to the anterior borders of the sternocleidomastoid muscle laterally, and the thyroid notch inferiorly. Caution must be exercised not to advance the tip of the cannula deep to the platysma muscle to prevent inadvertent injury to the deep structures of the neck.

B

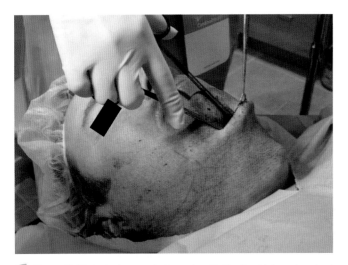

Figure 14-13 In the layer technique, the skin flap is widely undermined with Metzenbaum scissors across the submental region to just inferior (1 to 2 cm) to the jawline. Dissection is carried in a subcutaneous plane to the anterior borders of the sternocleidomastoid muscle and thyroid notch, with the tip of the scissors tenting the skin upward to prevent injury to the deeper structures of the neck. Sharp dissection should not be carried directly over the mandible to protect the marginal mandibular nerve. Placement of a double-hook at the incision provides counter-retraction on the skin flap.

tissue. The suction aperture should always face the deeper tissue, as aspiration of the skin flap may lead to dermal scarring. As in the tunneling technique, the surgeon uses the nondominant hand to fold the skin over the cannula tip, assessing the depth of adipose tissue (Fig. 14-14). To prevent a demarcation between the treated and untreated areas, undermining should extend beyond the aspiration site and feathering should be performed at the perimeters.

Although the authors do not advocate sharp lipectomy on a routine basis, direct excision may be used in select situations. Some patients have persistent midline adipose deposits even after suction lipectomy has been performed. These patients benefit from careful direct lipectomy, but direct excision may result in a submental depression if performed in an overly aggressive manner. The medial borders of the platysma may also be identified during direct lipectomy when a concomitant plastysmaplasty is planned.

Even after broad liposuction and direct excision, some patients have persistent submental fullness due to subplatysmal fat. Although suction lipectomy has been performed for subplatysmal fat, the authors do not routinely advocate this practice, as the subplatysmal plane is replete with submental vessels and the risk of bleeding is significant. Bleeding in the subplatysmal plane may be brisk and obtaining control of the bleeding with limited

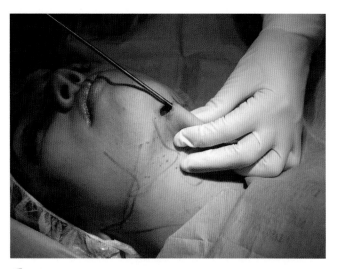

Figure 14-14 The surgeon drapes the skin over the cannula aperture with his or her nondominant hand to guide the passage of the cannula as well as to constantly assess the depth of adipose tissue. The cannula aperture should be directed away from the skin flap to prevent dermal scarring and contour irregularities. The cannula tip also helps tent the skin flap to prevent inadvertent injury to deeper structures.

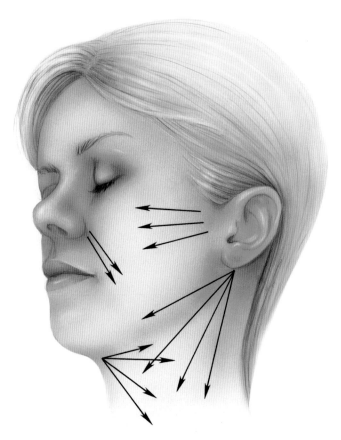

Figure 14-15 Cervicofacial liposuction may be achieved through a limited number of incisions. The submental incision allows excellent access to the central neck. The lateral neck and jowls may be approached from the infra- or retroauricular incisions, and the preauricular incision allows liposuction over the parotid bed and midface region. An incision in the nasal vestibule or nasolabial groove is used for the melolabial folds.

exposure and visualization using electrocautery places the marginal mandibular nerve at risk.

The jowls, lateral neck, and submandibular regions may be approached from postauricular or infralobular incisions (Fig. 14-15). The jowl is an unforgiving area for contour irregularities. When contouring the jowl, the cannula may extend to the oral commissure anteriorly and the margin of the mandible inferiorly. Thus, smaller cannulas (1 to 2 mm) are useful for delicate sculpting and creating a smooth transition with nonaspirated regions. Suction should be released upon withdrawal from the jowl to prevent inadvertent aspiration of tissue in the posterior facial tissue and creation of an unsightly divot. If a small volume of fat is to be removed, occasional release of the vacuum allows the fat to reach the collection canister. In this way, the surgeon may accurately assess the amount of fat that has been removed. The postauricular or infralobular incisions also provide excellent access to the submandibular area and allow overlap with the areas aspirated via the submental approach.

The prominent melolabial fold continues to be a challenge. Liposuction can be used to contour this region and begins with a small incision placed in the nasal vestibule. An incision may also be made in the nasolabial groove but risks a visible scar. A 1-mm cannula is placed through the incision, and tunnels are created in an arc-like fashion from the prominence of the fold to the antral fat. The authors do not routinely treat the melolabial folds primarily with liposuction, as the results are variable and often transient.[30,31] However, when performed to complement another procedure, such as rhytidectomy, liposuction of the melolabial fold may add to the overall improvement of the face.[32]

Lipocontouring alone may be inadequate for many patients seeking rejuvenation of the neck. Liposuction will not benefit patients with lax skin or platysmal banding. Liposuction is frequently combined with platysmaplasty for neck recontouring in these cases. The platysmaplasty may be performed after liposuction is completed, allowing the surgeon visualization of the platysma. Using a headlight and a converse retractor, the surgeon may evaluate the integrity of the platysma. The medial edges are lifted with forceps. If laxity exists, the medial strip of platysma is sharply resected. If there is wide separation between the medial edges, a long fine-pronged hemostat is used to undermine the platysmal edges to facilitate subsequent closure. Again, caution is exercised any time dissection is carried deep to the platysmal layer to prevent injury to the submental vascular plexus. Furthermore, any dissection or resection of muscle will increase the likelihood of bleeding. A long-handled bipolar forceps and suction should be available to obtain hemostasis. Backcuts are made on the platysma at the level of the cervicomental angle to decrease blunting of the angle from realignment of the medial edges of the platysma muscle. The medial edges of the exposed platysma muscle are reapproximated with a running 4-0 polydioxanone suture (PDS, Ethicon, Somerville, NJ; Maxon, US Surgical/Davis and Geck, Norwalk, CT) starting at the point superior to the back cuts. The incision is closed with a 6-0 polypropylene suture, placed in a running, interlocked fashion. Some have advocated the use of synthetic fibrin sealant on the superficial layer of the platysmal muscle followed by pressure for 5 minutes to aid with hemostasis and adhesion of the skin flap to underlying muscle.[3]

Concomitant chin augmentation may significantly enhance the results of submental liposuction in some patients (Fig. 14-16). The chin implant places anterior stretch on the cervical skin, creating a tighter cervicomental angle. In the preoperative assessment, patients with microgenia should be identified, and the benefits of a chin implant discussed. The chin implant should be placed after submental liposuction has been completed to accurately assess the projection of the implant. Implantation may be performed using the same submental incision described above. Some patients with microgenia may also have an occlusal deformity, most commonly a class II occlusion. The addition of a chin implant will not correct an occlusal mismatch, and this should be discussed with the patient preoperatively.

Liposuction may be combined with rhytidectomy to optimize aesthetic results (Fig. 14-17). This combination effectively removes undesirable collections of fat, highlights natural angles and contours of the face and neck, and removes redundant skin. Submental liposuction and platysmaplasty are such integral components of lower facial rejuvenation that they are practically considered part of complete rhytidectomy.[33] Submental liposuction and platysmaplasty usually precedes rhytidectomy. Even in lean necks that do not require submental liposuction, undermining of cervical skin promotes favorable skin contracture.[33] After liposuction, direct assessment and treatment of the platysma is possible. Plastysmaplasty only enhances neck contour when combined with posterior pull of the SMAS. Obviously, if a patient presents for a short-flap facelift (S-lift) for minimal jowl formation, submental liposuction and platysmaplasty are not indicated. After the submental incision is closed, attention is turned to the rhytidectomy.

The authors begin with a standard rhytidectomy incision. Skin flaps are elevated and facial liposuction is performed after SMAS plication. Other types of rhytidectomy (e.g., SMAS imbrication, deep-plane rhytidectomy) may be performed, depending on surgeon preference, and these techniques are further discussed in other chapters in this textbook. A 4-mm spatula-tip cannula may be used to aspirate fat from the pretragal region, jowl, and midface under direct vision (Fig. 14-18). In this manner, "cross-hatching" may be performed evenly to prevent overtreatment of any one area. A small 1-mm cannula is used for fine contouring over the jowl. Through the rhytidectomy incision, the lateral neck and the submandibular region may also be aspirated. This provides overlap with the central neck areas treated from the submental incision and promotes a smooth, overall contour. A "cobra" deformity, which may arise if the central neck receives aggressive liposuction, may thus be avoided.

The importance of a proper postoperative dressing cannot be overstated. A pressure dressing assists in decreasing edema, reducing the risk of hematoma formation, and allowing the skin to adhere to the underlying musculature. Equally important, a pressure dressing aids in the proper draping of the skin. A host of dressings are commercially available. Whichever is selected, it should be adjustable and comfortable (Fig. 14-19). Foam padding may also be used beneath the dressing to apply evenly distributed pressure on the surgical site. The pressure dressing is worn continuously for 1 week, followed by 2 to 4 weeks of additional nighttime wear.

Recently, there has been interest in applying ultrasound technology to techniques of liposuction.[5,34,35] Based upon the physics of sound transmission, ultrasonic energy may be targeted to specific tissues according to differences in tissue density. Denser tissues, such as tendons, ligaments, and skin, contain more collagen and elastin and are resistant to fragmentation when subjected to ultrasound treatment. Conversely, ultrasonic energy is more readily absorbed by less dense parenchymal tissues, such as adipose.[36] This results in both micromechanical disruption and cavitation of adipose tissue. In micromechanical disruption, ultrasonic waves affect intracellular components, leading to progressive structural rearrangements and ultimately cell death. Cavitation refers to the effect of the oscillatory activity of vapor-filled bubbles or microneuclei within cells. Ultrasound causes micronuclei to expand until a critical size is reached, at which time they implode, causing cell membrane disruption and diffusion of fatty acids into the extracellular matrix. Of these two phenomena, cavitation results in more significant tissue destruction, which results in easier fatty aspiration. Clinically, ultrasonic energy may be delivered internally through a cannula or by external application. Studies have found little benefit of external ultrasonic liposuction (XUAL) over traditional liposuction techniques.[37,38] Conversely, the advantage of internal ultrasound-assisted liposuction is well documented in areas of high fibrous content.[34,39,40] Although UAL confers an advantage for body contouring in areas of high fibrous content and larger volumes of fat, these are not usually concerns in the cervicofacial region.

Proponents of UAL assert that that this technology offers additional advantages in the cervicofacial region. Ultrasonic energy stimulates an inflammatory response in the skin, causing it to retract. Some believe that this retraction is greater than that achieved with traditional

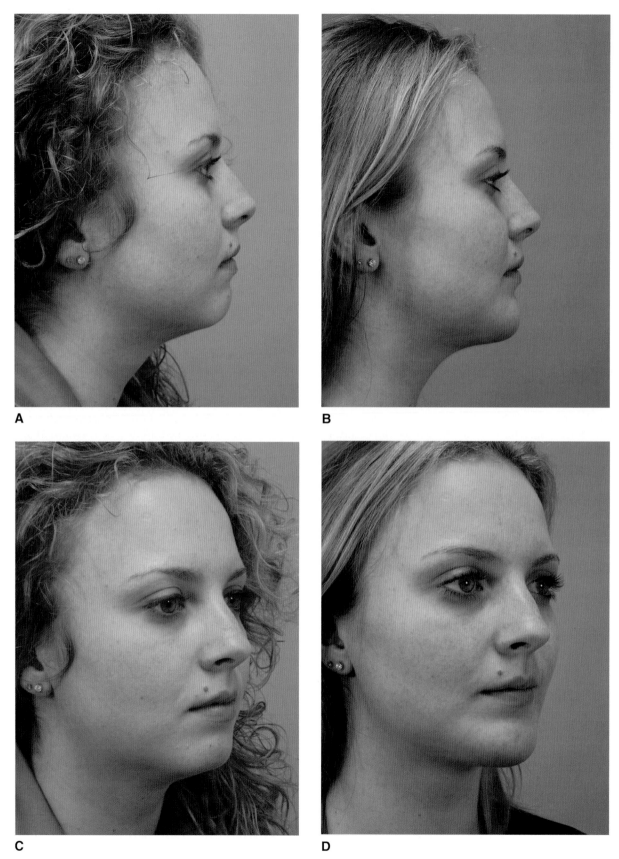

A

B

C

D

Figure 14-16 Preoperative (**A**) and 6-month postoperative (**B**) lateral and preoperative (**C**) and 6-month postoperative (**D**) oblique views of a 25-year-old patient with submental fullness, microgenia, and elastic skin who underwent submental liposuction and Gore-Tex chin augmentation. The chin implant serves as an excellent adjunct to submental liposuction by placing anterior stretch on the skin, resulting in a tighter cervicomental angle.

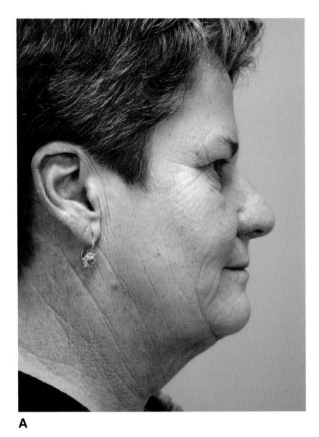

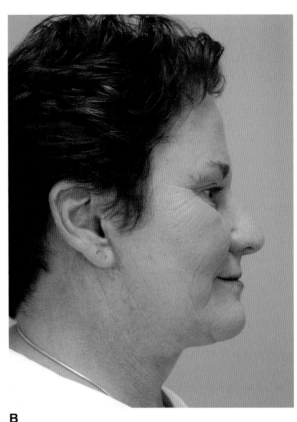

A   **B**

Figure 14-17   Preoperative lateral view (**A**) of a 64-year-old patient who was primarily concerned with the appearance of her neck. Submental liposuction alone would not significantly improve the cervicomental angle given the laxity and inelasticity of her skin. Postoperative lateral view (**B**) at 4 months following submental liposuction, rhytidectomy, and endoscopic brow/midface lift with notable improvement in her cervicomental angle.

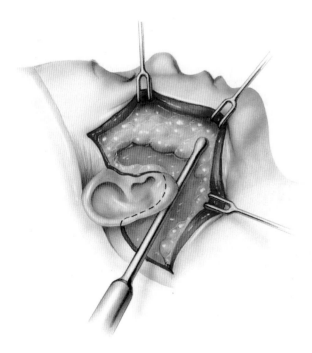

Figure 14-18   Liposuction over the parotid bed, jowls, and midface region may be facilitated under direct vision through the facelift incision. The authors prefer to elevate the rhytidectomy skin flaps in the traditional manner with sharp dissection, followed by liposuction. However, pretunneling may be performed initially with or without suction to facilitate skin flap elevation.

liposuction.[5] Thus, ultrasound advocates believe that UAL may accomplish more than what can be achieved by suction lipectomy alone, particularly in patients with more advanced signs of aging. Furthermore, internal ultrasound is thought to remove superficial fat more readily and more evenly, as the probe approaches the subdermal fat internally and thus reduces the risk of avulsion. Ultrasonic energy delivered internally facilitates liposuction through the emulsification and evacuation of fat. Pretunneling is performed, followed by the introduction of the ultrasound probe. The surrounding fat is emulsified, and a suction cannula is used to evacuate the emulsified fat, which takes on the consistency of a creamy liquid. The end point is reached when resistance is encountered from the overlying skin collapsing down into the cannula.

Internal ultrasonography, however, poses several inherent dangers. Given the proximity of the probe to the overlying dermis, extreme caution is recommended to prevent thermal injury to the skin or neurovascular embarrassment.[41,42] The probe should be used with constant motion in a consistently moist environment. Although many studies have enumerated the dangers of thermal-related injuries from internal ultrasonography, no large controlled studies have been performed comparing the

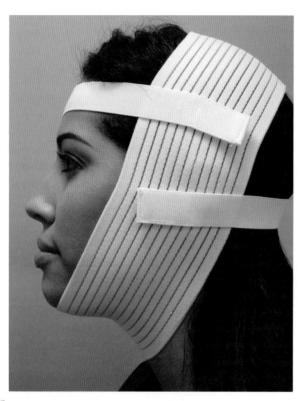

Figure 14-19 A large pressure dressing with cotton batting may be used on the first postoperative day following facial suction lipectomy, but a lighter pressure dressing as pictured above is worn continuously thereafter for 1 week, and then nightly for an additional 2 to 4 weeks to facilitate skin draping and to reduce postoperative swelling. This dressing is elastic, reusable, and adjustable with Velcro straps.

safety or efficacy of this technique to traditional suction lipectomy. As with the introduction of any new technology, the surgeon must develop appropriate experience and comfort to ensure comparable results and patient safety. Finally, the costs for new equipment and additional operative time should be taken into consideration.

The soft tissue shaving procedure has been introduced as another alternative to conventional liposuction. Soft tissue shaving, touted by some to be more precise and less traumatic, is based upon a completely different mechanism of soft tissue extraction. The liposhaver is thought to be less traumatic because it utilizes lower suction pressures and does not rely on the back-and-forth movements for fat extraction. Instead, current liposhavers utilize an oscillating cutting blade within a blunt cannula, which cuts tissue immediately adjacent to the blade and subsequently extracts it with low suction. The liposhaver may also be used as a conventional liposuction cannula with lower vacuum pressures. Soft tissue shavers have been used since the 1970s for removal of acoustic neuromas and have subsequently been employed for endonasal polypectomy and orthopedic arthroscopic surgery. In 1995, Gross and associates introduced liposhaving for facial plastic surgery.[43] Since then, the liposhaver has been utilized to remove fat from the submental region, beneath the facelift flap, and for the nasolabial folds via the submental, facelift, or intranasal incisions, respectively.[43-45] Multi-institutional studies have demonstrated that liposhaving contours fat evenly without dimpling or asymmetry.[44,45] These studies also established the safety profile of these techniques, with particular reference to facial nerve injury and postoperative hematoma formation. However, meticulous technique is critical, as the liposhaver can incise muscle and other soft tissues. The surgeons in the multi-institutional studies maintain that the light touch without firm pressure was critical in avoiding injury to the platysma. Most surgeons preferred the open approach with this device because of increased precision and safety.

POSTOPERATIVE CARE

Patients benefit from receiving a detailed description of their planned postoperative course prior to any procedure. Written information is helpful, and these instructions serve to minimize apprehension about their appearance and postoperative care. Patients are seen on the first postoperative day, when their pressure dressing is removed. The surgical site is inspected for hematoma, and the skin flaps are examined for proper redraping. If the skin flap is not properly redraped, gentle digital pressure and sweeping may serve to redirect the skin. Local wound care should be performed with the application of hydrogen peroxide and topical antibiotic ointment to the incisions. The pressure dressing is then reapplied, and patients are instructed to wear the compression garment continuously for 1 week. At 1 week, the submental sutures may be removed. The compression garment is then worn nightly for up to 4 additional weeks. Younger patients may require less time with the compression dressing, as youthful elastic skin will adhere and redrape more quickly than in older patients.

Patients should be counseled that postoperative edema may take months to resolve completely. Proper preoperative counseling will avoid confusion of typical postoperative swelling for failure to change the preoperative contour. Diligent use of the compression garment will hasten the resolution of edema. Ecchymosis and discoloration may also take up to 2 weeks to resolve. As postoperative swelling diminishes, subtle submental contour irregularities may appear; these typically soften and dissipate over time. Postoperative antibiotics are usually unnecessary unless a chin implant was placed. Postoperative discomfort is usually minimal.

COMPLICATIONS

Long-term experience with facial suction lipectomy has shown it to be a safe surgical modality with relatively few complications. Unlike whole-body liposuction, facial liposuction does not have the capacity to produce major fluid shifts typically seen with removal of large quantities of adipose tissue. Furthermore, even though bleeding can be brisk in the face and neck, blood loss is usually of negligible consequence and certainly much less than in body liposuction. Hematoma and seroma formation is rare (<1%) and may usually be evacuated by needle aspiration and pressure dressing.[46] A rapidly expanding hematoma, however, requires exploration and drainage in the operating room. Although primary infections occur in less than 1% cases, infections occurring in existing hematomas should be managed aggressively.[47] Fortunately, most reported cases of facial nerve neuropraxia are transient palsies arising from contusion or stretch injuries and resolve within a few weeks.[8,48] The marginal mandibular nerve is the most commonly affected, followed in frequency by the buccal branches of the facial nerve.

Other complications may result from overzealous liposuction. In the neck, aggressive liposuction may expose platysmal bands not previously apparent, creating a "cobra" deformity (Fig. 14-20). This may require platysmaplasty to correct. Conservative aspiration in the face will reduce the risk of "skeletonizaton," a phenomenon which may not be appreciated in the immediate postoperative period but which may become more pronounced with advancing age and subsequent loss of facial volume. When significant, the hollowed areas may be augmented with autologous fat injections. Misguided aspiration of the skin flap may result in dermal scarring with limited options for correction.

Contour irregularities and asymmetries may manifest once edema resolves. One study reported that 10% of patients were undertreated, necessitating touch-up treatments.[2] Touch-up liposuction may be performed in the office under local anesthesia with microcannulas. Corticosteroid injections may also be used to induce fat atrophy for subtle areas too small for microcannula aspiration. This technique should be used conservatively, with 1 to 3 mg triamcinolone acetate solution injected at 4- to 6-week intervals for 2 to 3 months. Overtreatment will result in dermal atrophy and depression as well as the formation of spider telangiectasias.

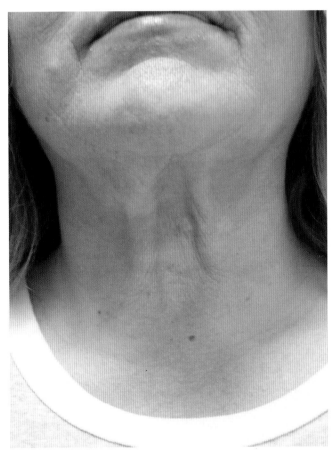

Figure 14-20 Platysmal bands were unmasked in this patient after aggressive liposuction and subdermal scarring is evident from poor technique of liposuction on the underside of the skin flap.

Future Considerations

Liposuction has experienced tremendous growth in popularity since the 1980s. It is now widely accepted as an effective and safe method of removing undesirable fat. In addition, though liposuction was initially developed for aesthetic purposes, its applications have expanded beyond the realm of cosmetic surgery. Liposuction has been used to remove lipomas[49] and to recontour bulky myocutaneous and cutaneous flaps via minimally invasive techniques.[50] Indeed, some have proposed using liposuction as a treatment for obesity-associated metabolic abnormalities, such as high plasma levels of glucose, insulin, and lipids; however, recent data show that reducing adipose tissue mass alone will not achieve the same metabolic benefits as weight loss.[51] Liposuction has also been advocated as a treatment for gynecomastia,[52] hyperhidrosis,[53] and upper extremity lymphedema for breast cancer patients following mastectomy and axillary node dissection.[54] Further research is needed to substantiate these and other proposed applications. Certainly the next decade will continue to see much change in the field of liposuction as has occurred since its introduction to the United States in 1982. The prospects for noncosmetic applications are exciting, though more clinical and basic science research needs to be done. It is our hope and expectation that with continued innovation, liposuction will increasingly improve the quality of life for our patients.

REFERENCES

1. American Society for Aesthetic Plastic Surgery Statistics, 2003, accessed at www.surgery.org.

2. Gryskiewicz JM: Submental suction-assisted lipectomy without platysmaplasty: Pushing the (skin) envelope to avoid a face lift for unsuitable candidates. Plast Reconstr Surg 2003;112(5):1393-1405; discussion 1406-1407.

3. Fattahi TT: Management of isolated neck deformity. Atlas Oral Maxillofac Surg Clin North Am 2004;12(2):261-270.

4. Guerrerosantos J: Liposuction in the cheek, chin, and neck: A clinical study. Facial Plast Surg 1986;4(1):25-34.

5. Grotting JC, Beckenstein MS: Cervicofacial rejuvenation using ultrasound-assisted lipectomy. Plast Reconstr Surg 2001;107(3):847-855.

6. Schaeffer BT: Endoscopic liposhaving for neck recontouring. Arch Facial Plast Surg 2000;2(4):264-268.

7. Goodstein WA: Superficial liposculpture of the face and neck. Plast Reconstr Surg 1996;98(6):988-996; discussion 997-998.

8. Knize DM: Limited incision submental lipectomy and platysmaplasty. Plast Reconstr Surg 2004;113(4):1275-1278.

9. Coleman WP: The history of dermatologic liposuction. Dermatol Clin 1990;8:381-383.

10. Schrudde J: Lipoexeresis as a means of eliminating local adiposity. International Society of Aesthetic Plastic Surgery. New York: Springer-Verlag, 1980;4:215-226.

11. Fischer A, Fischer G: First surgical treatment for molding body's cellulite with three 5 mm. incisions. Bull Int Acad Cosmet Surg 1976;3:35.

12. Fischer A, Fischer G: Revised techniques for cellulites fat reduction in riding breeches deformity. Bull Int Acad Cosmet Surg 1977;2:40.

13. Kesselring UK, Meyer R: A suction curette for removal of excessive local deposits of subcutaneous fat. Plast Reconstr Surg 1978;62(2):305-306.

14. Illouz YG: Body contouring by lipolysis: A 5-year experience with over 3000 cases. Plast Reconstr Surg 1983;72(5):591-597.

15. Fournier PF: Why the syringe and not the suction machine? J Dermatol Surg Oncol 1988;14(10):1062-1071.

16. Flynn TC, Coleman WP II, Field LM, et al: History of liposuction. Dermatol Surg 2000;26(6):515-520.

17. Ellenbogen R, Karlin JV: Visual criteria for success in restoring the youthful neck. Plast Reconstr Surg 1980;66(6):826-837.

18. Billings E Jr, May JW Jr: Historical review and present status of free fat graft autotransplantation in plastic and reconstructive surgery. Plast Reconstr Surg 1989;83(2):368-381.

19. Krotkiewski M, Bjorntorp P, Sjostrom L, et al: Impact of obesity on metabolism in men and women. Importance of regional adipose tissue distribution. J Clin Invest 1983;72(3):1150-1162.

20. Vasselli JR, Cleary MP, Van Itallie TB: Modern concepts of obesity. Nutr Rev 1983;41(12):361-373.

21. Hetter GP: Improved results with closed facial suction. Clin Plast Surg 1989;16(2):319-332.

22. Dedo DD: Management of the platysma muscle after open and closed liposuction of the neck in facelift surgery. Facial Plast Surg 1986;4(1):45-56.

23. Morrison W, Salisbury M, Beckham P, et al: The minimal facelift: Liposuction of the neck and jowls. Aesthet Plast Surg 2001;25(2):949-9.

24. Kamer FM, Lefkoff LA: Submental surgery. A graduated approach to the aging neck. Arch Otolaryngol Head Neck Surg 1991;117(1):40-46.

25. Klein JA: The tumescent technique for liposuction surgery. Am J Cosmet Surg 1987;4:263-267.

26. Klein JA: Tumescent technique for regional anesthesia permits lidocaine doses of 35 mg/kg for liposuction. J Dermatol Surg Oncol 1990;16(3):248-263.

27. Klein JA: The tumescent technique. Anesthesia and modified liposuction technique. Dermatol Clin 1990;8(3):425-437.

28. Teimourian B, Kroll SS: Subcutaneous endoscopy in suction lipectomy. Plast Reconstr Surg 1984;74(5):708-711.

29. Kesselring UK: Facial liposuction. Facial Plast Surg 1986;4(1):1-4.

30. Velazquez JM: Improving the labial commissurae and paralabial folds with minimally invasive procedures: A useful method for midfacial rejuvenation. Aesthet Plast Surg 2004;28(2):100-107.

31. Guyuron B, Michelow B: The nasolabial fold: A challenge, a solution. Plast Reconstr Surg 1994;93(3):522-529; discussion 530-532.

32. McKinney P, Cook JQ: Liposuction and the treatment of nasolabial folds. Aesthet Plast Surg 1989;13(3):167-171.

33. Williams EF, Lam SM: Comprehensive facial rejuvenation. Philadelphia: Lippincott Williams & Wilkins, 2004.

34. Omranifard M: Ultrasonic liposuction versus surgical lipectomy. Aesthet Plast Surg 2003;27(2):143-145.

35. Graf R, Auersvald A, Damasio RC, et al: Ultrasound-assisted liposuction: An analysis of 348 cases. Aesthet Plast Surg 2003;27(2):146-153.

36. Lawrence N, Coleman WP 3rd: The biologic basis of ultrasonic liposuction. Dermatol Surg 1997;23(12):1197-1200.

37. Lawrence N, Cox SE: The efficacy of external ultrasound-assisted liposuction: A randomized controlled trial. Dermtatol Surg 2000;26(4):329-332.

38. Cardenas-Camarena L, Cardenas A, Fajardo-Barajas D: Clinical and histopathological analysis of tissue retraction in tumescent liposuction assisted by external ultrasound. Ann Plast Surg 2001;46(3):287-292

39. Cardenas-Camarena L, Andino-Ulloa R, Mora RC, et al: Laboratory and histopathologic comparative study of internal ultrasound-assisted lipoplasty and tumescent lipoplasty. Plast Reconstr Surg 2002;110(4):1158-1164; discussion 1165-1166.

40. Rohrich RJ, Morales DE, Krueger JE, et al: Comparative lipoplasty analysis of in vivo-treated adipose tissue. Plast Reconstr Surg 2000;105(6):2152-2158; discussion 2159-2160.

41. Igra H, Satur NM: Tumescent liposuction versus internal ultrasonic-assisted tumescent liposuction. A side-to-side comparison. Dermatol Surg 1997;23(12):1213-1218.

42. Howard BK, Beran SJ, Kenkel JM, et al: The effects of ultrasonic energy on peripheral nerves: Implications for ultrasound-assisted liposuction. Plast Reconstr Surg 1999;103(3):984-989.

43. Gross CW, Becker DG, Lindsey WH, et al: The soft-tissue shaving procedure for removal of adipose tissue. A new, less traumatic approach than liposuction. Arch Otolaryngol Head Neck Surg 1995;121(10):1117-1120.

44. Becker DG, Cook TA, Wang TD, et al: A 3-year multi-institutional experience with the liposhaver. Arch Facial Plast Surg 1999;1(3):171-176.

45. Becker DG, Weinberger MS, Miller PJ, et al: The liposhaver in facial plastic surgery. A multi-institutional experience. Arch Otolaryngol Head Neck Surg 1996;122(11):1161-1167.

46. Jasin ME: Submentoplasty as an isolated rejuvenative procedure for the neck. Arch Facial Plast Surg 2003;5(2):180-183.

47. Kridel RWH, Pacella BL: Complications of liposuction. In

Eisele D (ed): Complications of Head and Neck Surgery. St. Louis: Mosby-Year Book, 1992, pp 791-803.

48. Tapia A, Ferreira B, Eng R: Liposuction in cervical rejuvenation. Aesthet Plast Surg 1987;11(2):95-100.

49. Al-basti HA, El-Khatib HA: The use of suction-assisted surgical extraction of moderate and large lipomas: Long-term follow-up. Aesthet Plast Surg 2002;26(2):114-117.

50. Mowlavi A, Brown RE: Suction lipectomy during flap reconstruction provides immediate and safe debulking of the skin island. Ann Plast Surg 2003;51(2):189-193.

51. Klein S, Fontana L, Young VL, et al: Absence of an effect of liposuction on insulin action and risk factors for coronary heart disease. N Engl J Med 2004;350(25):2549-2557.

52. Gasperoni C, Salgarello M, Gasperoni P: Technical refinements in the surgical treatment of gynecomastia. Ann Plast Surg 2000;44(4):455-458.

53. Atkins JL, Butler PE: Hyperhidrosis: A review of current management. Plast Reconstr Surg 2002;110(1):222-228.

54. Brorson H: Liposuction in arm lymphedema treatment. Scand J Surg 2003;92(4):287-295.

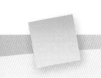

CHAPTER FIFTEEN

Complementary Fat Grafting

Samuel M. Lam, MD • Mark J. Glasgold, MD • Robert A. Glasgold, MD

HISTORY

The history of autologous fat transfer stretches back over an entire century. The first clinical case of fat transfer was described by Neuber in 1893 who reported the use of parcels of fat harvested from the upper extremity to reconstruct a facial defect engendered by tuberculous osteitis.[1] Two years later, Czerny commented on filling a breast deformity created by removal of a benign mass with an excised lipoma.[2] In 1910, Lexer described fat transplantation with larger pieces of fat and found that doing so resulted in improved survival.[3] The following year, Bruning injected harvested fat into a postrhinoplasty defect successfully[4] and Tuffier used fat placed into the extrapleural space to manage pulmonary conditions.[5] In 1932, Straatsma and Peer used fat to plug fistulas that arose after frontal sinus surgery.[6] Two years later, Cotton finely morselized and inserted fat into various defects. In 1956, Peer remarked that walnut-sized fat transplanted fared better than smaller morselized grafts, noting that free fat grafts lose almost half their weight and volume after a year.[7,8]

The rise of liposuction in 1974 stimulated renewed interest in autologous fat transfer.[9] In 1982, Bircoll reported using liposuctioned fat for contouring a range of defects.[10] In the 1980s, Illouz,[11] Krulig,[12] and Newman,[13] based on Pierre Fournier's work, continued the trend of using aspirated fat for recontouring the face and body. Despite these efforts at autologous fat transfer, the question of viability remained and limited the widespread adoption of this technique. Renewed interest in fat grafting took root as reports of long-term viability began to surface with the use of more gentle harvesting techniques utilizing hand rather than machine suction and improvements in fat processing with the use of straining and centrifugation.[14,15] Despite older claims to the contrary, injection of very small parcels of fat appeared to improve survival, as the nourishment of each fat cell is increased by the surrounding neighboring tissue.

Today, proponents of autologous fat transfer have shown the long-term efficacy of fat transfer as well as its importance in facial rejuvenation. Sydney Coleman revolutionized the field of aesthetic facial surgery by putting forth the idea that volume depletion and not gravitational descent represents the primary mechanism of facial aging.[16] He has demonstrated sustained 5-and 10-year facial enhancement results after "lipostructure" fat grafting. Roger Amar has meticulously analyzed the face in terms of the intricate underlying musculature and has based his fat grafting method on using injections into the respective muscle bellies to achieve aesthetic volume enhancement, calling his unique protocol "fat autograft muscle injection" (FAMI).[17]

PERSONAL PHILOSOPHY

Autologous fat transfer has become increasingly recognized as an important technique for facial rejuvenation. Traditional rejuvenative procedures, such as blepharoplasty and facelifts, have been predicated on tissue excision. However, many of these efforts have failed to truly rejuvenate the aging face, resulting in an unnaturally pulled and lifted appearance. Furthermore, traditional procedures may result in an exaggeration or accentuation of age-related volume loss. A new paradigm has shaken the way we approach the aging face. The aging face suffers principally from volume depletion over time like a grape that shrinks into a raisin. Therefore, removal of apparent skin and tissue redundancy can unnaturally transform the face. On the other hand, reinflation of the collapsed face with much-needed volume can restore the face to its natural and youthful form. Autologous fat transfer can play a crucial role in facial rejuvenation as a stand-alone procedure or in combination with traditional lifting procedures[18] (Fig. 15-1).

Like all rejuvenative procedures, the aim of facial fat grafting is threefold: achieve a natural appearance by restoring a youthful vibrancy, avoid complications, and attain long-lasting aesthetic benefit. As the modern era of facial fat grafting is only now emerging, a paucity of scientific literature exists to describe an effective strategy for facial rejuvenation with autologous fat. This chapter will attempt to outline a systematic approach toward facial fat enhancement that emphasizes simplicity, consistency, and safety and has been culled through a decade of clinical experience with ongoing technique refinements.

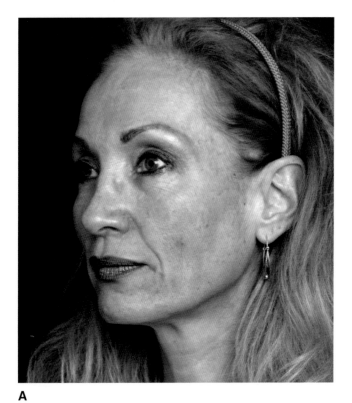

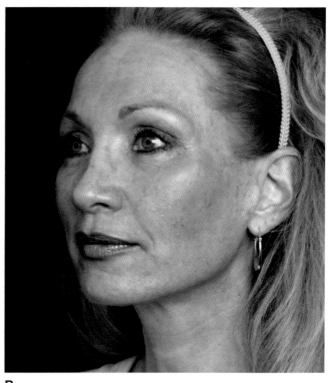

A

B

Figure 15-1 Preoperatively this patient displays midfacial volume loss (**A**). Postoperative photo 1 year after autologous fat transfer (21 mL to cheek, periorbital, and buccal regions, 15 mL to the perioral region, 10 mL to jawline) and a lower facelift (**B**). (From Lam S, Glasgold MJ, Glasgold RA: Complementary Fat Grafting. Philadelphia, Lippincott Williams & Wilkins, 2007. Copyright Lippincott Williams & Wilkins.)

The use of fat grafting requires the surgeon to acquire a new aesthetic appreciation of the aging process. A new set of skills is required, including fat harvesting and infiltration as well as management of unique complications. Consequently, we advocate a conservative approach when beginning to incorporate facial fat transfer in one's practice. In our experience, the postoperative surgical morbidity rate increases as one pushes the limits of fat transfer to obtain ideal results, particularly in the periorbital region. Additional fat transfer in cases of undercorrection is an easier task when compared to the difficulty of managing complications such as visible contour irregularity or an overcorrected face. Conservatism, particularly in the lower periorbital region, should be the rule, especially for the surgeon inexperienced with facial fat grafting.

The new aesthetic principles utilized in volume restoration mandate a different approach to the patient. Rather than arbitrarily defining an aesthetic objective, the surgeon should try to aim at regaining the patient's youthful appearance. Many surgeons today evaluate a patient during consultation and attempt to define what areas of the face require improvement without reference to how the patient actually looked when younger. For instance, browlifting is usually recommended when the brow appears ptotic. However, a patient may never have had a well-defined upper-eyelid sulcus or arched eyebrow

position. At times, overelevating a brow can look unnatural and may not return a patient to the way that he or she looked when younger.[19] Volume restoration may be all that is necessary for a patient who always had a low-lying brow that has lost its fullness with age. If the patient's brow was relatively higher in youth and now has fallen, concurrent browlifting and fat grafting may be emphasized. Patients are encouraged to bring in photographs of themselves when they were younger. These photographs help the surgeon to learn more about the patient's youthful appearance and the patient to understand the importance of volume loss in the aging process. In any case, reviewing a patient's old photographs has particular relevance and importance in order to appreciate the role of fat grafting and help the surgeon conceptualize the surgical plan.

Our approach for facial rejuvenation does not rely solely on autologous fat transfer. We have entitled this chapter "Complementary Fat Grafting" to emphasize the complementary role that fat grafting plays in our clinical practices (i.e., a patient's aesthetic result and satisfaction can be greatly enhanced by using a combination of approaches such as fat grafting, facelifting, and blepharoplasty to attain the desired level of improvement). Patients may be considerably more pleased when each procedure adds to the tally of aesthetic improvement (Fig. 15-2). Traditional procedures and fat transfer need not be

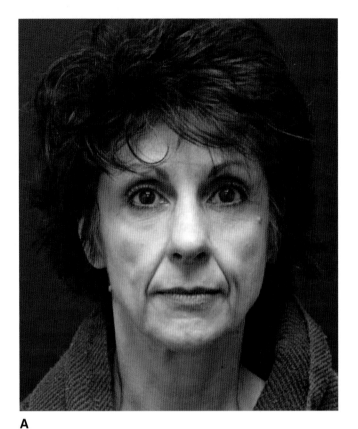

A

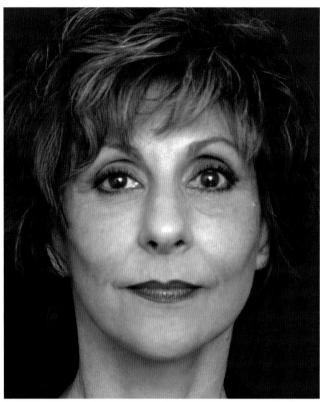

B

Figure 15-2 Preoperative (**A**) and 3-year postoperative (**B**) photos of a patient who underwent autologous fat transfer (27 mL to the cheek, periorbital, and buccal regions) and facelift. (From Lam S, Glasgold MJ, Glasgold RA: Complementary Fat Grafting. Philadelphia, Lippincott Williams & Wilkins, 2007. Copyright Lippincott Williams & Wilkins.)

exclusive of one another. We can embrace two ideologies: autologous fat transfer for volume depletion and lifting procedures for gravitational descent. Judicious use of fat grafting with select lifting procedures can constitute a very potent mixture for correcting specific flaws of aging. For example, prominently descended jowls and loose platysmal bands cannot be adequately improved with fat grafting alone. Standard cervicofacial rhytidectomy combined with fat grafting of the prejowl sulcus is needed to obtain the ideal aesthetic results. Combining procedures can also diminish perioperative morbidity; fat grafting alone in areas that could be more easily targeted with facelift procedures requires considerable volume, adding to the already long recovery period necessitated by fat grafting. The periorbital region is particularly unforgiving. Selective blepharoplasty to reduce pseudoherniated fat combined with fat grafting along the hollow orbital rim provides the optimal balance of safety and aesthetic benefit. In patients with considerable pseudoherniated fat, the significant volume needed for fat grafting can lead to patient dissatisfaction secondary to increased likelihood for contour irregularity and overcorrection of the region. With ongoing clinical experience, a surgeon will begin to perceive the complementary role

that volume enhancement can play in facial rejuvenation.

Although autologous fat has been used successfully to manage hypoplastic lips and depressed facial lines (like the nasolabial and labiomandibular folds), we strongly believe that the rejuvenative benefit for these areas is limited. Fat enhancement of the lips often requires significant fat deposition with marked, prolonged ecchymosis and edema with limited longevity. Similarly, augmentation of the deeper lines in the perioral region often fails to achieve adequate patient satisfaction. We do infiltrate fat into the nasolabial folds when performing fat augmentation of the cheek to ensure that the newly augmented cheek does not exaggerate the apparent depth of the nasolabial folds. Patients whose primary goal is lip augmentation or effacement of facial lines are best treated with one of the many available injectable fillers.

ANATOMY

The understanding of facial topography is the most important aspect of anatomy as it relates to fat grafting. The soft tissue loss that is associated with the aging process is accentuated by the presence of facial retaining ligaments, which create unfavorable depressions (Fig. 15-3). Hills and valleys develop across the surface of the face, contrasting the convexity associated with a youthful appearance.

The face is usually divided into thirds for better anatomic understanding. The upper third comprises the brow and temple area and the middle third corresponds to the cheek and midface. The lower third constitutes the chin, prejowl, jowl, and lateral mandible. This systematic appraisal will provide a concrete formula for specific volume enhancement based on each individual anatomic territory. Clinically relevant regions of each anatomic zone will be emphasized with pearls to guide surgical strategy.

THE UPPER THIRD

The upper third of the face comprises three main constituent elements: the brow, upper eyelid, and temple. The brow remains one of the most easily targeted areas for rejuvenation. The brow is defined by the hair-bearing portion of the eyebrow and, more important, the soft tissue that envelopes the lateral half of the superior orbital rim. Placement of fat along this lateral half can restore the desirable fullness that is lost during the aging process. The upper eyelid and temple can also significantly hollow with aging. In appropriate candidates, these areas can be significantly enhanced with autologous fat grafting. Surgical manipulation of this region should be reserved for experienced fat-transplant surgeons due to the complex anatomy and increased potential for complications.

THE MIDDLE THIRD

The middle third of the face is the most complex subunit and perhaps the most important area for facial rejuvenation with autologous fat grafting. This region encompasses the lower eyelid and the malar and submalar areas. A youthful face is characterized by a confluence of the lower eyelid and cheek regions, which becomes separated into visually distinct regions during the aging process. The orbital rim is more clearly observed as a separate entity from the cheek with aging due to the orbital fat bulging superiorly and the cheek fat receding. The voluminous lateral cheek mound of youth dissipates to reveal the smaller, flatter contour of the malar bony eminence that lacks any notable soft tissue coverage. The anterior cheek begins to separate, often with a linear depression that courses from the nasojugal depression down inferolaterally to the buccal recess that corresponds with the ligamentous attachment known as the malar septum.[20] Finally, the buccal region can exhibit marked atrophy and should be reconstituted along with the discussed anterior and lateral malar regions to achieve better confluence and to avoid an exaggeration of buccal hollowing following malar augmentation. As an extension of the midface, the nasolabial fold should be deemed part of midfacial volume enhancement.

THE LOWER THIRD

The lower third of the face is principally focused on the labiomandibular fold, prejowl sulcus, labiomental sulcus, and chin. The chin undergoes volume recession as opposed to the volume gain that can be appreciated in the jowl region. For very early jowling, volume enhancement with autologous fat in the prejowl sulcus can be sufficient to straighten the jawline. Even markedly conspicuous jowling is often accompanied by proportionate volume contraction along the prejowl region. Accordingly, face-lifting to correct significant jowling can still fail to

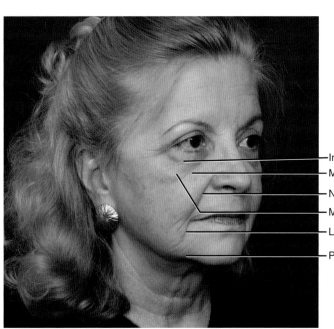

Infraorbital rim
Midface depression/malar septum
Nasolabial fold
Malar mound
Labiomandibular fold
Prejowl sulcus

Figure 15-3 The important anatomic landmarks for fat injections are depicted in this photograph. (From Lam S, Glasgold MJ, Glasgold RA: Complementary Fat Grafting. Philadelphia, Lippincott Williams & Wilkins, 2007. Copyright Lippincott Williams & Wilkins.)

straighten the jawline if prejowl augmentation is not performed. Volume deficiency in the lateral mandible, posterior to the jowl, may be age related or congenitally absent. The addition of volume to the lateral mandible can help diminish the appearance of the jowl and restore the youthful jaw contour.

PREOPERATIVE ASSESSMENT

The consultation for patients considering autologous fat grafting is primarily based on sound facial analysis and understanding the desires of the patient. Owing to the complex and unconventional nature of autologous fat grafting, patients may not entirely appreciate the benefits of the procedure if they are more accustomed to traditional surgical procedures such as facelifts and blepharoplasty. Examining photographs from a patient's youth can significantly aid the surgeon in explaining the aesthetic objectives of autologous fat grafting. Reviewing with the patient each decade of change and showing the gradual dissipation of soft tissue volume can be informative to most patients. Before-and-after photographs of other patients who exhibit similar anatomy can also be quite illuminating for a prospective patient. Digital morphing technology often falls short of the intended mark, as it is very difficult to convey volumetric changes.

After establishing realistic aesthetic objectives, the surgeon must ensure that the patient fully comprehends the benefits and limitations of the procedure. For instance, fat grafting has proved to be less than ideal to manage hypoplastic lips and deep nasolabial/labiomandibular folds. In these areas, soft tissue fillers may be a better solution.

SURGICAL TECHNIQUE

GENERAL CONSIDERATIONS

Autologous fat transfer can be undertaken with relatively light intravenous sedation and infiltration of local anesthesia. Preoperatively the patient's face should be marked carefully to delineate the recipient sites for fat grafting. Markings should be made with the patient in an upright position so that dependent tissues can help accentuate the highlights and shadows of the face. Determination of the appropriate donor site should also be made in the preoperative area. In deciding on the donor site, it is often helpful to ask patients where they feel they accumulate the most fat or which area has been the most recalcitrant to fat loss despite exercise. Prior surgery, especially liposuction, can preclude the harvesting of usable fat from an area. Finally, the prohibitive presence of occult or visible ventral hernias should be ascertained before embarking on harvesting from the lower abdomen.

FAT HARVESTING

The areas that are typically available for fat harvesting include the lower abdomen, inner thigh, outer thigh, anterior thigh, lower lateral buttock, lateral waist, lower back, inner knee, and triceps. The lower abdomen and inner thigh tend to be the most favored sites for fat harvesting, as the patient does not need to be repositioned (Fig. 15-4A and B). With 10-mL Luer-Lok syringes outfitted with a harvesting cannula, manual extraction of the fat should be performed with only 1 to 2 mL of negative pressure held on the plunger (Fig. 15-5). Entry sites for cannula insertion through the skin are made with a 16-gauge Nokor needle or a No. 11 blade in discreet areas such as the umbilicus for the lower abdomen and the inguinal line for the inner thigh. A gentle motion should be carried out to harvest the fat and the depth of the cannula should be at the midlevel of the fat pad. If tenting of the skin is noted, then the surgeon is most likely too superficial and risks the potential for a contour irregularity at the donor site. Passage of the cannula too deeply can elicit significant discomfort, especially in the lower abdomen, when the cannula abrades the rectus fascia. Harvesting uniformly over the entire area can maximize fat yield and minimize contour irregularities. Typically, owing to the presence of lidocaine, blood, and lysed fat cells in the preprocessed syringe, the amount of harvested fat should be anticipated to be about half the collected volume, that is, 5 mL of fat per 10-mL syringe. These estimates are important when calculating how many milliliters of fat are needed for transfer. The total volume of fat needed for transplantation will depend on the surgeon's clinical judgment and should be modified for each patient. On average, 30 to 50 mL of fat is a common amount for a semiconservative full-face fat transfer, with over 60 mL representing a more aggressive strategy.

PROCESSING THE FAT

After each 10-mL syringe has been filled from harvesting, it is sterilely passed to the surgical assistant who prepares that syringe for fat infiltration. Although many techniques exist for processing fat, we have relied on centrifugation as our sole method. The assistant fastens a plug onto the Luer-Lok end of the 10-mL syringe, removes the plunger with the syringe in an upright position, and places a specialized cap into the plunger side of the syringe. These caps and plugs can be purchased from any reputable manufacturer, but the original plunger and miniplastic Luer-Lok cover that comes with the syringe should never be used for centrifugation. After a balanced number of syringes have been collected, they are inserted sterilely into the centrifuge machine. Various types of systems are available, each equipped with different inserts that can be sterilized. The centrifuge is turned on to rotate for approximately 3 minutes at 3000 rpm. A leeway of

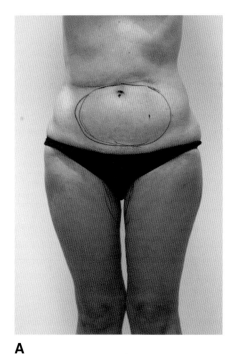

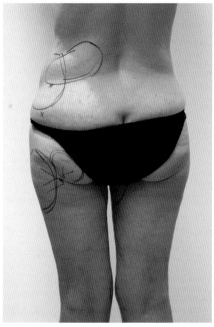

A   **B**

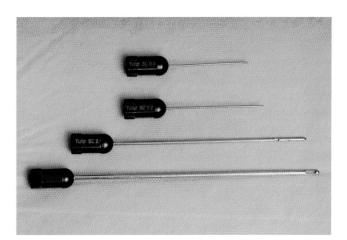

> **Figure 15-4** The donor sites for fat transfer are shown. The most easily accessible areas are in the abdominal and inner thigh regions (**A**). Additional sites include the lateral thigh and flank areas (**B**). (From Lam S, Glasgold MJ, Glasgold RA: Complementary Fat Grafting. Philadelphia, Lippincott Williams & Wilkins, 2007. Copyright Lippincott Williams & Wilkins.)

1 minute and 1000 rpm can usually be permitted without compromising the fat processing.

After the fat has been centrifuged, the syringe is removed again sterilely and placed into a test-tube rack resting on the sterile field. The processed syringe now appears separated into three distinct layers: a supranatant

> **Figure 15-5** Glasgold set of fat transfer instruments (Tulip Medical, Inc., San Diego, CA), from top to bottom: The 0.9-mm injecting cannula (4-cm length) is good for periorbital injections, particularly when placing fat superficially and for injection into the very fibrous recipient sites at the deep lateral inferior orbital rim and lateral canthal region. The 1.2-mm injecting cannula (6-cm length) is an all-purpose cannula that can be used for any other injections. The 2.1-mm multiport harvesting cannula (12-cm length) we have available as an alternative cannula for thin patients. The 3.0-mm bullet-tip harvesting cannula (15-cm length) is our primary harvesting cannula and can be used as one's sole harvesting cannula. (From Lam S, Glasgold MJ, Glasgold RA: Complementary Fat Grafting. Philadelphia, Lippincott Williams & Wilkins, 2007. Copyright Lippincott Williams & Wilkins.)

consisting principally of the oily residue of free fatty acids, the central core of viable fat, and the infranatant composed of blood and lidocaine (Fig. 15-6*A*). The cap from the plunger side is always removed first to pour out the supranatant (see Fig. 15-6*B*). Then, the plug is unscrewed from the Luer-Lok side and the infranatant is allowed to drain from below (see Fig. 15-6*C*). The syringe is returned to the test-tube rack without cap or plug and with the plunger side facing upward so that the fat does not spill. Additional supranatant is wicked away by placing an unfurled 4 × 4 cotton gauze into the exposed plunger side of the syringe to make contact with the column of fat (see Fig. 15-6*D*). It is very important that the 4 × 4 gauze pad not be trimmed so as to prevent introduction of particles of shorn cotton into the mixture of fat intended for infiltration. After a few minutes have transpired, the wicks are removed and the fat is transferred into the back end of a 20-mL syringe to facilitate transfer into the 1-mL infiltration syringes (Fig. 15-7*A*). The plunger of the 20-mL syringe is gently reinserted, and a transfer hub is used to join the 20-mL syringe with the 1-mL syringe via a Luer-Lok connection (see Fig. 15-7*B*). The fat is then transferred to each 1-mL syringe, one at a time. Generally, only four 1-mL syringes are required; as the surgeon constantly infiltrates fat, the assistant can reload the next syringe.

INFILTRATING THE FAT

The fat is always infiltrated with a 1-mL Luer-Lok syringe so as to ensure placement of a very limited parcel of fat per each passage of the cannula. Differential placement of fat will optimize its viability and minimize

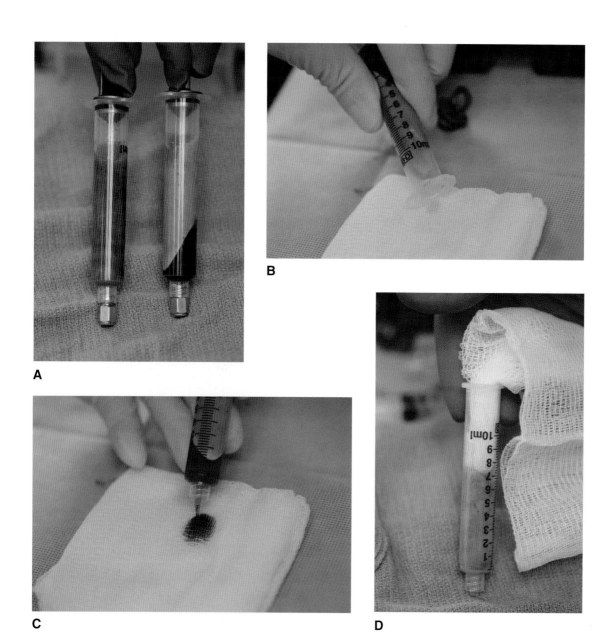

Figure 15-6 A shows harvested fat in 10 mL syringe pre- (*left*) and post- (*right*) centrifugation. In **B**, the surgeon pours off supranatant (free fatty acids). In **C**, the surgeon drains infranatant (primarily blood). In **D**, the fat is wicked with gauze to remove residual supranatant. (From Lam S, Glasgold MJ, Glasgold RA: Complementary Fat Grafting. Philadelphia, Lippincott Williams & Wilkins, 2007. Copyright Lippincott Williams & Wilkins.)

complications. In areas that are less forgiving, such as the periorbital region, 0.03 to 0.05 mL is injected per pass. In more robust regions, such as the prejowl sulcus and midface, 0.1-mL injections can be performed in each pass. Only blunt injection cannulas should be used in order to minimize the chance of nerve or vessel damage during infiltration (see Fig. 15-5). A standard 18-gauge needle is used to create the puncture site in the skin through which the cannula tip is introduced. If considerable resistance on the plunger is met when infiltrating fat, the cannula should be withdrawn from the patient and cleared to prevent inadvertent injection of a large bolus of fat.

Upper Third

The lateral half of the brow can be approached from an entry site that is lateral to the lateral canthal tendon, and filled to achieve a more robust, youthful contour (Fig. 15-8*A* and *B*). A sausage-like shape can arise after infiltration and should not raise alarm, as this will quickly resolve postoperatively. Placement of the fat should be relatively deep, ideally in the supraperiosteal plane. The upper-eyelid recess corresponds with the inferior aspect of the superior orbital rim. The "sunken eye" appearance occurs in individuals who exhibit a very hollow upper eyelid. This is an extremely difficult problem to correct.

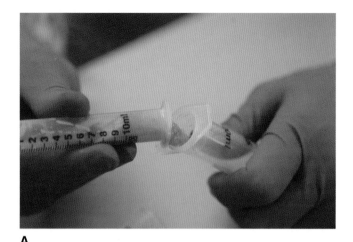

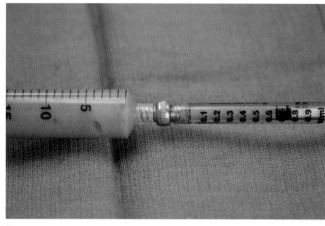

A   **B**

▨ **Figure 15-7** Processed fat is poured into a 20-mL syringe (**A**). The fat is then transferred to 1-mL Luer-Lok syringes through the attached transfer hub (**B**). (From Lam S, Glasgold MJ, Glasgold RA: Complementary Fat Grafting. Philadelphia, Lippincott Williams & Wilkins, 2007. Copyright Lippincott Williams & Wilkins.)

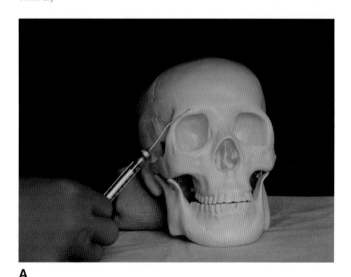

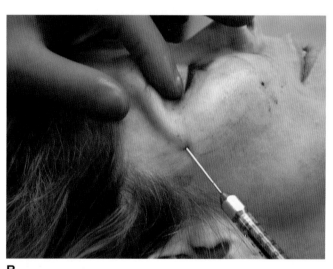

A   **B**

▨ **Figure 15-8** **A** shows placement of fat along the lateral brow. **B** shows an intraoperative view of fat placement in the lateral brow in a supraperiosteal plane. (**A** from Lam S, Glasgold MJ, Glasgold RA: Complementary Fat Grafting. Philadelphia, Lippincott Williams & Wilkins, 2007. Copyright Lippincott Williams & Wilkins.)

Placement of fat along the inferior aspect of the superior orbital rim can create a less hollowed-out appearance. This maneuver is often accompanied by a protracted period of swelling. Discussion with the patient about the anticipated postoperative period is important in order to establish realistic expectations.

The temple can also be an unforgiving area to augment; therefore, only very small amounts of fat should be delivered per cannula passage, as contour deformities can readily arise in this area. We advise venturing to correct the temple and hollow upper eyelid only after adequate clinical experience has been acquired with fat grafting elsewhere in the face.

Middle Third

Volume loss in the midface results in visible breakpoints along the malar septum and between the lower lid and

cheek, imparting an aged and tired appearance. Often, the midface is the most important region of the face to augment with fat. Reestablishing a uniform and seamless contour between the lower eyelid and cheek should be the principal objective in many cases. Although infiltration of fat into the precanine fossa and nasolabial fold is unlikely to efface a deep nasolabial fold, it can create a better transition between the newly augmented cheek and the upper lip.

The inferior orbital rim is one of the more difficult areas of the face to enhance with fat and constitutes a region where the majority of complications arise. Large volume fat injection (greater than the recommended 0.03 to 0.05 mL per cannula pass) or placement of fat in a superficial plane can increase the chance of a noticeable irregularity postoperatively. Our complication rates have dramatically reduced by approaching this region from an inferior-based entry site (Fig. 15-9*A* and *B*). Using this

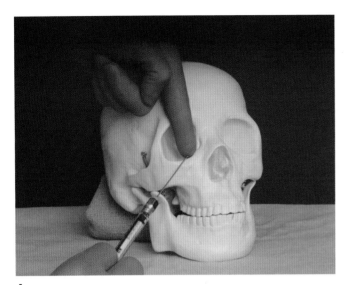

A

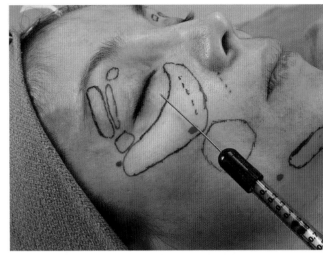

B

Figure 15-9 A shows placement of fat along the inferior orbital rim; the index finger of the surgeon's nondominant hand protects the globe. **B** shows an intraoperative view of fat placement along the inferior orbital rim. (From Lam S, Glasgold MJ, Glasgold RA: Complementary Fat Grafting. Philadelphia, Lippincott Williams & Wilkins, 2007. Copyright Lippincott Williams & Wilkins.)

approach, the cannula tip passes perpendicularly to the inferior orbital rim. This maneuver should be performed with the index finger of the surgeon's nondominant hand placed on the superior aspect of the inferior orbital rim in order to protect the globe. As one begins incorporating fat transfer it is recommended that a conservative amount of fat be placed along the inferior orbital rim (a total of 2 mL per side) in the supraperiosteal plane so as to minimize contour problems. Larger volumes of fat can be judiciously used in the more volume-deficient patients with additional fat placed in a more superficial plane.

The lateral and anterior cheeks are easier areas to augment. The cheeks can tolerate a more generous amount of fat (0.1 mL per pass) in more superficial planes without risking contour irregularities. The skeletonized lateral cheek should be augmented to restore a youthful, full, rounded contour that blends well with a full, anterior cheek. The anterior cheek is typically divided by a linear depression running from the superomedial nasojugal groove inferolaterally to the buccal region. Placement of fat into the anterior cheek should be principally situated into the greatest areas of tissue loss, the depression at the malar septum and the region inferomedial to the malar septum. Passage of the cannula to reach the anterior cheek can be made from a lateral cheek entry site, and the cannula often must be forcefully pushed through the fibrous malar septum to breach it (Fig. 15-10A and B). At times, the malar septum does not pose much resistance and can be easily traversed.

Patients should be evaluated for the presence of a malar mound, which appears as a protuberance at the junction of the anterior and lateral cheek lying just lateral to the upper portion of the malar septum. When this feature is present, the surgeon should attempt to avoid placement of excessive fat under the already prominent malar mound. Gentle contouring around the malar mound can help soften the appearance of the malar protuberance while at the same time rebuilding lost volume of the cheek. If patients note a history of fluctuating, cyclic edema of the malar mound, placement of fat immediately below this structure may only worsen the condition and lead to a protracted swelling in this area for several months.

In the thin patient, the buccal and submalar regions are often hollow and can tolerate a generous amount of fat with minimal concern of contour irregularity. Placement of fat into the subcutaneous tissue and somewhat more deeply will soften a gaunt appearance and provide a better transition between the malar and submalar regions. Finally, the precanine fossa (the triangular depression circumscribed by the nasal ala medially and the upper extent of the nasolabial fold laterally) and the nasolabial fold are augmented not with the expectation of effacement of the fold, but rather to achieve an improved transition between the newly augmented anterior cheek and the upper lip. A generous amount of fat can be placed into the precanine fossa deeply into the supraperiosteal plane to improve the hollowness in this area. The entire nasolabial fold including the precanine fossa can then be augmented from a perpendicular direction (i.e., from the lateral cheek) into a more superficial subcutaneous plane.

Lower Third

The principal areas of the lower face that benefit from fat augmentation are the prejowl sulcus, labiomandibular recess, labiomental sulcus, lateral jawline, and anterior central mentum. Of these three areas, the prejowl sulcus

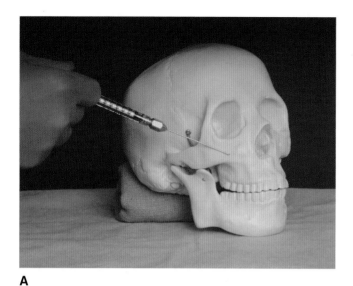

A

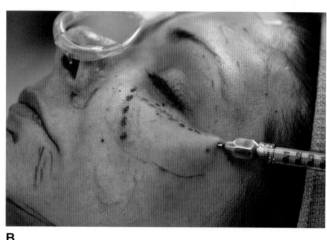

B

Figure 15-10 **A** shows the location and trajectory of the anterior cheek injection. In **B,** the intraoperative injection is performed. (**A** from Lam S, Glasgold MJ, Glasgold RA: Complementary Fat Grafting. Philadelphia, Lippincott Williams & Wilkins, 2007. Copyright Lippincott Williams & Wilkins.)

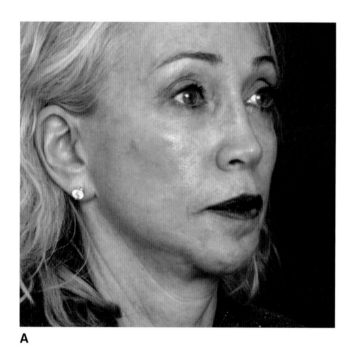

A

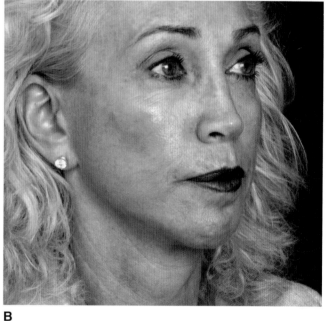

B

Figure 15-11 This patient had a facelift 7 years ago and is unhappy with her jawline (**A**). Her primary issue is volume loss in the prejowl sulcus. **B** shows the results 1 year after isolated volume augmentation to the prejowl sulcus. (From Lam S, Glasgold MJ, Glasgold RA: Complementary Fat Grafting. Philadelphia, Lippincott Williams & Wilkins, 2007. Copyright Lippincott Williams & Wilkins.)

can be considered the most important for enhancement in order to provide maximal straightening of a descended jawline (Fig. 15-11). A generous amount of fat can be placed into the prejowl sulcus without risking contour deformity. Placement of fat should be made along both the anterior and inferior aspects of the mandibular body in order to achieve a three-dimensional, cylindrical reshaping of the prejowl depression (Fig. 15-12A and B).

If the chin appears to benefit from mild projection, fat can also be placed along the anterior chin to achieve the effect of an augmentation mentoplasty. The lateral mandible is augmented as needed, with placement of fat posterior to the jowl so as not to accentuate the fullness. If a concurrent rhyitidectomy is planned, fat should not be distributed along the lateral mandible, as this area will be undermined regardless of the type of facelift performed.

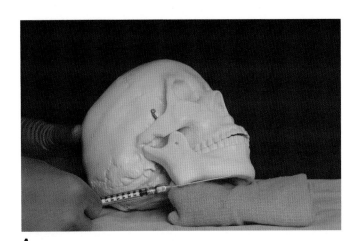

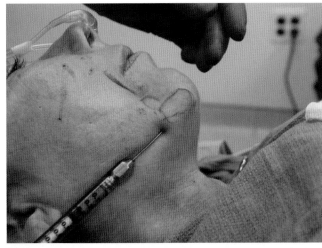

A

B

Figure 15-12 **A** depicts the location and trajectory of the prejowl injection. In **B,** the intraoperative injection is performed. (**A** from Lam S, Glasgold MJ, Glasgold RA: Complementary Fat Grafting. Philadelphia, Lippincott Williams & Wilkins, 2007. Copyright Lippincott Williams & Wilkins.)

POSTOPERATIVE CARE

At the end of the procedure, the patient does not require any sutures, bandages, or drains of any kind unless a concurrent lifting procedure was performed. The patient is discharged after the appropriate interval of post-anesthesia observance. Although some surgeons who practice fat transfer do not believe in immediate postoperative icing of transplanted regions owing to the risk of reducing fat-cell viability, we believe that doing so does not compromise the aesthetic result and can also expedite the recovery. We advocate icing intermittently for at least the first 48 to 72 hours postoperatively. Head elevation is stressed for the first several nights after surgery as it can reduce the extent of postoperative edema. Although heavy exercise, especially with increased intra-abdominal pressure and bending over, should be avoided, a light isometric weight-lifting regimen with one half to one third the typical weight and lighter cardiovascular exercise can be undertaken once the swelling has begun to recede usually by the fourth or fifth postoperative day. Besides these restrictions, there are no limitations per se that prevent exercising areas of the body that were used for donor harvesting. Finally, limiting salt intake may minimize and assist in the resolution of postoperative edema.

Although postoperative care is relatively simple and straightforward, management of postoperative expectations may be more involved. Patients may perceive that their face appears too inflated for their liking in the first several postoperative weeks and regard this outcome as an unintended result. Although the expected course of recovery is explained in detail preoperatively, constant reassurance should be proffered, with patients returning as often as necessary. Ecchymosis and edema that accom-

pany fat grafting can be more pronounced than in traditional surgical procedures, resulting in a social and professional encumbrance for a longer period of time. The periorbital region may be the most afflicted area with bruising and soreness. In contrast to the face, where the patient generally experiences very little discomfort, the fat harvesting sites are generally more painful for the first several days to weeks after surgery.

COMPLICATIONS

The complications that arise after fat grafting are relatively unique compared with those that may arise after traditional lifting procedures. Injuries to nerves or vascular structures are extremely rare. The more common problems with fat transfer arise from contour irregularities ("lumps" or "bulges") and over- or undercorrection. A systematic appraisal of the problem and targeted correction for each individual problem should be undertaken in every case.

"Lumps" present as small discrete areas of excessive fat, and are most likely to occur in the periorbital region. Conservative placement of fat in the periorbital region is an important step in avoiding this problem. When a lump does occur, treatment begins with steroid injections into the area of concern. If this fails to correct the problem, and there appears to be a relatively discrete lump of fat, directly excising this can alleviate the contour deformity (Fig. 15-13).

"Bulges" are wider areas of elevation and may represent persistent edema or induration, or in some cases a large uneven placement of fat. Bulges present as thickened areas, which can be palpated and seen along the inferior orbital rim. Injection with conservative amounts

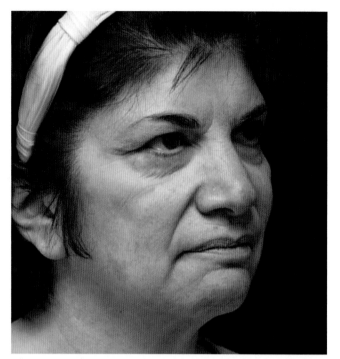

A

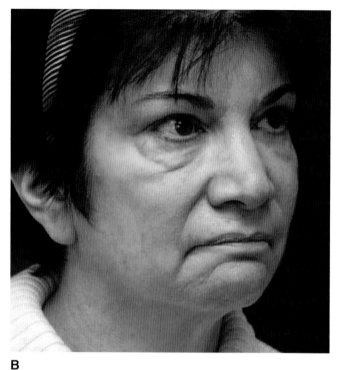

B

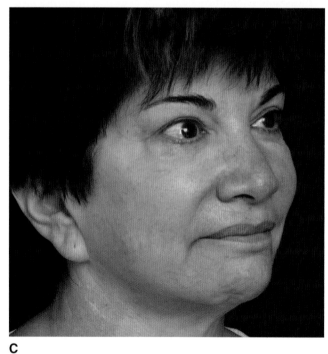

C

Figure 15-13 Preoperative view (**A**) of a patient who underwent fat transfer to the inferior orbital rim and cheek. Six months postoperatively, the patient has good malar augmentation but persistent visible lumps at the central inferior orbital rim (**B**). This patient was also unhappy with persistent lower lateral fat that had not been removed. After correction of these problems with direct excision of redundant lower lid skin and excess fat through an incision placed in the crease following the inferior orbital rim (**C**). The lateral fat pad was reduced through a transconjunctival approach. (From Lam S, Glasgold MJ, Glasgold RA: Complementary Fat Grafting. Philadelphia, Lippincott Williams & Wilkins, 2007. Copyright Lippincott Williams & Wilkins.)

of triamcinolone acetonide in increasing strengths from 10 mg/mL to 40 mg/mL have proved beneficial in most circumstances but must be repeated every 1 to 2 months until resolution. In our experience direct liposuction of these areas has not been successful.

Overcorrection implies that a generalized region has been overly inflated beyond the patient's expectations. As mentioned, the first several weeks to months are marked by ongoing resolution of tissue edema. Therefore, a conservative, expectant approach is advocated. If failure of timely resolution of the problem is encountered, then microliposuction with an 18-gauge Klein Capistrano cannula can be performed to reduce volume.

Undercorrection remains the most favorable complication, as it represents the most easily correctable condition. Additional fat harvesting and infiltration can be accomplished relatively quickly and without difficulty under local anesthesia or limited intravenous sedation.

Future Considerations

We are standing at the crossroads of a major paradigm shift from excision-based surgery to volume enhancement. Whether or not there will be an increasing shift away from excisional surgery in favor of volume correction is yet to be determined. We advocate a combination approach that requires judicious selection of lifting procedures and fat grafting tailored to each individual. Whatever the outcome, it appears that fat grafting and facial volume enhancement represent the present and future of facial rejuvenation, as we see it from the narrow vantage of today's prism.

As we still have yet to find the perfect facial filler, the field of synthetic facial injectables continues to advance at a dizzying pace. Just a few years ago, bovine collagen was the only Food and Drug Administration (FDA) approved synthetic filler. Today, we have a multitude of choices that continue to grow, as FDA approval marches forward. Every type of filler carries specific characteristics that make it more ideal for a certain clinical application and also drawbacks that may hinder implementation. The continuing change in the landscape of facial fillers offers the possibility for volume augmentation procedures with less downtime and without the need for harvesting fat. We predict that volume enhancement will continue to play an increasing role as both a complementary and a stand-alone procedure in facial rejuvenation.

REFERENCES

1. Neuber F: Fettransplantation. Chir Kongr Verh Dtsch Ges Chir 1893;22:66.
2. Czerny M: Plastischer ersatz der brusterlruse durch ein lipom. Verh Dtsch Ges Chir Zbl Chir 1985; 27:72–75.
3. Lexer E: Freie Fettransplantation. Dtsch Med Wochenschr 1910;36:640.
4. Bruning P: Cited by Broeckaert TJ, Steinhaus J: Contribution a l'étude des greffes adipueses. Bull Acad R Med Belg 1914;28:440.
5. Tuffier T: Abces gangreneux du pouman ouvert dans les bronches: hemoptysies repetee operation par decollement pleuro-parietal; guerison. Bull Mem Soc Chir Paris 1911;37:134.
6. Straatsma CR, Peer LA: Repair of postauricular fistula by means of a free fat graft. Arch Otolaryngol 1932;15:620-621.
7. Peer LA: The neglected free fat graft. Plast Reconstr Surg 1956;18:233.
8. Peer LA: Loss of weight and volume in human fat grafts. Plast Reconstr Surg 1950;5:217.
9. Shiffman MA (ed): Autologous Fat Transplantation. New York: Marcel Decker, 2001.
10. Bircoll M: Autologous fat transplantation. The Asian Congress of Plastic Surgery, February 1982.
11. Illouz YG: The fat cell graft: A new technique to fill depressions. Plast Reconstr Surg 1986;78:122-123.
12. Krulig E: Lipo-injection. Am J Cosmet Surg 1987;4:123-129.
13. Newman J, Levin J: Facial lipo-transplant surgery. Am J Cosmet Surg 1987;4:131-140.
14. Shu T, Lam SM: Liposuction and lipotransfer for facial rejuvenation in the Asian patient. Int J Cosmet Surg Aesthet Dermatol 2003;5:165-173.
15. McCurdy JA Jr, Lam SM: Cosmetic Surgery of the Asian Face, 2nd ed. New York: Thieme Medical Publishers, 2005.
16. Coleman SR: Structural Fat Grafting. St; Louis: Quality Medical Publishers, 2004.
17. Amar RE: Adipocyte microinfiltration in the face or tissue restructuration with fat tissue graft [In French]. Ann Chir Plast Esthet 1999;44:593-608.
18. Lam SM, Glasgold MJ, Glasgold RA: Complementary Fat Grafting. Philadelphia: Lippincott, Williams, & Wilkins, 2007.
19. Schreiber JE, Singh NK, Klatsky SA: Beauty lies in the "eyebrow" of the beholder: A public survey of eyebrow aesthetics. Aesthet Surg J 2005;25(4):348-352
20. Mendelson BC, Muzaffar AR, Adams WP: Surgical anatomy of the midcheek and malar mounds. Plastic Reconstr Surg 2002;110(3):885-896.

CHAPTER SIXTEEN

Nonsurgical Facial Rejuvenation

Douglas Hamilton, MD

HISTORY

Lasers and injectables are the two fulcra around which noninvasive facial rejuvenation navigate. Historically, the use of lasers in cosmetic medicine can be traced to Leon Goldman in the 1950s.[1-3] Although the ruby laser was the first medical laser developed, it was the argon laser that began a practical clinical application in the early 1970s with the removal of decorative tattoos.[4-7] These lasers did not achieve widespread use because of significant complications, but they heralded the modern era for noninvasive facial rejuvenation. Despite the exciting discoveries in the field, Goldman's national lectures did not draw copious attendees because of the lack of clinical relevance of these devices. In the ensuing 25 years, however, the carbon dioxide (CO_2) and erbium:yttrium aluminum garnet (Er:YAG) lasers have gained significant acceptance by allowing a well-controlled skin resurfacing modality with superior aesthetic outcome and limited complications. In the 1990s, "nonablative lasers" also became available, providing a no-downtime solution for treating minimal to moderate rhytids.

The birth of facial fillers could be dated back many decades to the use of fat and fascia lata transplants. The availability of bovine collagen (Zyderm and Zyplast, Inamed Aesthetics, Santa Barbara, CA), however, began the modern era of injectable fillers. These two products were designed in the mid-1970s and have been the "gold standard" to which other fillers are compared both in clinical practice and in Food and Drug Administration (FDA) trials. It is only since 2000 that other injectables have seriously challenged collagen's dominance with the availability of botulinum toxin type A (BTX-A), stabilized hyaluronic acid products, polymethyl methacrylate microspheres (PMMA), synthesized calcium hydroxylapatite (CaHA), and injectable poly-L-lactic acid (PLA). The continued popularity of BTX-A and longer-acting fillers have transformed our approach to facial rejuvenation. Unlike ablative laser and chemical resurfacing, these products truly allow the patients to obtain immediate facial enhancements with limited downtime.

PERSONAL PHILOSOPHY

The road to facial rejuvenation always starts with the diagnosis. Once the diagnosis is established, the therapy is naturally born. In evaluating the aging face one may see aesthetic pathology in three broad terms: laxity (type A), furrowing (type B), and rhytids (type C).[8] Rhytids are superficial cutaneous wrinkles, whereas furrows are deeper valley-like expression lines (Fig. 16-1). Other issues contributing to an aged appearance include color irregularity and loss of skin luster. The interplay among various aging processes often makes it impossible to obtain complete therapeutic effect from any one modality. Examples include unsightly nasolabial folds or marionette lines remaining after rhytidectomy or poor resolution of crow's-feet after periorbital laser resurfacing. Indeed, every face is unique with elements of aging and every area may have several pathologies contributing to the aging problem. As a result, noninvasive techniques are of great value for some aging defects but not for others. Skin and muscle laxity of more than a moderate degree requires surgical intervention whereas fine rhytids and furrowing are preferentially treated by lasers or noninvasive injectables, respectively. In this chapter, I will discuss my preferred nonsurgical techniques for facial rejuvenation.

ANATOMY

Different aesthetic deficiencies warrant distinctive therapies. Although a given area of the face can present with different issues in diverse individuals, there are recurrent patterns for each facial area. Figure 16-1 reveals the most frequently encountered aging changes in each area of the face. Periorbital aesthetic pathology includes crow's-feet furrows or rhytids, lower eyelid rhytids and furrows, lower lid laxity, fat pad herniation, tear-trough depression, darkness in the skin, dermatochalasia of the upper lids, and brow ptosis. The forehead most commonly ages with ptotic brows and the development of expression furrows. Horizontal forehead furrows develop secondary to

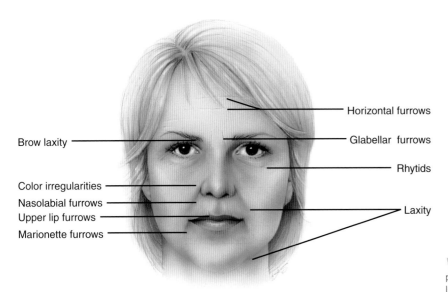

Horizontal furrows

Glabellar furrows

Rhytids

Brow laxity

Color irregularities
Nasolabial furrows
Upper lip furrows
Marionette furrows

Laxity

Figure 16-1 The aging process. Three broad pathologic changes occur during the aging process: laxity (type A), furrowing (type B), and rhytids (type C).

frontalis muscle activity. Glabellar furrows occur because of corrugator and procerus muscle contraction. In females, these lines may be superficial enough to classify them as rhytids.

In the midface, laxity of the cheeks and progressive volume loss are often readily apparent. The salient manifestation of the cheek and facial tissue laxity is mandibular line blurring, jowl formation, and accentuation of nasolabial folds. Perioral changes due to bone and teeth movement along with recurrent facial expressions most often develop furrows: nasolabial, marionette (below the mouth commissure), and lip lines. True intracutaneous rhytids of the upper lip must be treated differently than furrows. Upper lip furrows are rarely seen in men whereas about 70% of women will exhibit significant muscle movement of the upper lip when speaking, therein leading to these musculocutaneous furrows. The cheek region may develop laxity as well as rhytids.

PREOPERATIVE ASSESSMENT

The preoperative analysis for noninvasive facial rejuvenation includes a thorough history and physical examination. Patients with history of collagen vascular disease (systemic lupus, scleroderma, and keloid formation), vitiligo, isotretinoin (Accutane, Roche, Nutley, NJ), and radiation therapy are cautioned about laser and chemical resurfacing. Isotretinoin and radiation therapy destroy the adnexal structures that are necessary for epithelial regeneration after skin resurfacing. We like to wait at least 12 months after the discontinuation of isotretinoin to proceed with laser resurfacing. Patient skin classification is also important in the preoperative analysis, especially for those who are being considered for laser resurfacing.

We utilize the Fitzpatrick scale (Table 16-1) to determine patient suitability for ablative laser resurfacing.[9,10] Generally, patients who are at the extremes of the Fitzpatrick scale are unsuitable candidates (types I, IV, V, and VI). Type I patients are at risk for hypopigmentation, which can be an extremely difficult complication to correct. Patients who are darker are at risk for hyperpigmentation that usually can be treated successfully with topical creams although the wait can be an anxious one for physician and patient alike. Nonablative lasers are suitable for all patients. The Glogau classification can also be useful for evaluating appropriate candidates (Box 16-1). This classification system focuses on the degree and type of wrinkles and the effects of photoaging.[11]

After the general skin survey, we perform our facial analysis based upon three major categories of defects: laxity (type A), furrowing (type B), and rhytids (type C). Proper analysis allows us to bring patients into an understanding of what treatments will be required for their type of facial aging. The categorization firmly roots the credibility of the physician's choice of procedure and

Table 16-1   Fitzpatrick Classification System

Skin Type	Skin Color	Reaction to Sun
Type I	Very white or freckled	Always burns
Type II	White	Usually burns
Type III	White to olive	Sometimes burns
Type IV	Brown	Rarely burns
Type V	Dark brown	Very rarely burns
Type VI	Black	Never burns

Type I: Mild
- 28–35 years old
- "No wrinkles"
- No keratosis
- Requires little or no makeup

Type II: Moderate
- 35–50 years old
- "Wrinkling in motion"
- Shallow complexion with early actinic keratosis
- Requires minimal makeup

Type III: Advanced
- 50–60 years old
- "Wrinkles at rest"
- Discoloration of the skin with telangectasias and actinic keratosis
- Always wears makeup

Type IV: Severe
- Over 60 years old
- "Only wrinkles"
- Photoaging, gravitational and dynamic forces affecting skin
- Actinic keratosis with or without cancer
- Wears makeup with poor coverage

the patient's confidence in the decision. Moderate to severe facial laxity, brow ptosis, and eyelid dermatochalasia require surgical intervention. Periorbital dynamic furrows generally require chemodenervation of the offending muscles with BTX-A. Occasionally, deep furrows in the glabellar region will require BTX-A and fillers to enhance the overall results. Perioral furrows such as nasolabial folds, marionette lines, and smoker's lines can be successfully treated with fillers. In appropriate patients, periorbital and perioral rhytids can also be treated successfully with laser resurfacing. Chemical peels can play an important role in nonsurgical facial rejuvenation in a similar manner to laser resurfacing.

ABLATIVE LASER RESURFACING

Laser resurfacing is a powerful tool that gives the surgeon precise control over the depth of ablation and the potential outcome. Laser facial rejuvenation can be broadly classified into two major divisions: ablative and nonablative. Ablative laser resurfacing techniques most commonly utilize the CO_2 and Er:YAG lasers (Fig. 16-2). The CO_2 laser (10,600 nm wavelength) vaporizes water containing skin tissue, resulting in thermal injury and tissue vaporization. By pulsing the delivery of the CO_2 laser, newer systems are able to vaporize the epidermal and dermal region without causing significant residual thermal damage.[12] Each pass of the CO_2 laser will ablate 20 to 100 μm of tissue (depending on the fluence) with 150 μm of residual thermal damage. The Er:YAG laser (2940 nm wavelength) is also absorbed by water, albeit at 12 to 18 times the efficiency of the CO_2 laser. At a fluence of 5 J/cm^2, the Er:YAG laser will vaporize about 5 to 20 μm with minimal residual thermal injury. As a result, the skin reepithelializes more rapidly and the postoperative course is shorter with Er:YAG laser resurfacing.

Clinically, I have seen two phases of rejuvenation with ablative laser resurfacing. The first phase is the immediate improvement in wrinkles that disappears within 2 to 3 months. A second phase begins in the ensuing months with "reimprovement" of rhytids and tightening of the skin. My experience with ablative lasers over the past decade in close to 1000 patients suggests that CO_2 and Er:YAG achieve comparable results. If Er:YAG treatment entails a high number of passes (greater than five), its depth of injury is similar to that of CO_2 lasers.

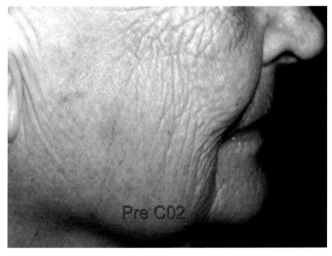

A

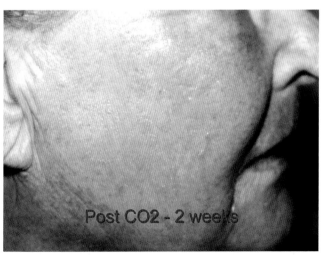

B

Figure 16-2 Preoperative (**A**) and postoperative (**B**) photographs of a patient who received ablative laser resurfacing.

Laser resurfacing is indicated for patients with perioral and periorbital rhytids, furrows, mild lower eyelid dermatochalasia, actinic changes, and facial elastosis. Preoperative preparations include 2 to 4 weeks of tretinoin (Retin-A) and hydroquinone application to speed epidermal migration and reduce postoperative hyperpigmentation. Patients are routinely prescribed acyclovir 3 days before and cefuroxime beginning 12 hours before surgery. Full face procedures are performed under conscious sedation with regional nerve blocks. Halcion has been used orally in place of IV sedation in some cases. Regional procedures generally require only nerve blocks.

The CO_2 laser is performed on surgically prepped skin that is then immaculately dried. With the Ultrapulse CO_2 laser (Lumenis, Santa Clara, CA), I use a setting of 300 mJ at a fluence of 5 J/cm^2 with a rectangular pattern. The white char is removed using wet gauze and the face is dried again. The first pass generally removes about 60 to 100 μm of tissue reaching the superficial dermis. Pinpoint bleeding may begin depending upon the area of the face. A second pass at this setting is required if collagen remodeling and substantial long-term benefits are to be achieved. It is on the second pass that the long-term aesthetic results of laser resurfacing are observed with the ablation of the shoulders of the wrinkles and collagen contraction. The latter can be quite dramatic to any observer. Even though further beneficial effects may be achieved by a third pass, many experienced laser surgeons avoid further passes while treating the eyelids or upper lips. I have routinely used a spot third pass in both of these areas without adverse sequelae. One wants to avoid a grayish hue, which indicates imminent penetration of subcutaneous fat. After a final removal of char, I apply refrigerated Vigilon (C.R. Bard, Murray Hill, NJ) and the patient is discharged. The Vigilon is removed in 24 to 48 hours by the nursing staff.

Postoperative care after bandage removal entails alternating cold vinegar and water soaks with the application of plain Aquaphor (Beiersdorf AG, Hamburg, Germany). Local débridement of crusts and copious use of Aquaphor create a clean and moist environment, which speeds up the healing process and epidermal cell migration. The patients are able to apply make-up once the skin has re-epithelialized within 7 to 10 days. Patients must be warned about postoperative erythema, which can persist up to 6 to 8 weeks.

Adverse sequelae resulting from ablative laser resurfacing include infection (usually candidiasis), hypopigmentation, persistent erythema, and elevated scars (normally seen after extended erythema). Hyperpigmentation, which occurs more frequently in darker-skinned (Fitzpatrick type IV to VI) individuals, usually resolves with medical management. Hypopigmentation more frequently affects individuals with fair skin (Fitzpatrick type I). Hypopigmentation, a less common complication, can be a serious adverse outcome, as the skin rarely repigments to its normal color. Therefore, the higher risk candidates for adverse pigmentation issues are lighter skinned individuals. Strict perioperative protocols virtually eliminate persistent postoperative erythema and elevated scars.

Although the introduction of collagen provided a foreshadowing of nonsurgical procedures, it was the advent of the CO_2 laser resurfacing that ushered in the modern era of noninvasive technologies by the virtue of its remarkable aesthetic outcome. The demand of laser resurfacing has waned over the past few years, as it is now perceived by patients as being too invasive.

NONABLATIVE LASER RESURFACING

Nonablative lasers such as the N-lite (ICN Photonics, UK) and Cool Touch (Cool Touch Corp., Roseville, CA) have been developed with the intent to stimulate and remodel collagen without significantly injuring the epidermis. With multiple treatments, nonablative lasers can clinically reproduce in a limited manner the second phase of skin remodeling that is seen with ablative lasers. Nonablative lasers do not produce any collagen contraction and therefore cannot cause localized tightening of tissue (e.g., lower eyelids). The most clinically studied nonablative laser is the Cool Touch. Cool Touch is a pulsed neodymium:yttrium-aluminum-garnet laser (Nd:YAG; 1320 nm wavelength) that has a fiberoptic hand piece coupled to a thermal sensing cryogenic spray. The coupling of Nd:YAG to a cooling system allows delivery of thermal energy to the dermis while preventing epidermal thermal damage.[13]

This laser can be used on all skin types.[14] Preoperative preparation is not necessary, although local anesthesia may be required for certain patients. The treatment technique is very simple. The laser utilizes minimally overlapping nonstacking pulses. Stacking the pulses will abort the desired collagen synthesis. The patients will typically require multiple treatments. Each additional treatment improves the depth of the wrinkles, which may be seen as early as 1 month after the first treatment. Treatment intervals can be as short as 2 weeks, although 3 to 6 months is the most common, because collagen synthesis appears to continue for 6 weeks after each session. The most common indication for this treatment modality is improvement of fine periorbital and perioral rhytids. There is no associated pain and minimal postoperative care and complication (Fig. 16-3).

CHEMICAL PEELS

In the 1990s chemical peeling relinquished much of its application to the CO_2 and erbium lasers. Lasers are perceived to provide superior control to the physician,

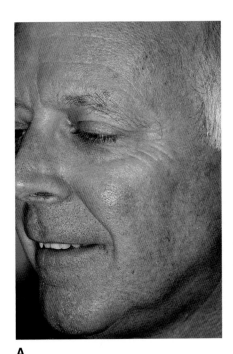

A

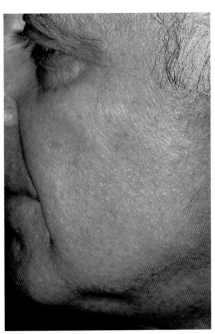

B

Figure 16-3 Preoperative (**A**) and postoperative (**B**) photographs of the periorbital region of a man who received three treatments of N-lite nonablative laser resurfacing.

resulting in more predictable results. Chemical peels, however, do have certain well-clarified indications and can serve as an important tool in an aesthetic practice. Medium to deep peels cause a chemical necrosis at the papillary to reticular dermal level, while the superficial peels generally affect the epidermal stratum corneum.

SUPERFICIAL PEELS

Superficial peels include glycolic (alpha hydroxy) and beta hydroxy acids. They function in a similar manner to microdermabrasion by improving the skin's overall appearance. Superficial peels remove stratum corneum and even out cutaneous pigmentation. Glycolic peel preparations vary widely, and one should become accustomed to a single brand because variations in concentration and pH cannot be readily transposed from one proprietary peel to another. Additionally, practitioners must understand the other variables that would affect the depth of penetration and the ultimate outcome (i.e., pre-peel treatment with retinoic acid, duration of application, the physical pressure of the Q-tip at the time of peel, length of time that chemical is left on before dilution with water or bicarbonate).

MEDIUM PEELS

The classic medium-depth peel is trichloracetic acid (TCA). Previously, 50% concentration was used but in recent years a 35% concentration immediately following a superficial peel (CO_2 ice or Jessner's peel) has become popular because it reduces side effects while maintaining efficacy. Rhytids can be improved by medium-depth peels

but not superficial peels. The histologic effects of medium-depth peels extend just short of the junction of the papillary and reticular dermis.

DEEP PEELS

Deep peels are performed with phenol, usually 88% mixed with croton oil (Baker's formula). The croton oil may play more of an active role than previously suspected. Injury extends to the reticular dermis with a healing period of 7 to 10 days. Phenol peels can significantly improve rhytids. Pigmentation changes however are common. Deep peels must be performed by experienced physicians in a controlled environment and under sedation. Phenol peels can potentially cause significant cardiac and renal toxicity. Cardiac complications can be avoided by hydrating the patient perioperatively, providing close cardiac monitoring, and allowing 20 minutes between applications to each facial subunit.

INJECTABLE SUBSTANCES

Bovine collagen dominated the U.S. market for over two decades while the availability of filler substances in Europe approached 100 different compounds. The early years of the new millennium brought several new injectables onto the U.S. market. We will classify them into broad clinical categories of temporary and long-acting (Box 16-2). Each injectable substance has to be placed in an appropriate skin location to maximize aesthetic outcome while limiting potential complications (Fig. 16-4).

Box 16-2   Temporary and Long-Acting Injectables

Temporary

Collagen
Trade names: Zyplast, Zyderm, CosmoDerm, CosmoPlast
Category: filler
Duration: 2–4 months
Allergy testing: Zyplast and Zyderm only
Injection site: superficial/mid-dermis

Stabilized hyaluronic acid
Trade names: Restylane, Hylaform, Captique, Perlane, Juvederm
Category: filler
Duration: 4–8 months
Allergy testing: no
Injection site: mid-dermis

Botulinum toxin type A
Trade name: Botox
Category: neurotoxin paralytic agent
Duration: 3–4 months
Allergy testing: no
Injection site: muscle
Notes: only product in its category, best choice for crow's-feet and dynamic rhytids/furrows of forehead

Long-acting

Calcium hydroxylapatite
Trade names: Radiesse, Radiance FN
Category: filler
Duration: 2–5 years
Allergy testing: no
Injection site: deep dermis
Notes: FDA approval for vocal cord augmentation, higher incidence of nodules in lips

Polymethyl methacrylate
Trade name: Artefill
Category: filler
Duration: permanent
Allergy testing: yes
Injection site: deep dermis

Silicone
Trade names: Silikon 1000, Adato Silol 500
Category: filler/collagen stimulator
Duration: Permanent
Allergy testing: no
Injection site: deep dermis
Notes: FDA approved for ophthalmic use, excellent natural lip contour, newer silicone oils have much better safety profile, limited clinical experience with newer products

Poly-L-lactic acid
Trade names: Sculptra, New-fill
Category: volumizer
Duration: 1–2 years
Allergy testing: no
Injection site: dermal-subcutaneous junction
Notes: FDA approved for HIV lipoatrophy, only product in its class that produces significant volume enhancement

COLLAGEN

Bovine collagen was the first filler on the market, heralding the modern era of noninvasive facial rejuvenation in the 1980s. Even with the advent of longer acting fillers, bovine- and human-derived collagen products continue to be used extensively in the clinical setting. Collagen products are delivered with lidocaine and therefore do not require local anesthetic. Duration of activity for most collagen fillers is generally 2 to 3 months. Zyderm and Zyplast are bovine derived and require skin testing. Many physicians will require two skin tests with 1-month and 2-week delays to decrease the rate of false negative results. The newer generation of collagen products such as CosmoDerm and CosmoPlast (Inamed Aesthetics, Santa Barbara, CA) are human derived and do not require skin testing.

Zyderm is typically injected in the superficial dermis; Zyplast is placed in the mid-dermis using a 30-gauge needle, which I bend to between a 90- and 150-degree angle. One advantage of collagen over other fillers is the absence of significant stinging and swelling. Because there is very limited inflammation and edema, the results are more evident at the time of injection. The post-treatment edema is minimal and patients are able to return to work immediately. As longer lasting fillers become more popular, the role of collagen will likely diminish. Collagen may continue to have a role for lip augmentation as well as improving very fine furrows.

STABILIZED HYALURONIC ACID

There are currently several stabilized hyaluronic acid dermal fillers on the market, including Restylane (Medicis Aesthetics, Scottsdale, AZ), Hylaform (Inamed Aesthetics, Santa Barbara, CA), and Captique (Inamed Aesthetics, Santa Barbara, CA). Restylane is a cross-linked nonanimal stabilized hyaluronic acid that had long been available in Canada and Europe. It was first marketed in the United States in 2003 and has achieved rapid acceptance (Fig. 16-5). It does not require skin testing but does induce some stinging for several minutes and more swelling than collagen. Duration of therapeutic effects is up to twice that of collagen in most cases (4 to 6 months). It is usually injected into the mid-dermis using a 30-gauge needle, which I bevel up, as with collagen injections. Restylane has a tendency to diffuse into a wider area than Zyplast, making precision placement a little more difficult. On the other hand, it is clear and therefore nodularity on the lip is not as readily seen. The aftercare for Restylane is limited to the avoidance of extreme heat and sun for a few days. Most of the fillers are fragile in the presence of extreme heat. Hylaform is an animal-based hyaluronic acid which has not gained significant following in the United States. Perlane (Medicis Aesthetics, Scottsdale, AZ), which is longer acting than the other hyaluronic acids, will probably replace Restylane as the preferred filler for lip augmentation as well as other aesthetic applications. Juvederm (Inamed Aesthetics, Santa Barbara, CA), another cross-linked hyaluronic acid filler, was approved by the FDA in June 2006.

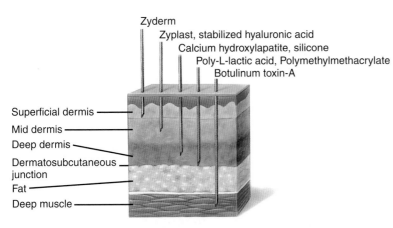

Zyderm
Zyplast, stabilized hyaluronic acid
Calcium hydroxylapatite, silicone
Poly-L-lactic acid, Polymethylmethacrylate
Botulinum toxin-A

Superficial dermis
Mid dermis
Deep dermis
Dermatosubcutaneous junction
Fat
Deep muscle

Figure 16-4 Each injectable product needs to be placed in an appropriate location in the skin: superficial dermis—Zyderm; mid dermis—Zyplast, stabilized hyaluronic acid; deep dermis—calcium hydroxylapatite, polymethyl methacrylate, silicone; dermal-subcutaneous junction—injectable poly-L-lactic acid; deep muscle—botulinum toxin type A

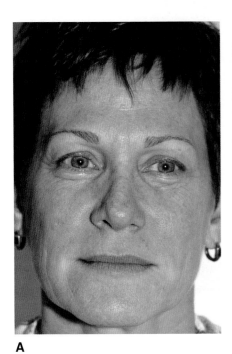

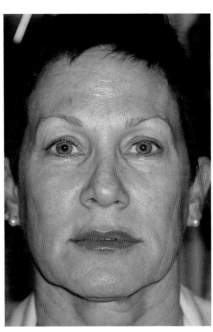

A   **B**

Figure 16-5 Preoperative (**A**) and postoperative (**B**) photographs of lip augmentation in a woman using hyaluronic acid.

BOTULINUM TOXIN TYPE A

BTX-A is a polypeptide neurotoxin derived from the anaerobic bacterium, *Clostridium botulinum*. Botox (Allergan, Irvine, CA) is currently the only FDA-approved BTX-A on the market. The mechanism of action for BTX-A is to prevent the release of acetylcholine from the presynaptic neuron at the neuromuscular end plate, thereby producing temporary chemical denervation and muscle weakness.[15] BTX-A treats furrows differently than do fillers; it reduces the muscle-induced elevations and thereby effects a flattening of the defect. Therein, BTX-A flattens the mountains while fillers raise the valleys. Originally produced in the 1970s and used for several years for strabismus and blepharospasm,[16-20] its cosmetic use began in the early 1990s for glabellar and frown furrows.[21-25] It was approved for such use in the United States in 2002. BTX-A remains, in my opinion, the treatment of choice among all for crow's-feet and female

forehead furrows (Fig. 16-6). In the case of greater muscular hypertrophy, such as the changes often seen in males, other fillers may also be required. Lower face rejuvenation with BTX-A has not gained significant popularity because of the complex anatomy and higher risks of unwanted complications. The administration of the toxin appears disarmingly simple in the periorbital region and in the vast majority of cases is administered without side effects and with substantial therapeutic benefit. It is when exceptional results occur that an understanding of both the physiology and facial anatomy can separate the technician from the physician.

Botox should be stored prior to and after reconstitution at 2° to 8° C. Botox can probably be stored up to 2 weeks after reconstitution without loss of vitality. During the preparation phase, avoid vigorous shaking, air bubbles, or contact with alcohol through the stopper (do not insert needle when wet). The manufacturer recom-

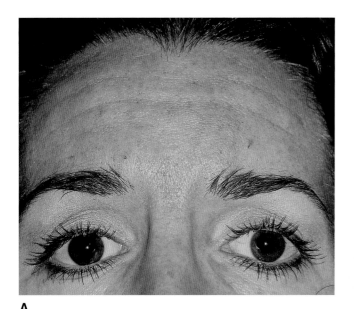

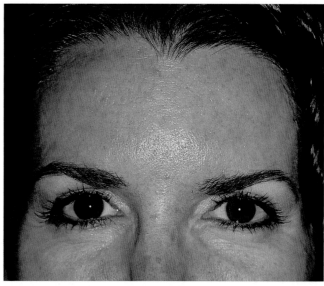

A

B

Figure 16-6 Preoperative (**A**) and postoperative (**B**) photographs of a patient with improvement of forehead rhytids after botulinum toxin type A injection.

mends a 2.5:1 dilution. I usually use 2:1 or 3:1 dilution. Dilutions up to 10:1 have shown equal effectiveness, but duration and precision of delivery may be compromised at higher dilutions.

The clinical approach varies from physician to physician. The typical patient is injected for horizontal forehead lines with a total of 9 units divided equally among three injection sites superficially along the frontalis: midway between the frontal hairline and the

eyebrow at both midpupillary lines and center of the forehead (Fig. 16-7). In patients whose lines are deeper or extended further laterally, I will use 16 units divided into a total of four injection sites with the furthest lateral being above the midpupillary line. Sometimes I may divide the 16 units with 5 units at each of the far lateral sites and 3 units each in the two more medial sites. One may "chase," with 1 to 2 units either at the time of the initial session or in 2 weeks, lines that may have been missed just

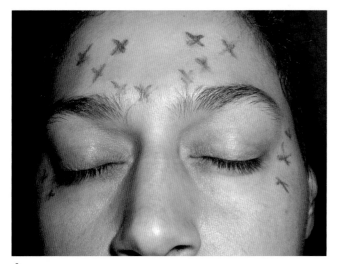

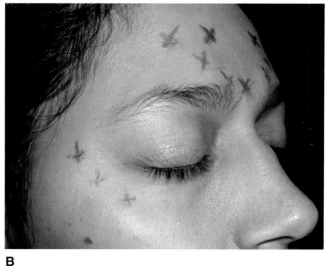

A

B

Figure 16-7 Botulinum toxin type A injection sites in the periorbital region. In patients with deep forehead rhytids, four injection sites (4 units per site) are utilized halfway between the hairline and eyebrow (**A**). The most lateral injection is placed above the midpupillary line. For glabellar rhytids, five deep injections are used in females. In a typical female 6 units are injected into the mid procerus just below a line joining the eyebrows. Four units are then injected into each corrugator supercilii on a line vertically above the medial canthus and above the superior orbital rim. An additional 3 units is injected about 1 cm above this area, and slightly laterally, thereby producing a "V" injection pattern. For the crow's-feet, 12 units are typically injected superficially at three sites on each side (**B**). It is important to stay at least 1 cm lateral to the orbital rim and above the inferior zygomatic rim in order to avoid complications.

above the eyebrows. Brow ptosis may occur if corrugators and procerus muscle are not treated. This is usually avoided if one stays at least 1.5 cm above the superior orbital rim. In fact, where ptosis has occurred previously in a patient, it is judicious to treat the frown area first and wait 2 weeks to treat the horizontal forehead furrows. I use 20 units to treat the glabellar area in women and, generally, 30 units for men. The needle is directed upward to avoid downward migration into the orbicularis oculi with resultant lid ptosis. Five deep injections (frontalis fibers may run superficial to the corrugators) are used in women, and two additional 5-unit injections above the midpupillary area (1.5 cm above the eyebrow) are used in thick-furrowed men. In a typical woman, 6 units are injected into the midprocerus just below a line joining the eyebrows. Four units are then injected into each corrugator supercilii along a vertical line above the medial canthus and the superior orbital rim. An additional 3 units is injected 1 cm superior and lateral to this area, producing a "V" injection pattern. In patients with flat brows, a total of 10 additional units are injected as noted earlier. It should be noted that this is my personal approach; the FDA trials used seven injection sites on all patients for the glabellar area.

For the crow's-feet, a variable dosage is utilized, depending upon the muscle thickness and location of furrows; 12 units are generally injected superficially at two or three sites on each side. It is important to stay at least 1 cm lateral to the lateral orbital rim and above the inferior zygomatic rim in order to avoid diplopia or lid ptosis. For lower eyelid folds, 1 to 1.5 units can be injected in each lower lid about 3 mm below the lid margin along the midpupilary line. This may cause widening of the eyes in some patients, which can be aesthetically pleasing. Patients must have a normal snap test in order to avoid unwanted lower lid malposition.

BTX-A treatment of perioral furrows, which usually occur secondary to orbicularis oris hypertrophy, carries a higher risk of complication and inconsistent results. Perioral furrows that have not responded well to fillers can be treated with 0.5 unit of BTX-A in each furrow up to a maximum of 2 units for each half of the lip (maximum of 4 units per lip). Downward turn of the oral commissure can be treated with 2 to 3 units into the extension of each nasolabial fold just above the ramus of the mandible, thereby paralyzing the depressor anguli oris. Excessive dosage and misplacement of toxin can lead to facial asymmetry in this region because perioral muscles have very complex and dynamic functions. Vertical platysmal lines in the neck can be successfully injected with up to 25 units in each vertical band (about 5 units every 1.0 cm). Two-unit injections at 1.0-cm intervals can also be placed into the dermis of horizontal "necklace" bands up to a total of 30 units.

Patients are advised to squint, raise their brows, or smile for 4 hours after treatment, depending upon the area treated, in order to facilitate movement of the toxin into the treated muscle groups. Touching of the area is strictly avoided, and patients with treated glabellar areas should probably not lie down for 3 to 4 hours to avoid ptosis. Contraindications to BTX-A are neuromuscular disease and pregnancy; relative contraindications are psychiatric disease with somatic manifestations, such as hysterical conversion reactions.

POLYMETHYL METHACRYLATE

PMMA was the first permanent filler approved for aesthetic use in the United States for treatment of nasolabial furrows under the trade name of Artefill (Artes Medical, San Diego, CA). PMMA microspheres are 30 to 40 μm and therefore probably are not taken up by macrophages. Collagen skin testing is required because Artefill consists of PMMA suspended in 3.5% bovine collagen and 0.3% lidocaine. Experience with PMMA began in the early 1990s in Germany.[26] Outside the United States, this product uses closed German herd hides for its collagen source; the U.S. product utilizes American hides.

I treated the first patient in the United States beginning FDA trials in 1998 and discovered that there is a distinct learning curve.[27] The material is injected into the dermis at the dermal-subcutaneous junction. This area is assessed by both visual and tactile guidelines: lack of visible needle tip and absence of reduced resistance of adipose tissue. Overcorrection should be avoided. Twenty percent of the fill will be with the PMMA granules and 80% with the temporary bovine collagen. This latter 80% is eventually replaced by the patient's own collagen in response to the presence of plastic PMMA microspheres. There is a quick dissipation of Artefill bovine collagen. After the treatment, there is a tapering of aesthetic improvement at about 1 month with "reimprovement" occurring over the next 2 to 3 months. At 4 months the histology is normally stabilized.

PMMA must be reserved for expression furrows and atrophic acne and varicella scars. The product should not be used for the treatment of fine rhytids. Initially, undercorrection is often achieved when the practitioner is concerned with producing irregularities. Once a more appropriate quantity is delivered, re-treatment incidences approach those reported by the inventor of Artefill, Professor Gottfried Lemperle.[28] My experience with Artefill has demonstrated excellent long-term resolution of nasolabial folds, upper lip furrows, marionette lines, and glabellar furrows for periods of over 5 years (Fig. 16-8). It offers a valuable alternative to temporary fillers. As of this writing, Artefill is still not approved for release in the United States. It is expected that any use other than for nasolabial folds will be considered "off label."

Early experience with PMMA was compromised by frequent granuloma development. This appeared to have been related to manufacturing issues. Since 1994, the

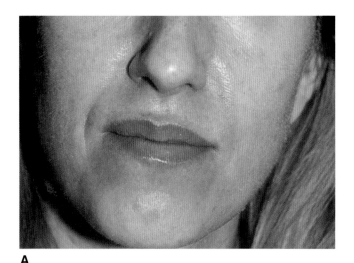
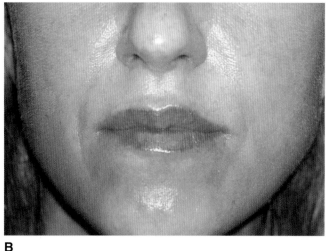

A

B

Figure 16-8 Preoperative (**A**) and postoperative (**B**) photographs of a 47-year-old woman who had long-term nasolabial fold improvement (4 years) with polymethyl methacrylate (Artefill).

reported incidence of granuloma formation has been below 0.01%. The cause of granuloma is unknown but seems to occur after the second and third treatments. Treating patients who have systemic infections also appears to raise the likelihood of granulomas.

CALCIUM HYDROXYLAPATITE

CaHA (Radiesse, BioForm Medical, San Mateo, CA) is a semipermanent filler that has enjoyed a quick surge of popularity since it was first introduced into the U.S. market in 2002.[29-32] Radiesse, formerly known as Radiance FN, is synthesized CaHA particles (25 to 45 μm) suspended in glycerin, water, and sodium carboxymethylcellulose. Because CaHA occurs naturally in bone and teeth, skin testing is not required. It is FDA approved for vocal fold augmentation and is used as a tissue marker because of its radiopaque characteristic. Presently, it is being used off label for facial aesthetic enhancement (Fig. 16-9). Published reports have been limited with regard to its use as a facial filler, but research in animals and its internal use suggests duration of 2 to 5 years.[29-32] We have seen duration of 18 to 24 months and counting. The material is injected into the lower dermis and overcorrection is avoided. I prefer to have two treatment sessions with a 1-month interval. There is a somewhat greater tendency toward edema and bruising with Radiesse than with other fillers. It should be used with caution in the lips as there is a higher tendency for nodule formation[32] (I have refrained from using it here). Because of the immediate tissue edema, there is a need for a more rapid injection so that one does not mistake swelling for correction. In case of overcorrection, simple surgical extirpation appears to be more effective than intralesional steroids because most of the augmentation is

secondary to the actual substance rather than the local collagen response. The overall risk of granuloma formation is very low (probably the lowest of all fillers) with this product.

SILICONE

Injectable silicone oil has experienced a comeback in aesthetic facial rejuvenation in the 2000s, although its use had never fully disappeared during its banned period of over 2 decades.[33-35] Two silicone oils, Adato SIL-ol 5000 (Bausch & Lomb Surgical, Rochester, NY) and Silikon 1000 (Alcon, Fort Worth, TX), were approved in 2000 for ophthalmic use. Silicone is polymerized dimethylsiloxane that can take the form of solid, gel, or liquid depending on its polymerization and cross-linkage. The highly viscous medical-grade liquid silicone products are presently being used off label for permanent lip augmentation and treatment of facial furrows.

For lip augmentation, multiple microinjections ("microdroplets") are given along the vermilion borders of the lips with additional two or three injections into the mucosal aspect of the mid-upper lip. Microdroplets consist of 0.01 mL injections separated by at least 2 to 10 mm. A total of approximately 0.1 mL is injected in each lip. The silicone functions solely as a collagen stimulator and not as a filler. The effects of silicone treatments are gradual. The regional edema is gone by the next day and patients must be apprised of the fact that the process occurs slowly. An inflammatory process occurs with subsequent fibrosis, creating delicate collagen strands around each microdroplet. Although patients are almost uniformly pleased, they must be made aware that there are limitations as to the size that can be achieved.

The use of medical grade silicone is still controversial.

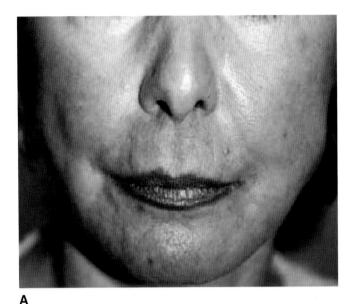

A

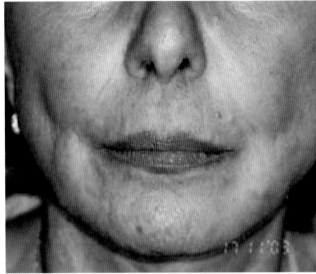

B

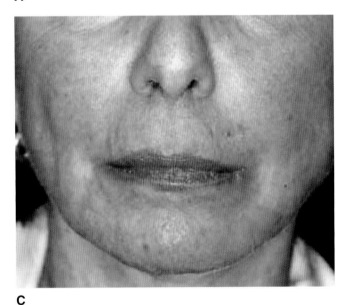

C

Figure 16-9 Long-term nasolabial fold and marionette furrow effacement with synthesized calcium hydroxylapatite (Radiesse). Preoperative (**A**), 10-month postoperative (**B**), and 2-year postoperative (**C**) photographs.

Webster reported minimal complication with the microdroplet technique in over 500 patients using pure medical-grade silicone.[36] Others have reported local and systemic complications such as chronic inflammation, migration, granuloma formation, hepatitis, pulmonary embolism, and pneumonitis.[37-39] These complications are most likely related to large-volume facial augmentation, poor-quality silicone, and improper technique. In my experience, silicone appears to yield the most natural lip augmentation results of any injectable with an extraordinarily low incidence of complications. I have, however, observed patients from other physicians with nodules resulting from silicone injected in the glabella, forehead, and nasolabial folds while not finding a similar circumstance in lip augmentation. I limit my use of silicone to lip augmentation only.

INJECTABLE POLY-L-LACTIC ACID

PLA (Sculptra, Dermik Aesthetics, Bridgewater, NJ) is a soft tissue filler that appears to be a valuable addition to our armamentarium. PLA, previously known as New-fill in Europe, is a compound that causes an inflammatory reaction to the overlying skin.[40,41] It is FDA approved for human immunodeficiency virus (HIV) patients with facial lipoatrophy and is currently being used as an off-label product for aesthetic facial rejuvenation. Lipoatrophy develops in 15% to 80% of individuals who are treated with antiretroviral therapy that contains protease inhibitors or nucleoside reverse transcriptase inhibitors.[42] PLA is slightly different from other fillers as it provides volume restoration to the treated area in a comparable manner as autologous fat injections. It usually requires three to six injections, depending on the degree of volume restoration. European studies have shown that it can last up to 2 years but usually requires annual touch-up injections.[40,41] PLA can be used for the treatment of HIV lipoatrophy, aesthetic facial volume restoration, and enhancement of deep rhytids and furrows.

Sculptra is typically mixed with 3.5 mL of saline and 1.5 mL of lidocaine (without epinephrine) 6 to 24 hours prior to the treatment. This regimen appears to have reduced the rate of granuloma formation and needle clumping. The injections are performed using a 25-gauge needle after topical anesthetic is applied. PLA is typically injected in the junction of dermis and subcutaneous fat. Special care is made not to overcorrect the area. The injection and immediate results are impressive as the plane of injection is extremely fluid. Ice is applied postoperatively, and the practitioner should aggressively massage the treated regions. The patients are encouraged to continue massaging the injected areas and must understand that the immediate correction dissipates over the ensuing 10 days. The dermal/epidermal thickening begins about 3 weeks later and the third session typically produces the most dramatic results. Complications include erythema, edema, granuloma formation, and irregularity. The product's complication profile has improved since its initial use in Europe. Overall, the complication rates are reported to be lower if the product is diluted appropriately and injected in the proper plane.[40,41] It should be understood by all physicians that all fillers may be associated with true granulomas with varying incidences.

Future Considerations

The future of nonsurgical facial rejuvenation will likely focus on longer-acting fillers and creating more effective nonablative laser technology. Several new classes of botulinum toxins are undergoing FDA trials and will likely increase the product line of neuromuscular paralytic injectables. Although surgical intervention will remain an important aspect of facial rejuvenation, nonsurgical alternatives will continue to gain acceptance as reliable alternatives for younger patients.

REFERENCES

1. Goldman L, Blaney DJ, Kindel J Jr, et al: Pathology of the effect of the laser beam on the skin. Nature 1963;197:912.
2. Goldman L, Blaney DJ, Freemond A, et al: The biomedical aspects of lasers. JAMA 1964;188(20):302.
3. Goldman L, Blaney DJ, Kindel DJ Jr, et al: Effect of the laser beam on the skin. Preliminary report. J Invest Dermatol 1963;40:121.
4. Laub DR, Yules RB, Arras M, et al: Preliminary histopathological observation of Q-switched ruby laser radiation on dermal tattoo pigment in man. J Surg Res 1968;8(5):220.
5. Goldman L, Wilson RG, Hornby P, et al: Radiation from a Q-switched ruby laser: Effect of repeated impacts of power output of 10 megawatts on a tattoo of a man. J Invest Dermatol 1965;44:69.
6. Dixon JA, Rotering RH, Huether SE: Patient's evaluation of argon laser therapy of port wine stain, decorative tattoo, and essential telangiectasia. Lasers Surg Med 1984;4(2):181.
7. Apfelberg DB, Maser MR, Lash H, et al: The argon laser for cutaneous lesions. JAMA 1981;245(20):2073.
8. Hamilton D: A classification of the aging face and its relationship to remedies. J Clin Dermatol 1998;3:35.
9. Fitzpatrick RA, Goldman MP, Satur NM, et al: Pulsed carbon dioxide laser resurfacing of photo-aged facial skin. Arch Dermatol 1996;132(4):395.
10. Fitzpatrick TB: The validity and practicality of sun-reactive skin types I through VI. Arch Dermatol 1988;124(6):869.
11. Glogau RG: Aesthetic and anatomic analysis of the aging skin. Semin Cutan Med Surg 1996;15(3):134.
12. Koch RJ: Laser skin resurfacing. Facial Plast Surg Clin North Am 2001;9(3):329.
13. Lask GL, Lee PK, Seyfadeh M, et al: Nonablative laser treatment of facial rhytids. SPIE Proc 1997;2970:338.
14. Newman J: Nonablative laser skin tightening. Facial Plast Surg Clin North Am 2001;9(3):343.
15. Brin MF: Botulinum toxin: Chemistry, pharmacology, toxicity, and immunology. Muscle Nerve 1997;6(suppl):X146.
16. Scott AB: Botulinum toxin injection into extraocular muscles as an alternative to strabismus surgery. J Pediatr Ophthalmol Strabismus 1980;17(1):21.
17. Scott AB, Rosenbaum A, Collins CC: Pharmacologic weakening of extraocular muscles. Invest Ophthalmol 1973;12(12):924.
18. Scott AB: Botulinum toxin injection of eye muscles to correct strabismus. Trans Am Ophthalmol Soc 1981;79:734.
19. Scott AB: Botulinum toxin injection into extraocular muscles as an alternative to strabismus surgery. Ophthalmology 1980;87(10):1044.
20. Clark RP, Berris CE: Botulinum toxin: A treatment for facial asymmetry caused by facial nerve paralysis. Plast Reconstr Surg 1989;84(2):353.
21. Blitzer A, Brin MF, Keen MS, et al: Botulinum toxin for the treatment of hyperfunctional lines of the face. Arch Otolaryngol Head Neck Surg 1993;119:1018.
22. Keen M, Blitzer A, Aviv J, et al: Botulinum toxin A for hyperkinetic facial lines: Results of a double-blind, placebo-controlled study. Plast Reconstr Surg 1994;94(1):94.
23. Carruthers A, Kiene K, Carruthers J: Botulinum A exotoxin use in clinical dermatology. J Am Acad Dermatol 1996;34(5 Pt 1):788.
24. Foster JA, Barnhorst D, Papay F, et al: The use of botulinum A toxin to ameliorate facial kinetic frown lines. Ophthalmology 1996;103(4):618.
25. Garcia A, Fulton JE Jr: Cosmetic denervation of the muscles of facial expression with botulinum toxin. A dose-response study. Dermatol Surg 1996;22(1):39.
26. Lemperle F, Hazan-Gauthier N, Lemperle M: PMMA microspheres (Artecoll) for skin and soft tissue augmentation. Part II: Clinical investigations. Plast Reconstr Surg 1995;96:627.
27. Hamilton D: A pilot study of the first patients treated in the United States with Artecoll implantations for the aging face. Cosmet Dermatol 2001;14(9):47.
28. Lemperle G, Hazan-Gauthier N, Lemperle M: PMMA microspheres (Artecoll) for long-lasting corrections of

wrinkles: Refinements and statistical results. Aesthet Plast Surg 1998;22:356.

29. Flaharty P: Radiance. Facial Plast Surg 2004;20(2):165.

30. Skylar JA, White SM: Radiance FN: A new soft tissue filler. Dermatol Surg 2004;30(5):764.

31. Tzikas TL: Evaluation of the Radiance FN soft tissue filler for facial soft tissue augmentation. Arch Facial Plast Surg 2004;6(4):234.

32. Kanchwala SK, Holloway L, Bucky LP: Reliable soft tissue augmentation: A clinical comparison of injectable soft-tissue fillers for facial-volume augmentation. Ann Plast Surg 2005;55(1):30.

33. Benedetto AV, Lewis AT: Injecting 1000 centistoke liquid silicone with ease and precision. Dermatol Surg 2003;29(3):211.

34. Orentreich D, Leone AS: A case of HIV-associated facial lipoatrophy treated with 1000-cs liquid injectable silicone. Dermatol Surg 2004;30(4 Pt 1):548.

35. Jones DH, Carruthers A, Orentreich D, et al: Highly purified 1000-cSt silicone oil for treatment of human immunodeficiency virus-associated facial lipoatrophy: An open pilot trial. Dermatol Surg 2004;30(10):1279.

36. Webster RC, Fuleihan NS, Gaunt JM, et al: Injectable silicone for small augmentation: Twenty year experience in humans. Am J Cosmet Surg 1984;1(4):1.

37. Bigata X, Ribera M, Bielsa I, et al: Adverse granulomatous reaction after cosmetic dermal silicone injection. Dermatol Surg 2001;27(2):198.

38. Ficarra G, Mosqueda-Taylor A, Carlos R: Silicone granuloma of the facial tissues: A report of seven cases. Oral Surg Oral Med Oral Pathol Oral Radiol Endod 2002;94(1):65.

39. Pearl RM, Laub DR, Kaplan EN: Complications following silicone injections for augmentation of the contours of the face. Plast Reconstr Surg 1978;61:888.

40. Vochelle D: The use of poly-L-lactic acid in the management of soft-tissue augmentation: A five-year experience. Semin Cutan Med Surg 2004;23(4):223.

41. Humble G, Mest D: Soft tissue augmentation using sculptra. Facial Plast Surg 2004;20(2):157.

42. Burgess CM, Quiroga RM: Assessment of the safety and efficacy of poly-L-lactic acid for the treatment of HIV-associated facial lipoatrophy. J Am Acad Dermatol 2005;52(2):233.

CHAPTER SEVENTEEN

Lateral Canthoplasty

Robert E. Levine, MD

HISTORY

Lateral canthal surgery was initially utilized for paralytic and functional ectropion.[1,2] In 1969, Tenzel[3] was the first to propose the lateral tarsal strip procedure as a method to repair lower lid malposition. In the 1970s, the rate of lower eyelid complications increased because of the rising popularity of skin-muscle flap blepharoplasty.[4-8] Subsequently, there has been a greater understanding of post-blepharoplasty complications as lateral canthal surgery is now routinely utilized for both the prevention and reconstruction of lower lid malposition.[9,10]

PERSONAL PHILOSOPHY

Lateral canthal surgery is an indispensable surgical tool for surgeons interested in performing aesthetic eyelid surgery. Lateral canthoplasty has a role in both preventing and correcting post-blepharoplasty eyelid malposition. Furthermore, it is an essential surgical tool for treating functional eyelid disorders such as paralytic, involutional, and cicatricial ectropion. Surgical treatment of the lateral canthus can allow adjustment of several lower eyelid variables such as the angle at which the lower lid meets the upper lid, tension on the lower lid, the position of the lower lid relative to the corneal limbus, and the anteroposterior position of the lower lid relative to the upper lid (Box 17-1). Ideally, the choice of procedure that is performed at the lateral canthus should allow the surgeon to tailor the procedure to accommodate all these variables. Currently, four lateral canthoplasty techniques are in common use[11]: the dermal orbicular pennant, the inferior retinacular lateral canthoplasty, the lateral retinacular suspension, and the lateral tarsal strip. The lateral tarsal strip is the only procedure that allows the surgeon to fully control all the important lower eyelid variables.

In my own experience, I have chosen to use three variations of the tarsal strip procedure to address the lateral canthus. By varying the basic tarsal strip procedure, the surgeon has a variety of options that can be adapted to solve a multiplicity of problems. The great advantage of this approach is that the surgeon has full control of the variables of lid position and tension as well as the angulation necessary to design the appropriate lateral canthus for a given patient. Because all these procedures are variations of a single technique, only one learning curve is required to master the full range of options. The surgeon can choose the least extensive procedure that will accomplish the desired lower lid repositioning. If the outcome is inadequate after attempting a lesser variant, the surgeon is still free to change to a variant that will give a greater effect. These three variations can be performed as isolated procedures or in combination with lower blepharoplasty and other reconstructive techniques.

ANATOMY

The anatomy of the eyelids has been discussed at length in Chapter 2. For the purposes of this section, the lower eyelid anatomy is separated into three functional layers, commonly referred to as lamellae (Fig. 17-1). The skin and orbicularis muscle make up the anterior lamella. The middle lamella is made up of the orbital septum, which originates from the inferior orbital rim and inserts onto the tarsal plate. The posterior lamella is composed of conjunctiva and lower lid retractors. The lower lid retractors are composed of the inferior rectus muscle as it extends into the capsulopalpebral fascia and surrounds the inferior oblique muscle.

The lower eyelid is suspended and supported by the medial and lateral canthi. The lateral canthal tendon extends from the pretarsal orbicularis oculi muscle and tarsus to the lateral orbital tubercle approximately 2 mm

---

Box 17-1 Lower Eyelid Variables that Can Be adjusted with Lateral Canthal Surgery

1. The angle at which the lower lid meets the upper lid, e.g., a sharp angle or a rounded canthal angle
2. Anterior posterior position of the lower lid relative to the upper lid, e.g., whether they meet in the same plane or whether the lower lid passes behind the upper lid
3. The tension on the lower lid
4. The position of the lower lid relative to the inferior corneal limbus in patients with lower lid retraction and scleral show

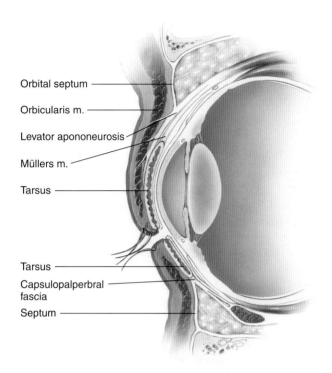

Orbital septum
Orbicularis m.
Levator apononeurosis
Müllers m.
Tarsus

Tarsus
Capsulopalperbral fascia
Septum

Figure 17-1 Eyelid anatomy. The lower eyelid is functionally composed of three lamellae. The skin and orbicularis muscle make up the anterior lamella. The middle lamella is made up of the orbital septum. The posterior lamella is composed of conjunctiva, capsulopalpebral fascia, and lower lid retractors.

inside the orbital rim.[12] The medial canthus is usually better suspended to the orbital rim than the lateral canthus and therefore medial ectropion occurs less frequently. The tarsus, canthal ligaments, and pretarsal orbicularis muscle provide upward support for the lid whereas the skin, orbital septum, and capsulopalpebral fascia exert an inferior pull.

Eyelid malposition can have two distinct components: ectropion and lid retraction. Ectropion arises when the lower eyelid margin turns away from the globe. Lid retraction with scleral show occurs when the eyelid is positioned inferiorly. The anatomic causes of lower lid malposition include vertical deficiencies in any of the three lamellae, generalized laxity of the canthal eyelid suspension complex, or weakness of the orbicularis oculi. Deficiency of the anterior lamella following aesthetic surgery is usually caused by aggressive skin and muscle resection, which may lead to lateral canthal rounding and ectropion. Lower lid retraction can result from middle lamellar insufficiency secondary to contracture and scarring of the septum. A shortened posterior lamella vertical deficiency usually results in entropion. Box 17-2 summarizes the issues related to post-blepharoplasty eyelid malposition.

PREOPERATIVE ASSESSMENT

Surgical manipulation of the upper eyelid is more forgiving than that for the lower eyelid. Post-blepharoplasty lower eyelid malposition such as ectropion and lid

Box 17-2   Blepharoplasty-related Eyelid Malposition

Etiology
1. Excess skin removal
2. Excess fat removal
3. Scar contracture
4. Orbicularis oculi muscle injury
5. Eyelid edema
6. Orbital septum adhesion
7. Hematoma
8. Lax lid margin
9. Proptosis
10. Unilateral high myopia

Predisposing factors
1. Involutional changes leading to hypotonicity
2. Malar hypoplasia
3. Shallow orbit
4. Graves' disease
5. Unilateral high myopia
6. Secondary blepharoplasty

Adapted from Cheney ML: Facial Surgery: Plastic & Reconstructive. Philadelphia: Williams & Wilkins, 1997.

retraction almost always occurs because of inadequate preoperative evaluation. Adequate eyelid assessment will allow the surgeon to select appropriate candidates for lower blepharoplasty. Patients who are at risk for postoperative eyelid malposition can then be appropriately managed with lateral canthal surgery. Careful preoperative analysis and judicious blepharoplasty techniques with lateral canthal surgery should virtually eliminate the long-term risk of post-blepharoplasty complications.

During the initial consultation, a complete history and physical examination are obtained. There are two patient populations that should be considered for lateral canthoplasty. The first group represents patients who are seeking surgical reconstruction for functional or post-blepharoplasty lower lid malposition. The second group represents aesthetic blepharoplasty patients who may require adjunctive procedures such as lateral canthoplasty. In the first group, the history and examination should focus on the cause and type of functional lid malposition in order to determine the appropriate surgical reconstruction. Post-blepharoplasty patients with lid malposition present with both aesthetic and functional complaints such as eye irritation, epiphora, blurry vision, and redness. In the second group, the surgeon should focus on key predisposing factors for post-blepharoplasty complications (see Box 17-2). A history of thyroid disorders, facial nerve paralysis, prior blepharoplasty, and trauma increase the risks of post-blepharoplasty eyelid retraction and ectropion. Patients with thyroid-related orbital disorders may present with scleral show, proptosis, lagophthalmos, and pseudoherniation of orbital fat. They should first be treated medically or by orbital decompression when appropriate.[13]

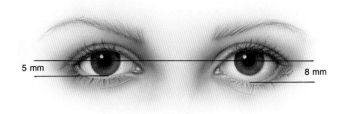

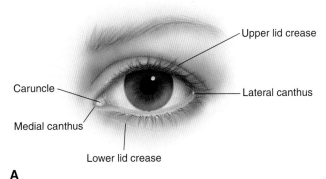

Figure 17-2 Marginal reflex distance-2. The Marginal reflex distance-2 (MRD$_2$) is measured from the corneal light reflex to the lower eyelid lash line when the patient is in a neutral gaze. The lash line should normally rest just above the lower limbus with an MRD$_2$ of 5 mm. In patients with lower lid retraction and scleral show, this distance is usually greater than 7 mm.

The physical examination usually begins with a thorough ophthalmologic evaluation including visual acuity and extraocular movement testing. Lower eyelid lash line should normally rest just above the inferior limbus in the neutral gaze (Fig. 17-2). A small amount of scleral show may be normal, but significant lid retraction is aesthetically and functionally disturbing. The marginal reflex distance-2 (MRD$_2$) can be used to objectively determine the significance of scleral show. MRD$_2$ is the distance between the corneal light reflex and the lower eyelid lash line, which is normally about 5 mm. The MRD$_2$ of patients with lower lid retraction and scleral show is usually greater than 7 mm.

The lateral canthal angle is formed by the junction of the upper and lower eyelid adjacent to the orbital rim. The lateral canthus in Caucasian patients should be approximately 2 mm superior to the medial canthus (Fig. 17-3). Lid laxity will reduce this difference. Snap test and lid distraction tests are performed to objectively evaluate the integrity of the lower eyelid canthal complex. The snap test is performed by pulling the lower eyelid down and away from the globe and asking the patient not to blink (Fig. 17-4). The eyelid should return to its normal resting position in less than 1 second. In the lid distraction test, the distance that the lower eyelid can be pulled away from the globe is measured (Fig. 17-5). A distance of greater than 7 to 10 mm represents a lax lid. Lateral canthal integrity can also be determined by grasping the lower eyelid and pulling it medially (Fig. 17-6). This maneuver can usually give the surgeon an understanding of the degree of laxity.

The orbitofacial vector must also be determined during the physical examination. A negative vector due to real or apparent exophthalmos is one of the main reasons patients develop postoperative eyelid complications.[14] A negative orbitofacial vector is diagnosed if a straight line drawn from the cornea falls anterior to the inferior orbital rim in the lateral view. This can result from malar hypoplasia or myopia as well as proptosis commonly present in Graves' ophthalmopathy.

After the examination, a surgical treatment plan must be established. In patients presenting for aesthetic ble-

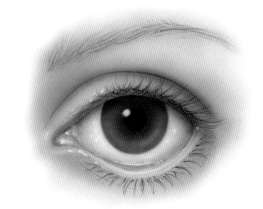

Figure 17-3 Lower lid malposition. The lateral canthus in Caucasian patients should be approximately 2 mm superior to the medial canthus (**A**). Ectropion arises when the lower eyelid margin turns away from the globe, and lid retraction with scleral show occurs when the eyelid is pulled inferiorly (**B**).

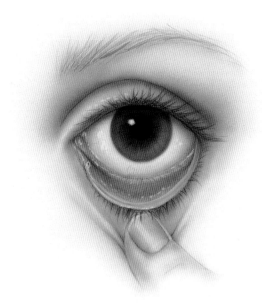

Figure 17-4 Snap test. The lower eyelid is pulled inferiorly and away from the globe. The eyelid should return to its normal resting position in less than 1 second.

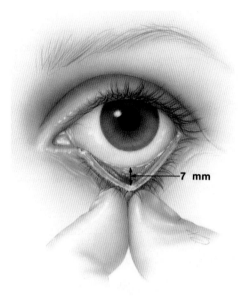

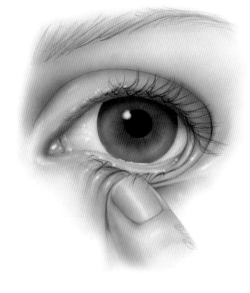

Figure 17-5 Lid distraction test. The lower eyelid is pulled away from the globe and the distance is measured. A distance of greater than 7 to 10 mm represents a lax lid.

Figure 17-6 Lateral canthal integrity. The degree of lateral canthal laxity can be determined by pulling the lower eyelid medially toward the medial canthal tendon.

pharoplasty, the history and examination will determine whether they will require simultaneous canthoplasty. In individuals who are diagnosed with ectropion or lower lid retraction, the type of canthoplasty must be determined. These patients may also require adjunctive procedures to reestablish the normal lower eyelid anatomy. Patients with middle lamellar contraction resulting in lower lid retraction may require spacers such as hard palate grafts[15] or high-density polyethylene (Medpor, Porex Surgical Products, Newnan, GA).[16,17] Patients with severe vertical deficiency of the anterior lamella (skin/orbicularis) may also require midface lifting or skin grafting.[18] Paralytic ectropion may necessitate spacers or slings with tensor fascia lata or palmaris longus.

SURGICAL TECHNIQUES

Lateral canthoplasty with or without blepharoplasty may be performed under local anesthesia with propofol sedation. This technique allows the surgeon to evaluate the surgical results and level of tightening with the patient in an upright position. Topical anesthetic in addition to 1% lidocaine with 1:100,000 epinephrine are utilized for the local anesthesia regimen.

TYPE I LATERAL CANTHOPLASTY: MAXIMUM LID REPOSITIONING

The first canthoplasty variant (Fig. 17-7) is similar to the tarsal strip procedure initially described by Tenzel in

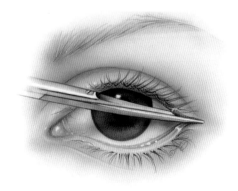

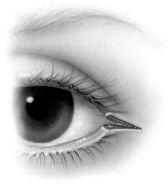

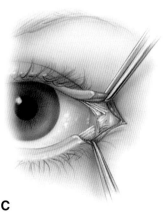

A **B** **C**

Figure 17-7 Type I lateral canthoplasty—maximum lid repositioning: A hemostat is used to clamp the lateral canthal angle (**A**). Lateral canthotomy is performed (**B**). The inferior canthal tendon and the inferolateral attachments of the lid are completely released so that the lid is freely movable (**C**).

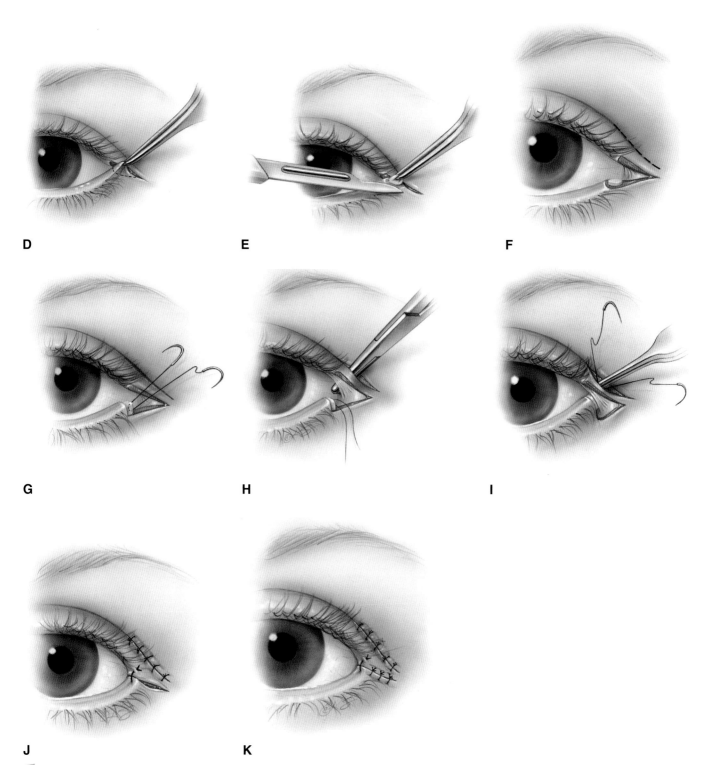

Figure 17-7 *Continued.* The lower lid is approximated to the desired position, with a slight overcorrection, and the extent of the proposed dissection marked (**D**). A tarsal tongue is created by excising the excess skin-muscle and mucocutaneous junction tissues (**E**). An incision is made to gain access to the upper arm of the lateral canthal tendon (**F**). A double-armed 4-0 Mersilene suture is sewn through the tarsus (**G**). Each arm is locked after undergoing a long and short pass. The lower arm is left longer for identification. A hemostat is passed under the upper arm of the lateral canthal tendon to create a tunnel (**H**). The sutures ends and tarsal tongue are brought into the tunnel (**I**). The ends of the suture are identified, and the superior suture placed superiorly, so as to not twist the tarsus. The Mersilene sutures are sewn into the lateral orbital rim periosteum after the desired lid position is determined (**J** and **K**). The sutures are always begun in the posterior periosteum so as to appose the lid well to the globe. A gray-line suture (5-0 plain gut) is placed to align the canthal angle. It is adjusted and tied simultaneously with the Mersilene sutures under appropriate tension. The Mersilene sutures are placed above the lateral raphe.

which the lateral end of the lid is freed entirely from its attachments, a tarsal strip is formed, and the strip is brought underneath the upper arm of the lateral canthal tendon. This variant is used when the maximal amount of lid tightening, lid elevation, or upward angulation of the canthus is required. It is also used when a canthal angle is desired wherein the lower lid passes behind the upper lid. It is important to keep in mind that if the lower lid is pulled too tightly over a prominent globe, the result will create a short chord that actually passes below the globe. In such instances, it is preferable to use a combination of other procedures together with the lateral canthoplasty, such as medial canthoplasty, fascia lata or palmaris longus suspension of the lid, or placement of a central stent to elevate the lid.

The maximal lid repositioning procedure begins with the clamping of the lateral canthal angle with a hemostat in order to improve surgical hemostasis. The clamp is removed and a lateral canthotomy performed. The inferior canthal tendon and the inferolateral attachments of the lid are completely released in order to allow the lid to freely move. The lower lid is approximated to the desired position, with a slight overcorrection, and the extent of the proposed dissection marked. Excess skin-muscle and mucocutaneous junction tissues are excised, leaving a tarsal tongue.

An incision is then made to gain access to the upper arm of the lateral canthal tendon. The lateral extension of an upper lid blepharoplasty incision may be utilized for this access. A double-armed 4-0 Mersilene suture is sewn through the tarsus. Each arm undergoes a long pass

followed by a short pass, and each arm is locked. The lower arm is left longer for identification. A tunnel is created by passing a hemostat under the upper arm of the lateral canthal tendon. The suture ends and tarsal tongue are brought under the tunnel and identified. The superior suture is placed superiorly in order not to twist the tarsus. A gray-line suture of 5-0 plain gut is placed to align the canthal angle. It is adjusted and tied simultaneous with the Mersilene sutures.

The Mersilene sutures are passed into the lateral orbital rim periosteum after determining the desired lid position. The sutures are always begun in the posterior periosteum, so as to appose the lid well to the globe. Sutures are tied under appropriate tension which can usually be ideally determined with the patient in the seated position on the operating table. Note that in this procedure, the sutures are placed above the lateral raphe.

TYPE II LATERAL CANTHOPLASTY: MODERATE LID TIGHTENING

The second canthoplasty variant differs from the type I canthoplasty; whereas the lid is still freed from the inferior arm of the lateral canthal tendon, it is not as completely released from its inferolateral attachments. The lower lid is therefore just free enough to be repositioned to the desired location. Additionally, instead of bringing the tarsal strip through a tunnel, it is sutured directly to the inner aspect orbital rim periosteum (Fig. 17-8). This variant is utilized when there is a moderate amount of lid laxity or preexisting eyelid malposition.

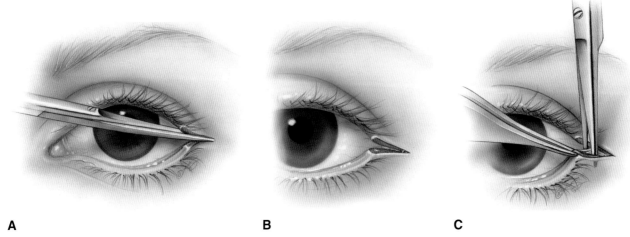

A   **B**   **C**

Figure 17-8 Type II lateral canthoplasty—moderate lid tightening. A hemostat is used to clamp the lateral canthal angle, and a lateral canthotomy is performed (**A**). Appearance of the lid after canthotomy (**B**). The inferior canthal tendon is cut, but the inferolateral attachments of the lid are only minimally released so that the lid is movable just enough for tightening (**C**).

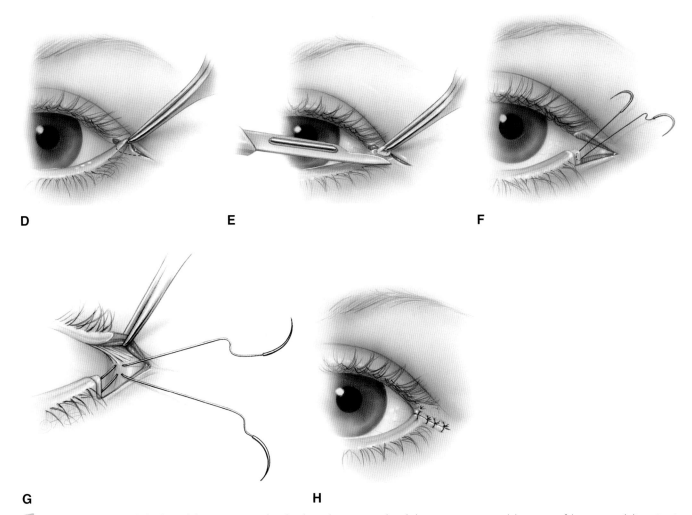

D   E   F

G   H

Figure 17-8 *Continued.* The lower lid is approximated to the desired position, with a slight overcorrection, and the extent of the proposed dissection is marked (**D**). Excess skin-muscle and mucocutaneous junction tissue are excised, leaving a tarsal tongue (**E**). A double-armed 4-0 Mersilene suture is sewn through tarsus (**F**). Each arm is locked after undergoing a long and short pass. The lower arm is left longer for identification. The sutures ends are passed directly into the orbital rim periosteum (**G**). No tunnels are made and the ends of the sutures are identified in order to place the superior suture cephalad so as to not twist the tarsus. The sutures are begun in the posterior periosteum in order to appose the lid and the globe. The sutures are placed at or below the lateral raphe. A gray-line suture of 5-0 plain gut is placed to align the canthal angle. It is adjusted and tied simultaneous with the Mersilene sutures (**H**).

The procedure is started by clamping the lateral canthal angle with a hemostat. Lateral canthotomy is then performed. The inferior canthal tendon is cut, but the inferolateral attachments of the lid are only minimally disturbed, allowing the lid to be mobile enough for tightening. The lower lid is approximated to the desired position, with a slight overcorrection, and the extent of the proposed dissection marked. Excess skin-muscle and mucocutaneous junction tissue are excised, leaving a tarsal strip. A double-armed 4-0 Mersilene suture is sewn through the tarsus undergoing a long pass followed by a short pass. The lower arm is left longer for identification. No tunnels are made, in contrast to the type I canthoplasty. The suture ends are passed directly onto the inner aspect of the orbital rim periosteum. The superior suture is placed superiorly in order not to twist the tarsus. A gray-line suture of 5-0 plain gut is placed to align the canthal angle. It is adjusted and tied simultaneously with

the Mersilene sutures. Sutures are tied under appropriate tension with the patient in a seated position on the operating table. Note that in this procedure, the sutures are placed at or below the lateral raphe.

TYPE III LATERAL CANTHOPLASTY: MINIMAL LID TIGHTENING

The third canthoplasty variation is utilized when only a minimal amount of lid tightening or elevation is required. This canthopexy procedure is accomplished by plicating the inferior arm of the lateral canthal tendon to the orbital rim periosteum without dissecting the lid free of its attachments (Fig. 17-9). Unlike the first two variations, the canthal angle is not opened. The procedure is performed by an internal approach, and access to the inferior arm of the lateral canthal tendon is gained through an incision at the lateral raphe. This may be the lateral

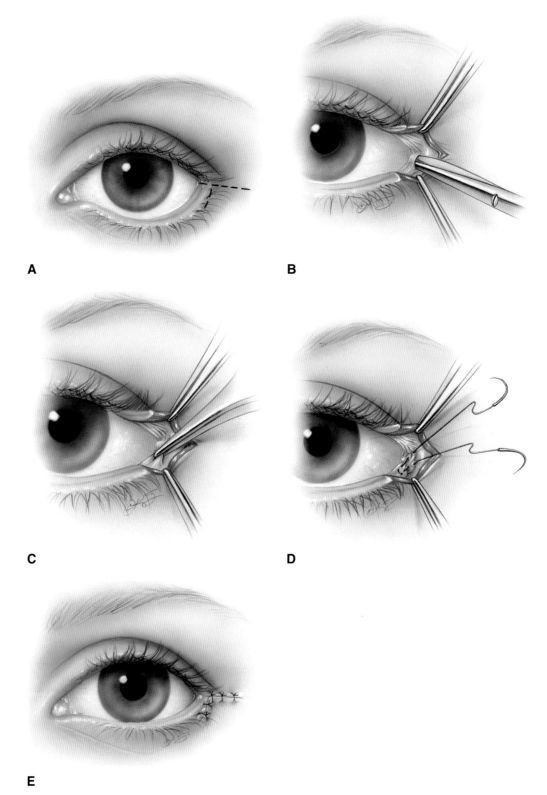

Figure 17-9 Type III lateral canthoplasty—minimal lid tightening. The canthal angle is not opened (**A**). Access to the inferior arm of the lateral canthal tendon is gained through an incision at the lateral raphe. This may be the lateral extension of a lower lid blepharoplasty incision. A tunnel is made with the scissors to the inferior arm of the lateral canthal tendon (**B**). The tendon is not cut. The medial end of the tendon is grasped with forceps and pulled out of the tunnel (**C**). A double-armed 4-0 Mersilene suture is sewn through the tendon (**D**). The lower arm is left longer for identification. The Mersilene sutures are passed into the lateral orbital rim periosteum (**E**). The sutures are always begun in posterior periosteum, so as to appose the lid well to the globe. Sutures are tied under appropriate tension.

extension of a lower lid blepharoplasty incision. A tunnel is made with the scissors to the inferior arm of the lateral canthal tendon. The medial end of the tendon is grasped with forceps and pulled out of the tunnel without cutting any attachments. A double-armed 4-0 Mersilene suture is sewn through the tendon with the lower arm left longer for identification. The Mersilene sutures are passed into the lateral orbital rim periosteum. As in the other variations, the sutures are always begun in the posterior periosteum so as to oppose the lid well to the globe. Sutures are then tied under appropriate tension with the patient in the seated position on the operating table. As with type II canthoplasty, the sutures are placed at or below the lateral raphe.

POSTOPERATIVE CARE

The patients are usually prescribed analgesics and antibiotics after the procedures. Ophthalmic antibiotic ointments are used on the incision line to keep the wound moist and clean. The patients are encouraged to use cold compresses in the first 2 to 3 postoperative days and asked to switch to warm compresses thereafter. The patients are seen on postoperative days 3 and 7 for examination and suture removal. The degree of postoperative edema is dependent on the extent of surgical manipulation.

COMPLICATIONS

The most common complication associated with lateral canthoplasty involves persistent or iatrogenic eyelid malposition requiring additional reconstructive procedures. These patients not only require revision canthoplasty but may also need adjunctive procedures such as middle lamellar stents, endoscopic midface lifts, fascia lata slings, or skin grafting. Other complications of canthal surgery include asymmetry, infection, corneal abrasion, and bleeding. As with all eyelid procedures, retrobulbar hematoma leading to vision loss is an extremely rare complication.

Future Considerations

The future of eyelid reconstruction will continue to converge on improving preoperative evaluation as well as increasing the patient and physician awareness of post-blepharoplasty eyelid malposition. The continued trend for utilizing the transconjunctival technique for lower blepharoplasty as well as preventive canthoplasty will result in fewer post-blepharoplasty complications.

REFERENCES

1. Converse JM, Smith B: Canthoplasty and dacrocystorhinostomy. Am J Ophthalmol 1952;35(8):1103.
2. Beard C: Canthoplasty and brow elevation for facial palsy. Arch Ophthalmol 1964;71:386.
3. Tenzel RR: Treatment of lagophthalmos of the lower eyelid. Arch Ophthalmol 1969;81:366.
4. Edgerton MT Jr: Causes and prevention of lower lid ectropion following blepharoplasty. Plast Reconstr Surg 1972;49(4):367.
5. Rees TD: Correction of ectropion resulting from blepharoplasty. Plast Reconstr Surg 1972;50(1):1.
6. Levine MR, Boynton J, Tenzel RR, et al: Complications of blepharoplasty. Ophthalm Surg 1975;6(2):53.
7. Tenzel RR: Surgical treatment of complications of cosmetic blepharoplasty. Clin Plast Surg 1978;5(4):517.
8. Friedman WH: Ectropion after blepharoplasty. Experimental and clinical observations. Arch Otolaryngol 1979;105(8):455.
9. Nowitzki T, Anderson RL: Advances in eyelid malposition. Ophthalmol Plast Reconstr Surg 1985;1:145.
10. Carraway JH, Mellow CG: The prevention and treatment of lower lid ectropion following blepharoplasty. Plast Reconstr Surg 1990;85(6):971.
11. Shorr N, Goldberg R, Eshagian B, Cook T: Lateral canthoplasty. Ophthal Plast Reconstr Surg 2003;19(5):345.
12. Dutton J: Clinical and surgical orbital anatomy. Philadelphia: WB Saunders, 1994, p 123.
13. Leone CR Jr: The management of ophthalmic Graves' disease. Ophthalmology 1984;91(7):770.
14. Shorr N, Enzer Y: Considerations in aesthetic eyelid surgery. J Dermatol Surg Oncol 1992;18:1081.
15. Shorr N: Madame butterfly procedure with hard palate graft: Management of post-blepharoplasty round eye and scleral show. Facial Plast Surg 1994;10(1):90.
16. Tan J, Olver J, Wright M, et al: The use of porous polyethylene (Medpor) lower eyelid spacers in lid heightening and stabilisation. Br J Ophthalmol 2004;88(9):1197.
17. Morton AD, Nelson C, Ikada Y, et al: Porous polyethylene as a spacer graft in the treatment of lower eyelid retraction. Ophthal Plast Reconstr Surg 2000;16(2):146.
18. Patel MP, Shapiro MD, Spinelli HM: Combined hard palate spacer graft, midface suspension, and lateral canthoplasty for lower eyelid retraction: a tripartite approach. Plast Reconstr Surg 2005;115(7):2105-2114; discussion 2115.

CHAPTER EIGHTEEN

Rhinoplasty in the Aging Patient

Ryan M. Greene, MD, PhD • Dean M. Toriumi, MD

HISTORY

Aesthetic and reconstructive rhinoplasty is commonly acknowledged as the most demanding and difficult of the plastic surgical procedures. Although many technical advances have occurred throughout the past century, its fundamental philosophy remains constant. This philosophy involves significant planning and conservative surgical changes to achieve a natural-appearing result. Initially, the operation generally involved a tissue reduction procedure with excision of various nasal anatomic components. More recently, rhinoplasty has evolved into a procedure that involves tissue reorientation and augmentation, with careful attention to long-term surgical outcome.

PERSONAL PHILOSOPHY

Rhinoplasty is a complex operation that requires precise preoperative diagnosis to select the appropriate surgical technique. Owing to variations in nasal anatomy and aesthetic expectations, no single technique is appropriate for all patients. Each rhinoplasty patient presents the surgeon with a diversity of nasal anatomy, contours, and proportions that require a series of organized maneuvers tailored to the patient's anatomic and functional needs. The surgeon must also be skilled at manipulating and controlling the dynamics of postoperative healing to attain optimal long-term aesthetic results. A necessary prerequisite is the skill to visualize the ultimate long-term healed result while manipulating the nasal structures.

ANATOMY

Aging of the nasal structures and external contour of the nose is influenced by a variety of genetic and environmental factors. Additionally, the nasal shape changes over time as well. In children, the nasal dorsum is typically concave, and assumes a more straight or convex shape in early adult life. This convexity is further enhanced in midlife by the development of a drooping, ptotic tip. In addition to these changes to the appearance of the nose, nasal function tends to deteriorate over time as the nasal airway changes.

As patients age, the skin thins with loss of elasticity, subcutaneous fat deposits resorb, and the underlying soft tissues atrophy. With these changes, the underlying support structures of the nose, such as the lower lateral cartilages and nasal bones, become skeletonized or visible. In addition, skin hydration is diminished, and the skin becomes less pliable.[1] This affects the skin's ability to contract and redrape after the cartilaginous and bony structures of the nose are reduced.

The most significant changes over time occur in the upper and lower lateral cartilages. These cartilages are connected by a fibrous union at the cephalic margin of the lateral crura, the scroll region.[1] As the nose ages, the upper and lower lateral cartilages begin to separate and fragment.[2,3] This may result in collapse of the internal nasal valve and lateral wall. As one ages, the middle nasal vault will tend to collapse as the upper lateral cartilages move inferomedially. Loss of support of the medial crura and stretching of the fibrous attachments from the posterior septal angle and nasal spine to the medial crural footplates result in their posterior movement and retraction of the columella.[3] These changes also occur by loss of the fat pad below the medial crura and resorption of the premaxilla.[2] With loss of support of the medial crura and separation of the lateral crura from the upper lateral cartilages, the nasal tip may become ptotic, with an appearance of increased length and a more acute nasolabial angle.

With aging, the nasal bones may become brittle and are more readily fractured.[4] Care must be taken during osteotomies to avoid excessive narrowing of the bony vault or comminuted fractures of the nasal bones. Periosteal elevation is not recommended in the aging patient and if used should not extend to the point of the intended lateral osteotomies, to avoid loss of periosteal support.[4] Although undesirable in the younger patient, greenstick fractures can be effective in the older patient.[4] Finally, dorsal hump reduction must be executed with great precision to minimize irregularities of the bony nasal vault as the skin over the dorsum tends to be very thin.

PREOPERATIVE ASSESSMENT

Preoperative assessment of the rhinoplasty patient includes not only the assessment of the anatomic and functional components, but also the emotional and psychological factors.[5] As with all facial aesthetic surgery, it is important for the physician to discuss motivation and aesthetic goals of rhinoplasty surgery with the patient. It is critical to elucidate what aesthetic changes the patient desires. Older patients have developed a self-image over many years, and must be prepared for the planned surgical changes. Many older patients do not want to look dramatically different, and thus conservative changes are generally most appropriate. Patients who desire dramatic changes warrant careful evaluation prior to consideration as surgical candidates.

In this age group, a thorough preoperative medical examination is mandatory. Many of these patients have co-morbid medical conditions. A careful medical history and physical examination are critical prior to performing this type of surgery. It is often a good idea to consult with the patient's primary care physician prior to scheduling surgery. Many of these patients take medications that can affect clotting. These medications should be stopped at least 2 weeks before surgery.

SURGICAL TECHNIQUE

PREOPERATIVE CONSIDERATIONS

The surgical approaches to the nose include nondelivery techniques (cartilage-splitting or retrograde approach), delivery of bilateral chondrocutaneous flaps, and the external rhinoplasty approach. Selection of the approach should be based on both operative objectives and surgical experience. When only conservative volume reduction of the lateral crura and dorsal hump reduction are planned, a nondelivery approach (cartilage-splitting or retrograde approach) will suffice. However, when more complex nasal tip work is required, delivery of bilateral chondrocutaneous flaps or the external rhinoplasty approach should be used. The external approach is preferred when complex tip grafting or middle nasal vault reconstruction is planned. Regardless, the surgeon should select the least invasive approach possible to avoid disruption of nasal support mechanisms and maximize the functional and aesthetic result.

External incisions can be used with greater frequency in older patients because the skin is less likely to scar unfavorably.[6] Nasal skin in the aging patient also has multiple rhytids that can aid in camouflage. Even though it is rarely necessary, direct excision of skin from the nasal dorsum or supratip can be performed to aid redraping of the skin or elevating the severely ptotic nasal tip.[7-9] Because of the thin skin found in the aging nose, even the smallest irregularities or asymmetries can become noticeable. As a result, debulking of underlying subcutaneous fat and muscle tissue should not be performed. This subcutaneous tissue should be preserved to maximize camouflage of the cartilage and bone. Tip grafts should also be limited unless the patient has medium to thick skin.[10] If they are used, they should be carefully sculpted and camouflaged to avoid visible edges. With thin skin, a thin layer of perichondrium or superficial temporal fascia can be applied over the graft, with an understanding that it will create temporary edema of the grafted area that should resolve over 6 to 12 months.

When treating the aging nose, the nasal tip should be managed first to set tip projection and rotation before completing profile alignment. After setting appropriate tip projection, dorsal hump reduction may not be needed. Frequently, older patients will also benefit from augmentation of the radix to create a straight profile. This strategy of increasing tip projection and raising the radix allows the surgeon to preserve a high dorsal profile while also creating a favorable tip-supratip relationship (Fig. 18-1). As mentioned earlier, only conservative changes should be made in the nasal contour because older patients tend to have a set self-image. The nose should also be in harmony with the patient's other facial features.

THE EXTERNAL APPROACH

The patient is first injected with 1% lidocaine with 1:100,000 epinephrine into the nasal tip, between and around the domes, down the columella, along the site of the marginal incision, and along the lateral wall of the nose. Additional injections high on the nasal septum and along the osteotomy sites are then placed. An inverted-V columellar incision is then marked, midway between the base of the nose and the top of the nostrils. A transcolumellar incision is executed with a No. 11 blade. Care must be taken to avoid damaging the caudal margin of the medial crura. Marginal incisions are then made along the caudal margin of the lateral crura, which are extended to meet the columellar incision.

After completing the incisions, angled Converse scissors are used to elevate the skin off the medial crura. Once the columellar flap is elevated off the medial crura, dissection is advanced laterally to expose the lateral crura. A thin layer of perichondrium is left on the surface of the lower lateral cartilages. The anterior septal angle is identified, with exposure of the middle nasal vault in the midline. Blunt dissection is continued to the rhinion, which may be followed by subperiosteal dissection of the skin off the nasal dorsum up to the nasion if profile alignment is necessary. If a radix graft is planned, then a narrow pocket should be dissected in the midline over the radix. This narrow pocket will prevent shifting of a radix graft if radix augmentation is necessary.

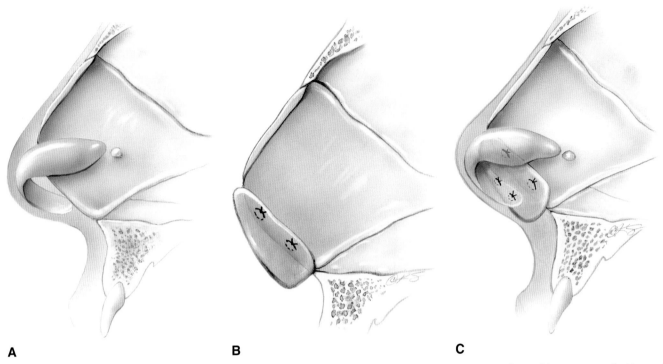

A   **B**   **C**

Figure 18-1 Part **A** shows a profile of an aging patient. Note the underprojection of the nasal tip. Placement of a caudal extension graft with septal cartilage overlapping the existing nasal dorsum is shown in **B**. Note the increased tip projection to create a straight dorsal profile in part **C**.

SEPTAL SURGERY

When performing septal surgery in the older patient, dissection of the mucosal flaps should be limited because the mucoperichondrium is thinner and drier. A substantial L-shaped septal strut should be preserved in order to support the lower two thirds of the nose. We prefer to leave at least a 2-cm anterior septal strut and 1.5-cm caudal strut for support. Extra cartilage should be left at the osseocartilaginous junction to avoid loss of dorsal septal support. A Killian incision is preferred because of its excellent exposure without compromise of the support attachments between the feet of the medial crura and the caudal septum. A hemitransfixion incision can be used if exposure of both sides of the caudal nasal septum is required. The hemitransfixion or full transfixion incision can sometimes lead to a loss of support due to disruption of some of the attachments between the medial crura and caudal septum. When a decrease in tip projection is desired, a full transfixion incision can be used to disrupt these attachments.

When exposing the septal cartilage in the aging patient, it is generally preferable to raise a mucoperichondrial flap on only one side of the septum, in order to preserve the vascular supply of the contralateral side and minimize chances of hematoma formation. After completion of the septal surgery, a running 4-0 plain catgut mattress suture is used to approximate the mucoperichondrial flaps and prevent fluid collection and hematoma formation. By limiting septal surgery, nasal packing can be minimized or

avoided. The surgeon should be aware that the septal cartilage may be partially calcified, which leaves the surgeon with less cartilage for harvesting or grafting.

In some patients it may be necessary to dissect between the medial crura to access the caudal septum. Patients with a deviated caudal septum may benefit from this approach to allow correction of the deformity. Other patients with poor tip support could benefit from stabilization of the nasal base through this approach.

PTOTIC NASAL TIP

As the nose ages, the nasal tip frequently droops, creating a ptotic nasal tip. This change in nasal contour gives an elongated appearance. Patients that have shorter medial crura are more likely to develop tip ptosis due to lack of support. Patients with long medial crura that wrap around the nasal spine and caudal septum are less likely to develop tip ptosis (Fig. 18-2). Severe ptosis of the nasal tip can also result in nasal airway compromise by altering the pathway of inspiratory air currents.[3] Correction of the ptotic nasal tip generally involves increasing nasal tip rotation and projection. As demonstrated by the tripod concept described by Anderson,[11] ptosis of the nasal tip can usually be corrected by supporting the medial and intermediate crura or by shortening the lateral crura.

We typically use a graduated approach for correction of the ptotic nasal tip by initially considering placing a

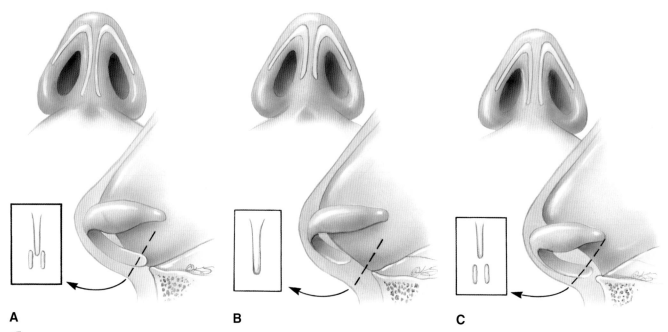

Figure 18-2 Relationship between medial crura and footplates to the caudal septum. Long strong medial crura extend to base of nose near posterior septal angle and wrap around caudal septum (**A**). This relationship provides excellent nasal tip support. Short medial crura do not extend to the nasal base and provide less tip support (**B**). Short caudal septum with separation of medial crura away from caudal septum results in loss of tip support (**C**).

sutured-in-place columellar strut between the medial crura. We have found this to be particularly effective if the dependent lobule is caused by buckling of the medial or intermediate crura. A sutured-in-place columellar strut both provides support and straightens buckled medial and intermediate crura. A straight rectangular piece of septal cartilage is placed in a precise pocket created between the medial and intermediate crura.[10] The columellar strut is fixed into position using a 5-0 plain catgut suture on a straight septal needle. The strut is easily applied using the external rhinoplasty approach, which allows maximal visualization, precise placement, and suture fixation of the graft. These struts can also be applied using a small endonasal incision placed just caudal to the caudal margin of the medial crura. Once the incision is made, a precise pocket is made between the medial crura for graft placement and suture fixation.

In many patients, a columellar strut will not provide sufficient support to the nasal base. These patients will require more significant structural support. One option is to suture the medial crura to the caudal septum. This maneuver will shorten the nose and support the nasal base. This technique should be used only when the caudal septum is long and would otherwise require shortening. Another option is to use a caudal extension graft. Such a graft is typically overlapped and sutured to the existing caudal septum. Then the medial crura are sutured to the caudal margin of the caudal extension graft to stabilize the nasal base and reposition the nasal tip. The caudal extension graft must be in the midline and oriented to increase tip rotation. Fixation of the medial crura to the

caudal septum or an extension graft provides increased tip support (Fig. 18-3). Such fixation creates moderate rigidity of the nasal tip that can be discussed with the patient preoperatively.

If stabilizing the nasal base does not adequately correct the ptotic nasal tip, then additional surgical maneuvers must be used to increase tip rotation. The objective of these maneuvers is to rotate the nasal tip by recruiting lateral crura medially. Placement of a transdomal suture recruits lateral crura medially to increase tip projection and rotation.[12,13] Without violating the underlying vestibular skin, a 5-0 clear nylon suture is placed in a horizontal mattress fashion across both domes. To recruit the lateral crura medially, the lateral bite of the suture extends lateral to the anatomic dome. This suture narrows the nasal tip by approximating the domes and creating a more acute domal angle, in addition to increasing tip projection and rotation. In some cases, the transdomal suture can further compromise the nasal airway if the lateral crura protrude into the airway. Such obstruction can be avoided by using an alar batten graft or lateral crural strut graft to lateralize the offending lateral segment of the lateral crus. If the transdomal suture does not correct the ptotic nasal tip, it may be necessary to perform a more aggressive maneuver that shortens the lateral crura.

The lateral crural overlay technique is a procedure that increases tip rotation by shortening the lateral crura. In this technique, the lateral crura are incised at the midpoint, and the medial segment is dissected from the underlying vestibular skin (Fig. 18-4). The cut ends of

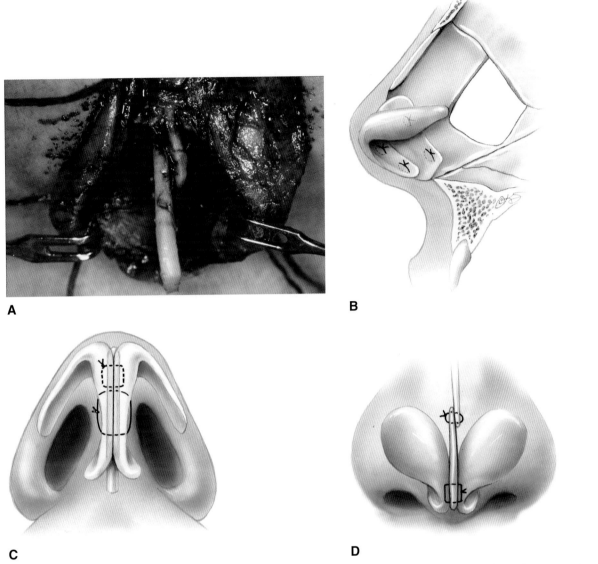

A

B

C

D

Figure 18-3 Caudal extension graft. The caudal extension graft is shown intraoperatively in part **A**. The graft then is shown sutured into place (**B**). Note the harvesting site, maintaining the L-shaped support. The caudal view of the graft sutured into position is shown in **C**. The superior view of the graft sutured into position is shown in **D**. Note how the caudal extension graft typically overlaps the existing caudal septum. It is critical that the caudal margin of the extension graft is in the midline.

cartilage are then overlapped (3 mm or 4 mm) and resutured with two 5-0 clear nylon mattress sutures to reconstitute the lateral crural segments into their shortened configuration. The degree of tip rotation is directly proportional to the degree of overlap (shortening) of the lateral crura. Symmetric alignment of the lateral crura must be achieved to avoid tip or alar margin asymmetry (Fig. 18-5).

Another technique employed in tip control involving the lower lateral cartilages is the lateral crural wedge technique (Fig. 18-6). The wedge resection of the lower laterals is made to rotate the tip cephalad. In most cases, adequate correction of the ptotic nasal tip requires the use of more than one of the aforementioned techniques. An

effective combination for correction of the ptotic tip is a lateral crural overlay with a caudal extension graft.

Once the ptosis of the nasal tip has been corrected, additional tip projection can be achieved by suturing a shield-shaped cartilage tip graft into position. A tip graft is sculpted from septal cartilage and sutured to the caudal margin of the medial and intermediate crura with 6-0 PDS (polydioxanone) suture (Ethicon, Somerville, NJ). The tip graft serves to provide additional tip projection, hide tip asymmetries, improve the shape of the lobule, and increase tip support.[14] The use of tip grafts should be limited in older patients, because maximal tip refinement is generally unnecessary. In addition, the leading edge of the tip graft will be more visible beneath the thinner skin

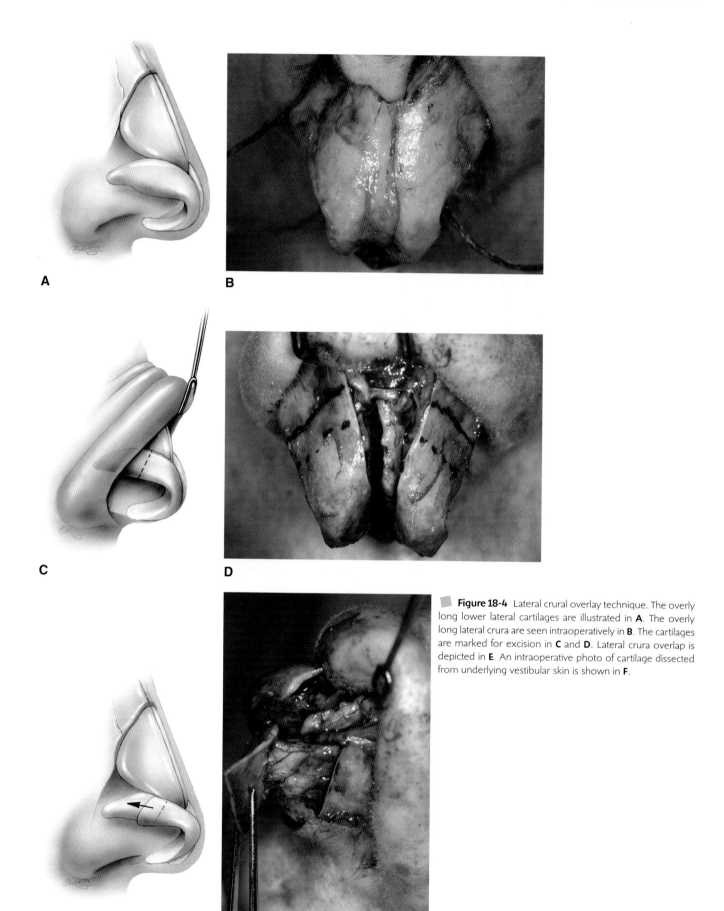

A

B

C

D

E

F

Figure 18-4 Lateral crural overlay technique. The overly long lower lateral cartilages are illustrated in **A**. The overly long lateral crura are seen intraoperatively in **B**. The cartilages are marked for excision in **C** and **D**. Lateral crura overlap is depicted in **E**. An intraoperative photo of cartilage dissected from underlying vestibular skin is shown in **F**.

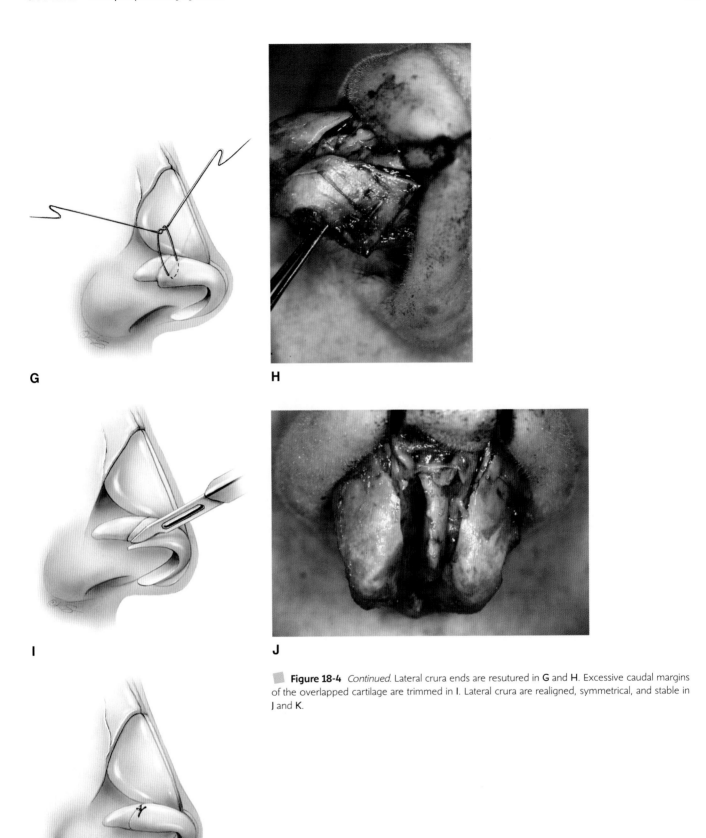

G

H

I

J

K

Figure 18-4 *Continued.* Lateral crura ends are resutured in **G** and **H**. Excessive caudal margins of the overlapped cartilage are trimmed in **I**. Lateral crura are realigned, symmetrical, and stable in **J** and **K**.

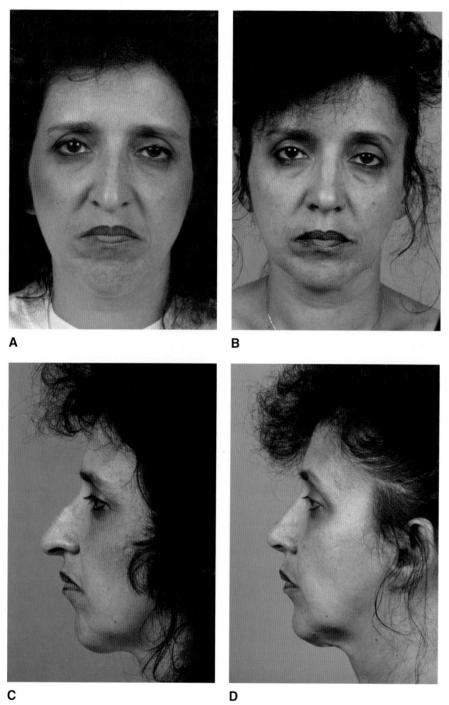

Figure 18-5 Patient with ptotic nasal tip. The lateral crural overlay technique was used to shorten the lateral crura and rotate the nasal tip. Preoperative (**A**, **C**, **E**, and **G**) and postoperative (**B**, **D**, **F**, and **H**) views.

of these patients and should be limited to patients with thicker skin. In thin-skinned patients, the leading edge of the tip graft should be camouflaged with crushed cartilage or soft tissue (perichondrium, fascia, etc.) (Fig. 18-7).

Other nasal tip problems, such as an underprojected or bulbous tip, can be managed by other techniques commonly used in younger patients. However, care must be taken to preserve as much of the cartilaginous framework as possible. Emphasis should be placed on repositioning existing cartilage structures, rather than excising them. The weaker cartilages of the aging nose are

also more prone to deformity (e.g., buckling, bossae) under the forces of scar contracture. When performing volume reduction of the lateral crura in the aging patient, resection should be primarily medial, leaving at least 8 to 10 mm of intact strip.

It is imperative that the surgeon anticipates the effects of scar contracture on the reduced cartilages. It is shortsighted to try to attain the ideal final result at the time of surgery, which neglects the additional refinement that occurs with resolution of edema and healing. Therefore, the surgeon can anticipate additional tip

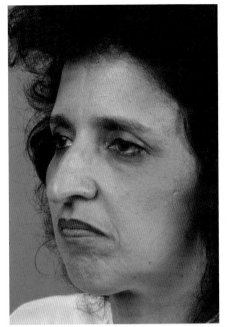

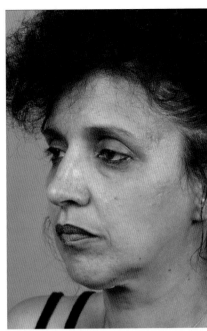

Figure 18-5 *Continued.*

E

F

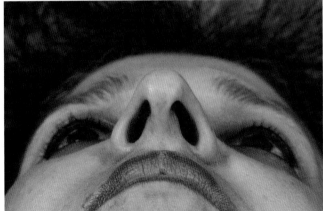

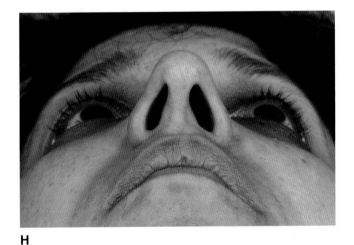

G

H

refinement that will result from postoperative forces of scar contracture. Finally, aesthetic changes should be conservative because older patients are more set in their self-image, as well as their perception of acceptable change in nasal contour.

NARROWED MIDDLE NASAL VAULT

In some older patients, an excessively narrow middle nasal vault can result when weak upper lateral cartilages collapse inferomedially. Severe collapse may also result in collapse of the internal nasal valve. These patients experience improvement in their nasal airway obstruction while performing the "Cottle maneuver" or with lateralization of the lateral nasal wall with an instrument. To correct this deformity, the surgeon can apply bilateral spreader grafts between the dorsal (anterior) margin of the nasal septum and the upper lateral cartilages.[14-16]

These grafts are rectangular in shape and measure approximately 5 to 15 mm in length, 3 to 5 mm in width, and 1 to 2 mm in thickness. The majority of spreader grafts extend from a point just cephalic to the anterior septal angle to the osseocartilaginous junction. In most older patients with a functional deficit at the internal nasal valve or lateral wall, spreader grafts will be insufficient, and alar batten grafts should be used. These cartilage grafts are placed caudal to the existing lateral crura to support the lateral wall.

Spreader grafts can be applied via an endonasal approach into precise submucosal tunnels[16] or may be applied directly between the upper lateral cartilages and the nasal septum via the external rhinoplasty approach.[6,15] In the external rhinoplasty approach, the upper lateral cartilages are freed from the nasal septum after the middle nasal vault is exposed. The rectangular spreader grafts are then applied between the upper lateral

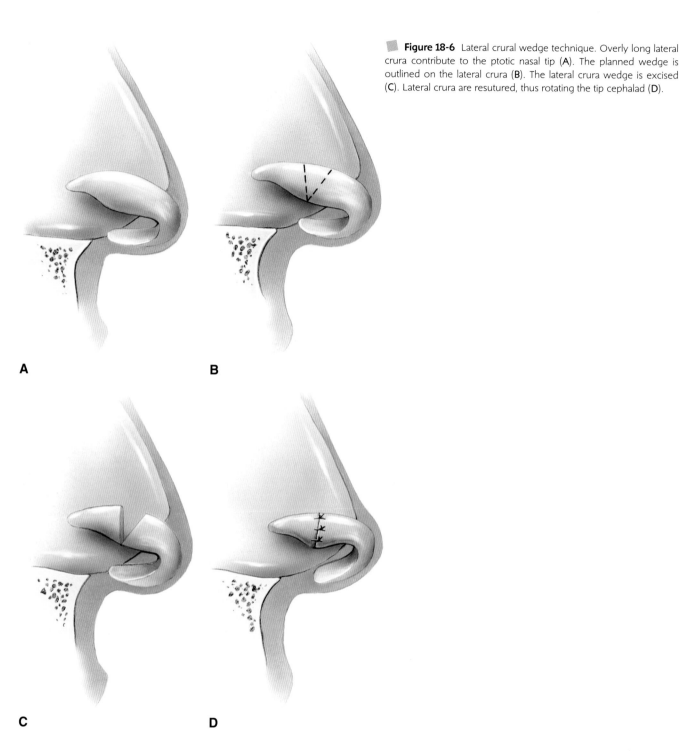

Figure 18-6 Lateral crural wedge technique. Overly long lateral crura contribute to the ptotic nasal tip (**A**). The planned wedge is outlined on the lateral crura (**B**). The lateral crura wedge is excised (**C**). Lateral crura are resutured, thus rotating the tip cephalad (**D**).

cartilages and septum, and sutured into place with a 5-0 PDS mattress suture. With incorporation of the upper lateral cartilages in the suture, the middle nasal vault width is set and inferomedial collapse of the upper lateral cartilages is avoided. Patients with short nasal bones are at higher risk of collapse and will need thicker and longer spreader grafts. Careful attention must be given to the width of the middle nasal vault to avoid creating excessive width with the spreader grafts. If possible, the surgeon should try to avoid dividing the upper lateral cartilages from the septum, in order to preserve support in the older

patient. Thus, if dorsal hump reduction is not needed, the spreader grafts may be placed into submucosal tunnels made via a small intranasal incision, with preservation of the attachment of the upper lateral cartilages to the septum.[6,16]

PROFILE ALIGNMENT AND NARROWING THE NOSE

Successful management of the bony nasal vault involves conservative dorsal hump reduction, preservation of a

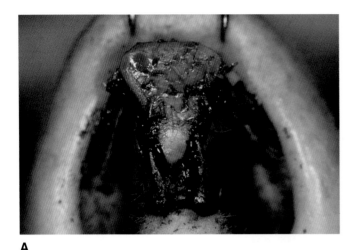

A

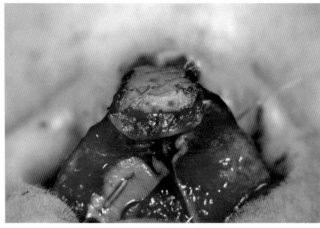

B

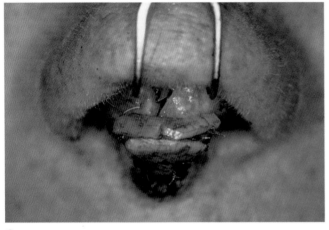

C

Figure 18-7 **A** and **B** show a tip graft camouflaged with a crushed cartilage graft behind the leading edge of the tip graft. **C** shows a tip graft from the anterior view sutured in position.

high dorsal profile, and avoidance of dorsal irregularities. Because the nasal bones in the aging patient can be thin and brittle, careful manipulation of the bony vault must be exercised in order to avoid comminuted fractures or excessive narrowing of the bony vault. Typically, conservative dorsal hump reduction is performed after tip position is set. In patients with a deep nasofrontal angle, small crushed-cartilage radix grafts can be placed above a dorsal hump to create a straight profile (Fig. 18-8). In many cases, dorsal hump reduction can be avoided if the profile can be corrected with the use of a radix graft in combination with an increase in tip projection and rotation. The surgeon should consider a radix graft in patients who demonstrate a deep nasofrontal angle with a low nasal starting point. The nasal starting point should be located at the level of the superior palpebral fold in female patients, with a slightly higher location in male patients.

For larger dorsal hump reductions, a Rubin osteotome can be used, while smaller dorsal humps can be managed with a fine rasp. With larger dorsal humps, wide undermining of the overlying skin-soft tissue envelope is necessary to accommodate for reduced skin elasticity and less rapid shrinkage and redraping. Because the thin skin

of older patients shows even the smallest dorsal irregularity, special care must be taken to ensure a smooth dorsum. Following profile alignment, lateral osteotomies can be performed using the smallest osteotome possible to minimize trauma and bleeding. Often a 2- or 3-mm straight osteotome can be used to fracture the thin bone.[6,16] In most aging patients, medial osteotomies can be avoided as the bones are readily fractured.

EXTERNAL NASAL VALVE COLLAPSE

Older patients often present to the surgeon with complaints of nasal airway obstruction located primarily at the entrance to the nose (nostril margin). The nostrils may collapse on moderate to deep inspiration, with inadequate support of the lateral nasal wall and alae secondary to weak lower lateral cartilages. In some cases, the lateral crura are in a cephalic position and provide little support to the alar side walls.[15,17,18] This deficiency has been described as "external nasal valve collapse" and can be diagnosed by observing alar collapse on deep inspiration. These patients will characteristically expe-

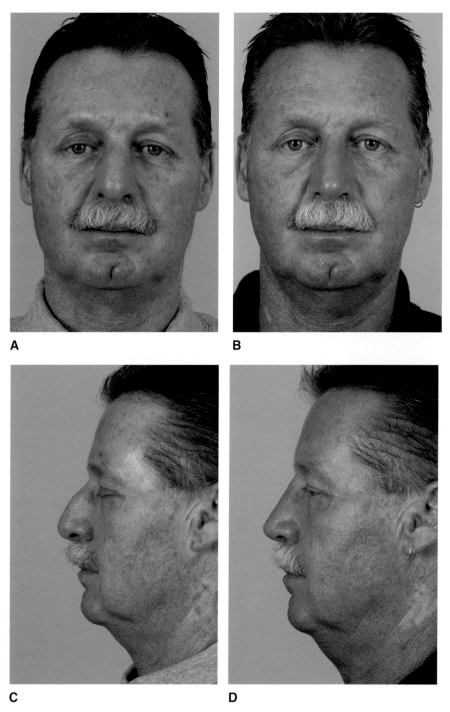

A

B

C

D

Figure 18-8 Patient with dorsal hump and deep radix. Double layer radix graft placed into narrow pocket over nasofrontal angle to augment the radix and help create a straight dorsal profile. Preoperative (**A**, **C**, **E**, and **G**) and postoperative (**B**, **D**, **F**, and **H**) views.

rience improved nasal airflow if the alae are supported during nasal breathing.

Internal or external nasal valve collapse can be surgically corrected by applying bilateral alar batten grafts at the site of maximal lateral nasal wall collapse or near the nostril margin, respectively.[15,17,18] Alar batten grafts can be fashioned from curved cartilage of the nasal septum or of the cavum or cymba conchae of the ear. The concave surface of the batten graft is oriented medially to support the collapsing segment of the nostril (external valve collapse) or lateral nasal wall (internal valve collapse). To

correct external valve collapse, the grafts are typically placed just caudal to the lateral crura and extend from the pyriform aperture to the lateral aspect of the lateral crura (Fig. 18-9). For internal valve collapse, the grafts are placed at the point of maximal lateral nasal wall collapse, usually at the point of the supra-alar groove. As with spreader grafts, these grafts can be applied through either an endonasal incision or via the external rhinoplasty approach. Once the graft is in position, there should be an immediate improvement in support of the alar side walls as well as diminution of alar collapse during inspiration

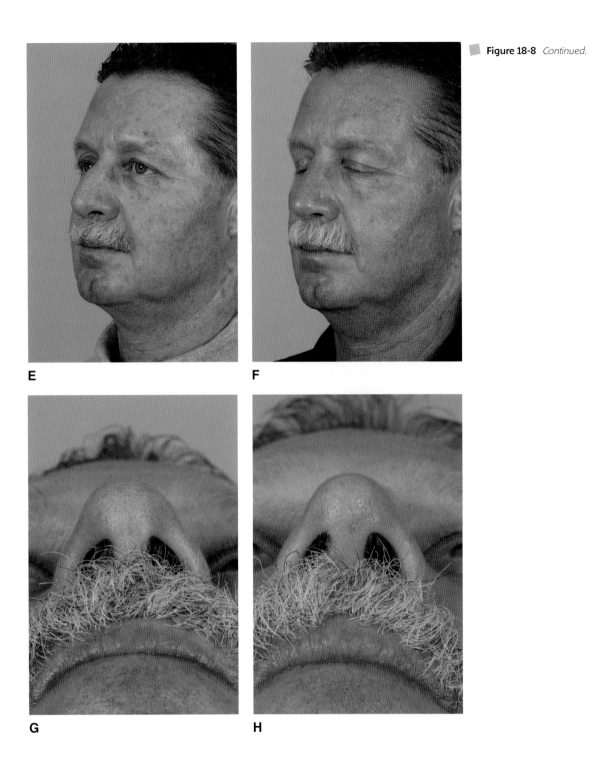

Figure 18-8 *Continued.*

E

F

G

H

through the nose. We use splints in the nasal vestibule to support the alar battens and to help them heal in a lateral position.

ACUTE NASOLABIAL ANGLE OR RETRACTED COLUMELLA

Owing to posterior positioning of the feet of the medial crura, the older patient frequently has an acute nasolabial angle. Correction of this deformity adds support to the medial crural component of the tripod complex and improves the aesthetic appearance on lateral view. For minor augmentation, 1- to 2-mm pieces of cartilage can be placed into a small pocket between the feet of the medial crura. This serves to support the lower lateral cartilages, preserve tip projection, and correct an acute nasolabial angle. With more significant deficiency of the medial crura, more aggressive maneuvers may be necessary. A sutured-in-place columellar strut may be sufficient. In most patients, however, a caudal extension graft will be necessary to support the nasal base and open the nasolabial angle.

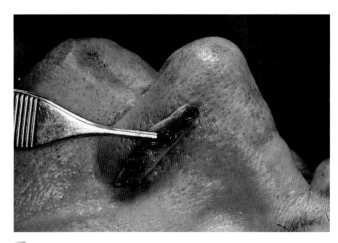

Figure 18-9 Alar batten graft applied into pocket caudal to existing lateral crura to support lateral wall.

The caudal extension graft is set in the midline and sutured between the medial crura. This maneuver moves the medial crura caudally and corrects the acute nasolabial angle or retracted columella.[19] A straight piece of septal cartilage is sutured to the stable caudal septum with 5-0 clear nylon mattress sutures (Fig. 18-10). This allows extension of the graft into a pocket between the medial crura. The graft is then sutured between the medial crura with 5-0 clear nylon sutures. During this maneuver, care must be taken to set the proper tip projection, rotation, and columellar show. A more rigid nasal tip with less recoil results due to fixation of the medial crura to the caudal extension graft. If this grafting technique is planned, this rigidity and lack of recoil should be explained to the patient prior to the procedure. In addition, this graft may alter the length of the upper lip, which could

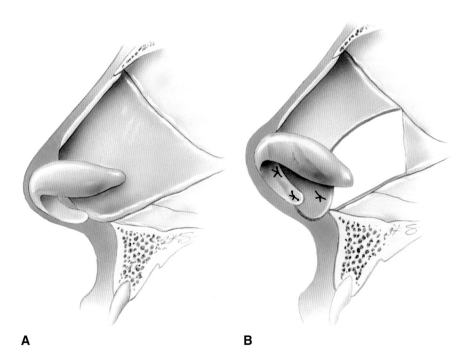

A   B

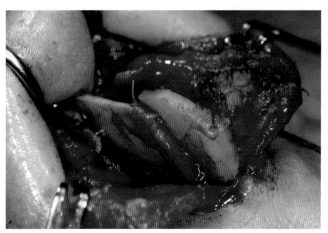

C

Figure 18-10 **A** shows a short caudal septum. **B** shows the caudal septal extension graft sutured in position. The graft is harvested with a standard septoplasty. **C** is an intraoperative photograph showing the graft sutured in place.

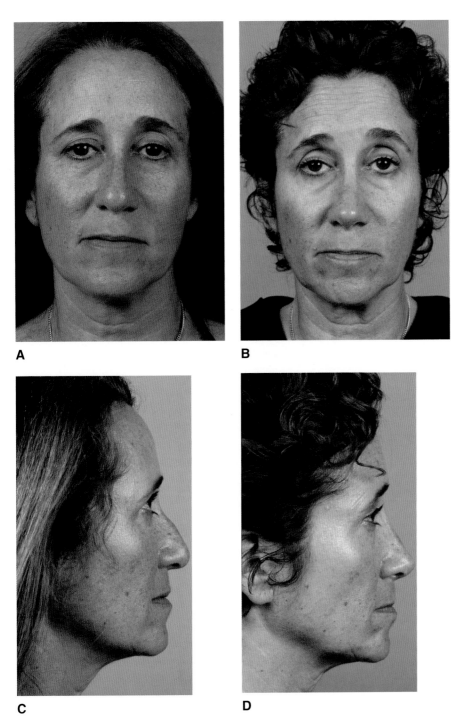

Figure 18-11 Patient with thick skin and bulbous nasal tip. In this patient, a tip graft was applied to increase tip projection. A caudal extension graft was used to support the nasal base. Preoperative (**A**, **C**, **E**, and **G**) and postoperative (**B**, **D**, **F**, and **H**) views.

A

B

C

D

change the upper lip posture during smiling. This technique may be coupled with a tip graft to optimize the overall appearance of the lower third of the nose (Fig. 18-11).

Many older patients present with a hanging columella deformity caused by loss of support or stretching of fibrous connections between the caudal septum and

medial crura. Correction of this deformity may entail trimming of the caudal margin of the nasal septum or medial crura. This can also include excision of excess vestibular skin between the caudal septum and medial crura as well. If the caudal nasal septum is trimmed, there may be a loss of nasal tip support. A better option to

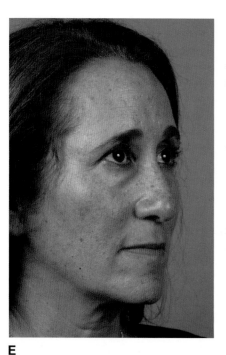

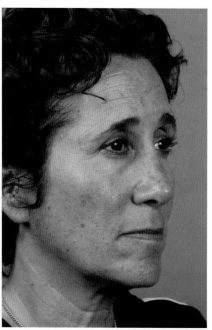

E

F

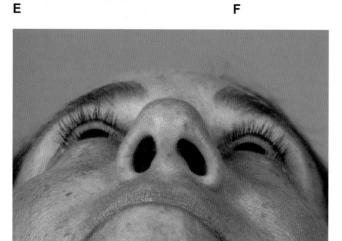

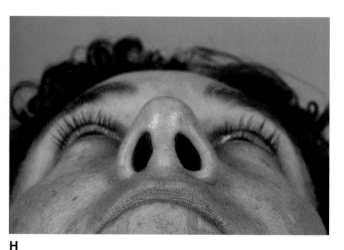

G

H

correct the hanging columella is set-back of the medial crura on the overly long caudal septum. After dissecting between the medial crura, the medial crura can be sutured to the caudal septum with 5-0 clear nylon suture to set tip projection and alar/columellar relationship.

POSTOPERATIVE CARE

Careful postoperative care is critical to achieve an optimal result following rhinoplasty. In addition, patients should be monitored closely during the immediate postoperative period to ensure adequate oxygenation and hemostasis. To avoid life-threatening complications, the cardiac and pulmonary status of the patient should also be monitored.

Finally, if nasal packing is used, it should be removed within 24 hours after surgery, with subsequent examination of the septal flaps to evaluate for a septal hematoma.

Columellar sutures should be removed on the seventh postoperative day. Postoperative edema that develops in the supratip region can be treated with taping of the supratip. On rare occasions, subdermal injections (0.1 to 0.2 mL) of triamcinolone acetonide (Kenalog, Westwood-Squibb, Buffalo, NY, 10 mg/mL) can be placed into the supratip. Such injections should only be used in patients with thick skin. These injections may be administered 2 weeks after surgery, with no more than one injection per month. Dermal atrophy may result from either intradermal injections or frequent injections of higher concentrations of Kenalog.

COMPLICATIONS

Because rhinoplasty is considered to be an elective surgery, complications in the postoperative period can be particularly distressing. It has been estimated that complications occur in approximately 10% of cases.[20] This figure may actually be much higher if sequelae such as persistent swelling, ecchymoses, and skin discoloration are considered. Postoperative sequelae and complications of rhinoplasty generally fall into five major categories: infection, trauma, necrosis, functional problems, and iatrogenic difficulties.[5]

Rhinoplasty is considered by many to be the most difficult facial plastic operation, largely due to the intricate and highly variable anatomy. In addition, any surgical modification is likely to change over the lifetime of the patient, secondary to postoperative scar contracture and healing. For these reasons, primary rhinoplasty is often associated with a suboptimal outcome. It has been estimated that 8% to 15% of primary rhinoplasty patients eventually undergo revision surgery.[21] There are a number of nasal deformities that can result from primary rhinoplasty, including middle vault collapse, supra-alar pinching, and pollybeak deformity. Every surgeon should become familiar with these deformities.

Future Considerations

The aging nose presents many unique challenges that must be considered to achieve a desirable result. In addition to addressing aesthetic changes, proper preoperative diagnosis is critical to identify all existing functional deficits. In this age group, aesthetic changes should be conservative, with extensive discussion prior to surgery. Because there is decreased structural support in the older patient, excision of supportive cartilaginous and bony structures should be minimized. Additional support should instead be provided with structural grafts to stabilize the nose and increase the likelihood of a favorable functional and aesthetic outcome.

REFERENCES

1. Janeke JB, Wright WK: Studies on the support of the nasal tip. Arch Otolaryngol 1971;93:458-464.

2. Krmpotic-Nemanic J, Kostovic I, Rudan P, et al: Morphological and histological changes responsible for the droop of the nasal tip in advanced age. Acta Otolaryngol 1971;71:278-281.

3. Patterson CN: The aging nose: Characteristics and correction. Otolaryngol Clin North Am 1980;13:275-288.

4. Tardy ME: Rhinoplasty in midlife. Otolaryngol Clin North Am 1980;13:289-303.

5. Holt GR, Garner ET, McLarey D: Postoperative sequelae and complications of rhinoplasty. Otolaryngol Clin North Am 1987;20:853-876.

6. Toriumi DM: Surgical correction of the aging nose. Facial Plast Surg 1996;12:205-214.

7. Larrabee WF: Rhinoplasty in the aging patient. In Krause CJ, Pastorek N, Mangat DS (eds): Aesthetic Facial Surgery. Philadelphia: JB Lippincott, 1991, pp 361-384.

8. Johnson CM, Anderson JR: Nose lift operation: An adjunct to aging face surgery. Arch Otolaryngol 1978;104:1-6.

9. Kabaker SS: An adjunctive technique to rhinoplasty of the aging nose. Head Neck Surg 1980;2:276-281.

10. Toriumi DM, Johnson CM: Open structure rhinoplasty: Featured technical points and long-term follow-up. Facial Plast Surg Clin North Am 1993;1:1-22.

11. Anderson JR: Surgery of the nasal base. Arch Otolaryngol 1984;110:349-358.

12. Tardy ME, Cheng E: Transdomal suture refinement of the nasal tip. Facial Plast Surg 1987;4:317-326.

13. Toriumi DM, Tardy ME: Cartilage suturing techniques for correction of nasal tip deformities. Op Tech Otolaryngol Head Neck Surg 1995;6:265-273.

14. Johnson CM, Toriumi DM: Open Structure Rhinoplasty. Philadelphia, WB Saunders, 1990.

15. Toriumi DM: Management of the middle nasal vault in rhinoplasty. Op Tech Plast Reconstr Surg 1995;2:16-30.

16. Sheen JH: Spreader graft: A method of reconstructing the roof of the middle nasal vault following rhinoplasty. Plast Reconstr Surg 1984;73:230-237.

17. Tardy ME, Garner ET: Inspiratory nasal obstruction secondary to alar and nasal valve collapse. Op Tech Otolaryngol Head Neck Surg 1990;1:215-217.

18. Constantian MB: The incompetent external nasal valve: Pathophysiology and treatment in primary and secondary rhinoplasty. Plast Reconstr Surg 1994;93:919-931.

19. Toriumi DM: Caudal extension graft for correction of the retracted columella. Op Tech Otolaryngol Head Neck Surg 1995;6:311-318.

20. Weimert TA, Yoder MG: Antibiotics and nasal surgery. Laryngoscope 1980;90:667-672.

21. Byrd HS, Hobar PC: Rhinoplasty: A practical guide for surgical planning. Plast Reconstr Surg 1993;91:642-656.

Index

Note: page numbers followed by b indicate boxed material; those followed by f indicate figures; those followed by t indicate tables.